Women's Health Problems - A Global Perspective

Edited by Russell Kabir, Ali Davod Parsa and Igor V. Lakhno

Published in London, United Kingdom

Women's Health Problems - A Global Perspective
http://dx.doi.org/10.5772/intechopen.104169
Edited by Russell Kabir, Ali Davod Parsa and Igor V. Lakhno

Contributors
Abigail L. Kohut-Jackson, Afifah Idris, Aise Chatzi Ismail Mouchterem, Alexios Alexiou, Ali Abbas, Ali Davod Parsa, Anastasia Bothou, Anna Chalkidou, Anna Maria Giammarioli, Ayehu Kassaw Asres, Bijaya Kumar Padhi, Brijesh Sathian, Dimitrios Kyriakou, Divya Vinnakota, Efthimios Oikonomou, Eloise Longo, Erika Schwartz, Fred Nunes, Georgios Iatrakis, Igor V. Lakhno, Ilias Mahmud, Jayanthi Rajendran, Jill Ketner Villa, Johnathan M. Borland, Kayla M. Joyce, Konstantinos Nikolettos, Leila Dehghani, Marema Jebessa Kumsa, Md Rakibul Hasan, Nektaria Kritsotaki, Nikolaos Nikolettos, Nor Jana Saim, Norulhuda Sarnon, Nur Saadah Mohamad Aun, Panagiotis Tsikouras, Patricia Sheerattan-Bisnauth, Raffaella Bucciardini, Robert L. Meisel, Russell Kabir, Sathiya Ramasamy, Sheikh Shamim Hasnain, Sherry H. Stewart, Sonia Kotanidou, Stefanos Zervoudis, Sumathi Saravanan, Theopi Nalbanti, Tonia Frame, Yirgalem Amogne, Yvette Delph, Zegeye Wubeshet Haile

First published in London, United Kingdom, 2024 by IntechOpen
IntechOpen is the global imprint of INTECHOPEN LIMITED, registered in England and Wales, registration number: 11086078, 167-169 Great Portland Street, London, W1W 5PF, United Kingdom

British Library Cataloguing-in-Publication Data
A catalogue record for this book is available from the British Library

Additional hard and PDF copies can be obtained from orders@intechopen.com

Women's Health Problems - A Global Perspective
Edited by Russell Kabir, Ali Davod Parsa and Igor V. Lakhno
p. cm.
Print ISBN 978-1-80356-839-3
Online ISBN 978-1-80356-840-9
eBook (PDF) ISBN 978-1-80356-841-6

For EU product safety concerns:
IN TECH d.o.o., Prolaz Marije Krucifikse Kozulić 3, 51000 Rijeka, Croatia,
info@intechopen.com or visit our website at intechopen.com.

Meet the editors

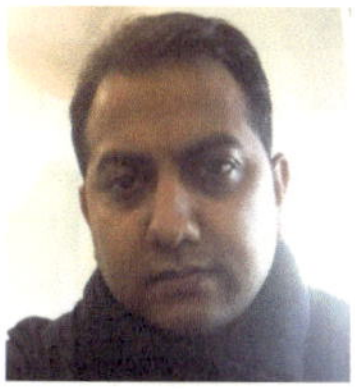

Dr. Russell Kabir is an Associate Professor of Public Health and Biostatistics at Anglia Ruskin University, UK. He leads the MSc Public Health and Community Wellbeing program at Chelmsford, Essex. He is the author of more than 150 peer-reviewed publications and has co-authored many edited book chapters. His books include *Learning SPSS Without Pain* (2021), *Data Analysis with STATA* (2022), *Panic Buying and Environmental Disasters* (2022), and *Basic Principles of Epidemiology* (2023). He has more than 15 years of research experience in public health. He teaches courses on Biostatistics, Epidemiology, and Research Methods to postgraduate and undergraduate public health students, leads the Epidemiology and Statistics module for postgraduate students in public health, and runs the Quantitative Methods sessions for the doctoral school. Dr. Kabir is an academic editor for *PLOS One*, *BMC Public Health*, and *Health and Social Care in the Community*. He is interested in collaborative and interdisciplinary research in public health issues with a special focus on suicide and mental health, dental public health, reproductive health issues, violence against women, and aging-related research. In particular, he has significant expertise and a proven track record in the field of violence against women. He is experienced in conducting secondary data analysis, systematic reviews, meta-analyses, and scoping reviews.

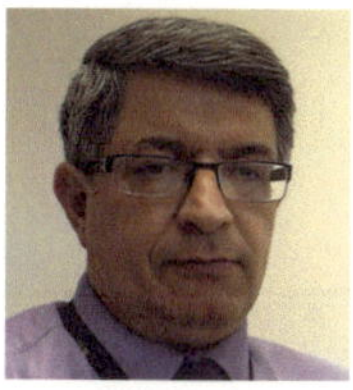

Dr. Ali Davod Parsa has more than 30 years of experience in research and teaching and has held senior national leadership roles in public health, health management, health economics, and health policy. He is an active researcher in medicine, public health policy, and management, and health economics. Dr. Parsa is an Associate Professor of Health Economics, Policy and Management in the Faculty of Health, Education, Medicine and Social Care, School of Allied Health, Anglia Ruskin University, UK. He has an established, proven track record of success in senior-level leadership, collaborative research, and teaching excellence at undergraduate, postgraduate, and doctoral levels. He held a series of high-profile governmental appointments in the Ministry of Health and Medical Education in Iran before joining Higher Education Institutions in the United Kingdom. Dr. Parsa graduated as a qualified general practitioner from the School of Medicine, Zanjan University of Medical Sciences and Health Services, Iran, in 1994. He worked for a decade as a clinician and then held senior management appointments, during which he developed an interest in policy and healthcare management research. Consequently, he was awarded a Ph.D. in Health Economics from the School of Clinical Sciences and a Postgraduate Diploma in Health Services Research (HSR) from the School of Community Health Sciences, the University of Nottingham, UK. Dr. Parsa is an experienced national-level health manager who has exercised health policymaking at the national strategic level.

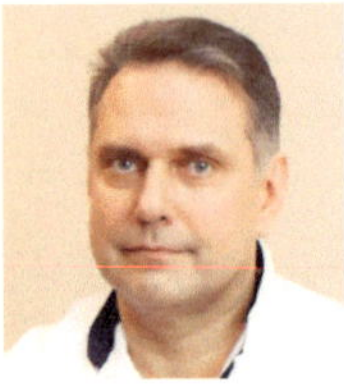

Dr. Igor Lakhno is a clinical professor and head of the Department of Obstetrics and Gynecology No. 3, Kharkiv National Medical University, Ukraine. He obtained his MD from the same university in 1994 specializing in obstetrics and gynecology in 1997. Additionally, he gained his Ph.D. in 1999 and his DSc from the PL Shupik National Academy of Postgraduate Education, Ukraine, in 2019. Dr. Lakhno is an author of about 230 published works. He is an associate editor for the *Cureus Medical Journal* and an editorial board member of *Reproductive Health of Woman*, *Emergency Medicine*, and *Technology Transfer: Innovative Solutions in Medicine*. He is also a consultant at the Kharkiv Municipal Perinatal Center, Ukraine. Dr. Lakhno has participated as a speaker at several international conferences and congresses. His main scientific interests are obstetrics, women's health, fetal medicine, and cardiovascular medicine.

Contents

Preface

Women's health issues constitute a multifaceted global challenge, encompassing a wide range of complex problems that impact millions of women around the world. This edited volume, *Women's Health Problems – A Global Perspective*, presents a comprehensive overview of the various health issues and societal challenges women face across different cultural, religious, and economic contexts.

Our expert contributors, from diverse fields, offer in-depth analyses and evidence-based insights into topics including reproductive health and sexual health matters, menstruation, health service utilization, violence against women, and inequalities experienced by women. By examining these topics from a global perspective, this book underscores both the shared and distinct challenges women face in various regions. We aim for this collection to not only inform and educate but also to inspire further research and policy initiatives to enhance women's health worldwide. This work is dedicated to all women, whose health and well-being are essential to the progress of our global society.

The health of a woman throughout her life, from childhood to menopause, is a key focus of this volume. The holistic approach postulates that the function of the female reproductive system is critically dependent on general health. Ultrasound is of great significance in the medical visualization and diagnosis of diseases in women. Social and psychological adaptation depends on hormonal regulation. Premenstrual disorders can disrupt the daily activities of adult women. Testosterone is responsible for some adverse effects in women with polycystic ovarian syndrome or adrenal gland hyperplasia. Transgender individuals are the target population for prolonged testosterone administration. However, androgens play a beneficial role in sexual desire. Marriage is a considerable step towards childbirth. Multinational marriage is not only an ethical dilemma but also an instrument for improving genetic disturbances. Pregnancy is a period of maximal adaptive changes in the female reproductive system. The system of antenatal screening using biochemical and biophysical markers can contribute to the early diagnosis of chromosomal disorders, pre-eclampsia, preterm birth, and fetal growth restriction. Pre-eclampsia is one of the major obstetric syndromes that plays a crucial role in the programming of fetal and maternal health. There is no efficient treatment for pre-eclampsia, thus the emphasis is on prevention.

Female endocrine regulation is an important part of homeostasis. Hypoestrogenicity is a trigger event for atherogenic vasculopathy. The activity of the ovaries impacts metabolic processes, vascular tone, and endothelial function. Hyperandrogenicity in polycystic ovarian disease is a trigger for adiposity, type 2 diabetes, and atherosclerosis. The increased level of testosterone persists even after menopause. Hormonal changes during menopause are discussed. Hormone replacement therapy has not shown an evident beneficial effect on the cardiovascular system. A possible therapeutic strategy for improved cardiovascular health during the transitional years of life is presented. The use of diet, L-arginine, and xylitol could be reasonable options for managing perimenopausal women. An alternative regimen of hormonal replacement therapy with herbal soy isoflavone extracts is presented as an efficient and safe option for women in their transitional years.

This book includes a preface by the editors, followed by 12 chapters written by international experts, arranged in four sections. It is a useful resource for social workers, psychologists, general practitioners, endocrinologists, and gynecologists.

Russell Kabir and Ali Davod Parsa
Faculty of Health,
Medicine and Social Care,
Anglia Ruskin University,
Chelmsford, UK

Igor V. Lakhno
Kharkiv National Medical University,
Kharkiv, Ukraine

Section 1

Violence and Inequality

Chapter 1

HIV and Violence among Female Sex Workers in India: A Scoping Review

Russell Kabir, Divya Vinnakota, Leila Dehghani, Brijesh Sathian, Bijaya Kumar Padhi, Md Rakibul Hasan, Sheikh Shamim Hasnain, Ilias Mahmud and Ali Davod Parsa

Abstract

Female sex workers (FSW) in India are highly stigmatised and discriminated against by the society. Additionally, this population faces public health issues, such as HIV, mental health challenges, and violence at work. Despite interventions being put in place, female sex workers continue to experience high HIV prevalence and violence. A scoping review of peer-reviewed articles was conducted by searching PubMed, PubMed Central, Embase, and CINAHL Plus using keywords. Using inclusion and exclusion criteria following Preferred Reporting Items for Systematic Reviews and Meta-Analyses (PRISMA) standards, the identified papers were screened. Twenty-four articles were selected for this review after critical appraisal. The data extracted from these articles regarding HIV and violence among female sex workers (FSWs) in India were analysed using narrative analysis. Most of the research looked at the prevalence of sexual violence and HIV infections and the factors contributing to these conditions. At the same time, the rest focused on mood disorders (e.g., depression) among FSWs. Client and intimate partner violence were common occurrences for FSWs. HIV infection was more prevalent among women who were forced into sex slavery than among those who entered sex work voluntarily. The increased HIV infections associated with sexual violence have become a crucial issue.

Keywords: India, HIV, female sex workers (FSWs), violence, scoping review, sex abuse, sex trafficking, child sexual abuse, sex slavery, AIDS (acquired immune deficiency syndrome)

1. Introduction

Sex work is one of the most longstanding professions [1]. According to a survey, there are about 10 million sex workers in India and Asia's largest sex trade hub. India's sex-work business value accounts for approximately 8.4 billion dollars. About 30% of sex workers are children [1]. Child sexual abuse is referred to the sexual activity that happens to an under the age of 18 reluctantly or involves pressure, manipulation, bullying, intimidation, threats, deception, or force. Nearly half a million children are dragged into the sex trade in India [1].

FSWs are a global reality regardless of whether it is localised in the community or not [2]. The high incidence of violence against female sex workers (FSWs) around the world, including sexual violence, makes them more susceptible to negative effects on their physical and mental health, particularly HIV infection [3].

The route of entry to the FSWs may have been different, with sex work as a chosen profession or as a result of sexual slavery and being a victim of sex trafficking or child sex abuse, but the consequences of all forms remain the same as FSW and all share the same type of mental and physical health risk and impact. According to a survey conducted by Rao et al. [4], two drivers that have forced Indian women into sex work were financial needs and broken families.

Gore and Patwardhan [2] argued that for Indian females the primary reasons for being a FSW are financial hardship and desperation. Broadly speaking these might include but are not limited to poverty due to widowhood or separation, family debt, lack of education, limited economic opportunities, lack of family support, lack of legal or social protection, negative social circumstances in life, vulnerabilities due to migration, sex trafficking, or even cultural tradition [2].

Although the exact number of female sex workers (FSWs) in India is not known it is estimated around 3million out of the 1.4 billion population [5, 6]; they are a highly stigmatised group [7]. Several other laws have caused some degree of restrictions on female sex work [8].

However, most FSWs personally are not willing to admit being sex workers [9]. Estimates show that about 1% of females in urban areas engage in sex work [9]. Most of these FSWs are between 15 and 54 years [9] and their mean age is 30 years [2].

Gore and Patwardhan [2] reported that on average an individual FSW in India would meet 7 to 9 clients per day which is higher than average in the USA or Thailand with 2 and 5.4, respectively. Therefore, this level of contact poses a higher health risk in particular HIV infection to them [2]. Additionally, this population faces other public health issues such as mental health issues and violence [10–13]. Notwithstanding interventions being implemented, FSWs continue to experience a surge in the prevalence of AIDS and the incidence of violence [12].

According to Ministry of Health and Family Welfare [14], more than 23 million of the Indian population are HIV patients (prevalence rate of 0.21%). Nevertheless, HIV infection among the general population has shown a decline from 1997 to 2021 [15].

However, the health challenge for the FSWs is overcoming health service access barriers such as access to HIV/AIDS treatment when needed, legal service, and protection. Therefore, these factors together make the FSWs highly vulnerable to HIV transmission [16].

According to the reports, Indian women accounted for 40% of annual new HIV infections in 2017 (see **Figure 1**) [17].

Rao et al. [4] found that FSWs' alcohol use has played as a negative factor in their ability to negotiate condom use during sex work and has increased their HIV vulnerability.

Research has identified that some of the sex buyers would bargain with the FSWs for paying a higher rate and having intercourse without contraception/protection [4].

FSWs in India live in an environment of risk and violence. For example, in a study of 200 sex workers, more than 95% of participants had experienced violence [12].

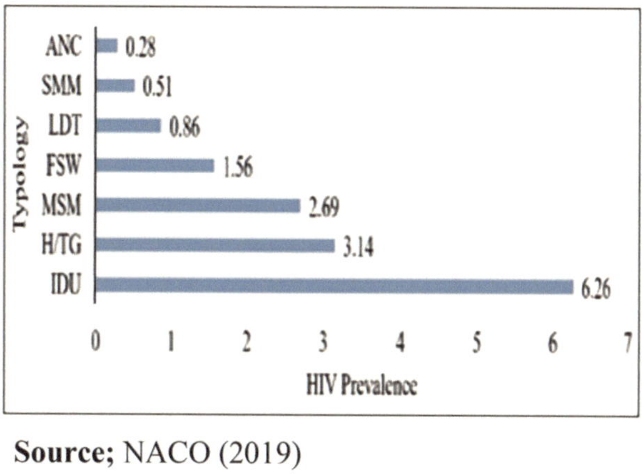

Figure 1.
HIV prevalence (%) among ANC client, FSW, MSM, IDU & other risk groups, India (HSS 2016–2017). Source: NACO [16].

This shows that most FSWs have been victims of some form of violence from men in the street or from the police [12]. The first weeks into entering sex work tend to be the most dangerous. The violence comes in various forms, including cutting or stabbing with knives, acid attacks, sexual harassment, and beating [12, 18]. Some have even lost their lives to violence [19].

India is ranked third in terms of the HIV burden worldwide [20]. According to the National AIDS Control Organisation (2012), about 2.1 million people were living with HIV/AIDs in the country [20]. The epidemic is concentrated among high-risk groups such as sex workers, especially women [10]. HIV prevalence among female sex workers differs from one state to another in India. Maharashtra tends to have a high burden, with a prevalence of 7.4% [12]. While there is a decline in prevalence, it is still significantly higher among female sex workers compared to the general population.

Nonetheless, there were few reviews on FSWs, while to the best of our knowledge, there was no review on HIV and violence among FSWs in India. Therefore, this scoping review aims to explore HIV and violence among female sex workers in India.

2. Methodology

2.1 Study design

This scoping review has included quantitative, qualitative, and mixed methods of primary research studies.

2.2 Search strategy

The databases used for the initial review of literature were PubMed, PubMed Central, Embase, and CINAHL Plus. Cochrane Database of Systematic Reviews was searched for existing or ongoing systematic reviews. Different systematic reviews were found related to FSWs; however, no review was conducted on HIV and violence among female sex workers in India.

A wide range of literature searches were conducted on published literature to identify different types of publications. The literature search was limited to India only because India is placed third for the global burden of HIV [20] and a publication period from 2000 to 2021 to confine the research to recent evidence. The text words and relevant indexing were used in the search strategy to capture the concept of HIV and violence among female sex workers in India.

2.3 Search tool

See **Table 1**.

The search terms were employed using Boolean operators (AND / OR), and the MeSH (Medical Subject Headings) browser was used for indexing articles.

The literature search in the databases used the following keywords:

- HIV/HIV infections/sexually transmitted infections
- Violence/client violence/Intimate Partner Violence (IPV)/sexual risk
- Female sex workers/sex work/sex workers/prostitution/sexual practices/sex trafficking/street-based female sex workers/FSWs, sex abuse, sex trafficking, child sexual abuse, sex slavery,
- India

The search was limited to the original research articles, English language articles and full-text articles.

In addition, reference lists of the included studies were searched to identify relevant studies, known as reference harvesting (**Figure 2**).

2.4 Study selection

See **Table 2**.

To avoid duplication bias, duplicate articles were removed before inclusion and exclusion criteria were implemented.

2.5 Implementation of inclusion and exclusion criteria

Initially, articles were screened for a study design that resulted after applying limitations. Further, titles and abstracts against inclusion criteria were scanned for the relevant articles, followed by the screening of complete articles identified in the initial

Population	**India female sex workers**
Exposure	Sex work
Outcome	HIV and violence

Table 1.
PEO.

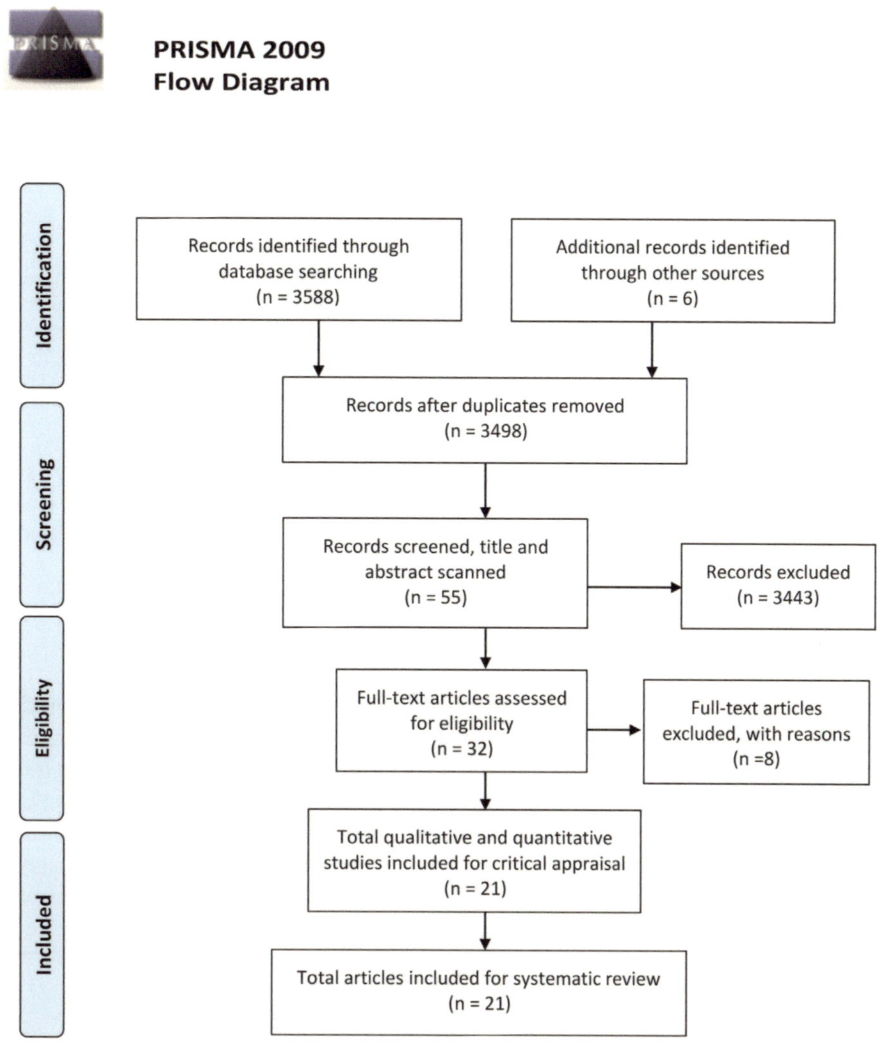

Figure 2.
Preferred reporting items for systematic reviews and meta-analyses (PRISMA) 2009 flow diagram.

Inclusion criteria	Exclusion criteria
• All research studies, including female sex workers in India • Articles about HIV among female sex workers • Research involving violence against female sex workers • Primary research articles, quantitative studies, qualitative studies, and articles published in the English language, including articles published from 2000 to 2021	• Any investigations that are not involving female sex workers in India • Research that is not related to HIV and violence • Review articles, commentaries, letters to the editors, and case studies, other than English language articles are not included

Table 2.
Inclusion and exclusion criteria.

screening as relevant potential articles. The articles with insufficient information regarding HIV and violence were excluded. Editorials, letters to the editors, review articles and commentaries were excluded. After the inclusion and exclusion criteria implementation, 21 Papers were chosen for the critical appraisal stage.

2.6 Data abstraction

Microsoft Excel was used to extract the data. The data extracted included the references of the article; research aim; the study setting, e.g., area, country; sample size; the study design, the key findings or the results related to HIV and Violence among female sex workers; the limitations of the study.

2.7 Analysis

As this scoping review includes data from both qualitative and quantitative studies, meta-analysis was not possible. The data taken from the included papers were organised and analysed using Microsoft Excel. After that, a textual narrative synthesis was performed.

2.8 Critical appraisal

The 21 studies were subjected to a critical assessment to determine their methodological strengths and shortcomings, the study's validity, the results' reliability, and the presence of biases. It was also done to see if the studies were designed, conducted, and published in a trustworthy manner, and if they provided a meaningful answer to the scoping review question. The studies were evaluated using a variety of appraisal methodologies, with the Critical Appraisal Skills Programme (CASP) being used to grade the qualitative research's quality. The AXIS critical appraisal instrument was, designed expressly, used to appraise cross-sectional studies.

2.9 Ethical consideration

No ethical approval is sought for this research as this scoping review retrieves and synthesises the data from already published articles.

3. Results

3.1 The outcome of the critical appraisal

The critical appraisal resulted in 21 studies that were included in the review.
See **Table 3**.
See **Table 4**.

3.2 Characteristics of the included studies

Table 5 presents the results of extracted summary information from the included studies. Characteristics of the included studies will be explored then.

Qualitative Studies: CASP tool	Section A: Are the results valid?					Section B: What are the consequences?				
Reference	Was there a clear statement of the aims of the research?	Is a qualitative methodology appropriate?	Was the research design appropriate to address the aims of the research?	Was the recruitment strategy appropriate to the aims of the research?	Was the data collected in a way that addresses the research issue?	Has the relationship between the researcher and participants been adequately considered	Have ethical issues been taken into consideration?	Was the data analysis sufficiently rigorous?	Is there a clear statement of findings?	How valuable is the research?
Blanchard et al. [21]	+	+/−	+	+	+	−	+/−	+/−	+	+

(+) = item adequately addressed, (−) = item not adequately addressed, and (+/−) = item partially addressed.

Table 3.
Critical appraisal for qualitative studies using the Critical Appraisal Skills Programme (CASP) tool.

	Introduction					Methods				Results					Discussion			
Reference	Were the Aims/ Objectives of the Study Clear?	Was the Study Design Appropriate for the Stated Aim (s)?	Was the Sample Size Justified?	Was the Target/ Reference Population Clearly Defined?	Was the Sample Frame Taken from an Appropriate Population Base So That It Closely Represented the Target/ Reference Population under Investigation?	Was the Selection Process Likely to Select Subjects/ Participants That Were Representative of the Target/ Reference Population under Investigation?	Were Measures Undertaken to Address and Categorise - non-Responders?	Were the Risk Factor and Outcome Variables Measured Appropriate to the Aims of the Study?	Were the Risk Factor and Outcome Variables Measured Correctly Using Instruments/ Measurements That Had Been Trialled, Piloted or Published Previously?	Is It Clear What was Used to Determine Statistical Significance and/or Precision Estimates? (e.g., *p*-Values, Confidence Intervals)	Were the Methods (Including Statistical Methods) Sufficiently Described to Enable Them to Be Repeated?	Were the basic data adequately described?	Does the response rate raise concerns about non-response bias?	Were the results internally consistent?	Were the results presented for all the analyses described in the methods?	Were the authors discussions and the conclusions justified by the results?	Were the limitations of the study discussed?	Was ethical approval or consent of participants attained?
Reed et al. [22]	+	+	+/–	+	+	+/–	NA	+	–	+	+/–	+	NA	+	+	+/–	+	+
Reed et al. [23]	+	+	+/–	+	+	+/–	NA	+	–	+	+	+	–	+	+	+/–	+	+
Swain et al. [24]	+	+	+	+	+	+	+	+	–	+	+	+	–	+	+	+	+	+
Ramesh et al. [25]	+/–	+	+/–	–	–	+	–	+	–	+	–	+	–	+	+	+	+	+
Blanchard et al. [26]	+	+	+	+/–	+	+	–	+	–	+	+	+	–	+	+	+	+	+
Travasso et al. [27]	+/–	+	–	+/–	–	+/–	–	+	+	+	+/–	+	–	+	+/–	+	+	+
Saggurti et al. [28]	+	+	+/–	+	+	+/–	–	+	–	+	+	+/–	NS	+	+	+	+	+
Javalakar et al. [19]	+	+	–	+	+	+	–	+	+	+	+	+	NS	+	+	+	+	+

	Introduction						Methods				Results					Discussion		
Patel et al. [29]	+	+	+	+	+	+/−	NS	+	+/−	+	+	+	NS	+	+	+	+	+
Sarkar et al. [30]	+/−	+	+/−	+/−	+/−	+/−	−	+	−	+	+/−	+	NS	+	+	+	+	+
Erausquin, Reed, and Blankenship [31]	+/−	+	+	+/−	+	+/−	−	+	−	+	+	+	−	+	+	+	+	+
George, Sabarwal, and Martin [32]	+/−	+	+	+	+	+	−	+	−	+	+/−	+	−	+	+	+/−	+	+
Wirth et al. [33]	+	+	+	+	+	+/−	−	+	−	+	+	+/−	−	+	+	+/−	+	−
Gupta et al. [34]	+	+	−	+	+	+/−	NS	+	+	+	+	−	NS	+	+	+/−	+	+
Heylen et al. [35]	+	+	+/−	+	+	+/−	NS	+	+	+	+	+		+	+	+	+	+
Mahapatra et al. [36]	+	+	+/−	+	+	+/−	NS	+	−	+	+/−	+	NS	+	+	+/−	+	+
Prakash et al. [37]	+	+	+	+	+	+/−	NS	+	+	+	+	+	NS	+	+	+	+	+
Reed et al. [38]	+	+	+/−	+	+	+	NS	+	−	+	+	+	NS	+	+	+	+	+
Patra et al. [39]	+	+	+	+	+	+/−	−	+	−	+	+	+	−	+	+	+	+	+
Deering et al. [40]	+	+	+	+	+	+/−	−	+	−	+	+	+	NS	+	+	+/−	+	+

(+) = item adequately addressed, (−) = item not adequately addressed, (+/−) = item partially addressed, NS = not stated or "I do not know", and NA = not applicable.

Table 4.
Critical appraisal for cross-sectional studies using the appraisal tool for cross-sectional studies (AXIS).

4. Characteristics of the included studies

Based on the inclusion criteria, overall, 21 articles were considered for this study. All the research was carried out between 2000 and 2021. The most often used scales for identifying sexual violence HIV infections were the Integrated Behavioural and Biological Assessments (IBBAs) and Polling Booth Surveys (PBS). Most research looked at the prevalence of sexual violence and HIV infections and the factors contributing to these conditions. At the same time, the rest focused on depression and mood disorders among sex workers. Around 11 papers emphasised both sexual violence and sexually transmitted infections, approximately seven papers depicted HIV infections solely among FSWs, and few papers prioritised depressive mood and emotional instability of the female sex workers. The characteristics of the included studies are presented in **Table 5**.

4.1 Design of Studies

The selected 21 papers comprised cross-sectional studies, descriptive studies, and some qualitative studies. The studies were undertaken by questionnaire, online survey, convenience sampling and in-person interviews to get consistent data.

4.2 Female sex workers and HIV infections

Client and intimate partner violence (CIPV) was an everyday occurrence for female sex workers. In the setting of alcohol use, harassment and forced group sex created intense obstacles to condom use negotiation. Furthermore, women's inability to negotiate condom use with intimate relationships was dictated by established gender conventions. However, there was evidence of women's positive views of their contributions to family well-being through sex work and the adoption of successful survival mechanisms in the face of risk. Sexual assault, physical violence, accepting more money for unprotected sex, and a recent sexually transmitted infections (STIs), including HIV infection symptoms were all more common among FSWs who reported household instability.

Domestic violence (DV) and unprotected sex with customers contributed to reported HIV infections, however, domestic instability remained strongly related to STIs (e.g., AIDS) even when both violence and unprotected sex with clients were considered. The studies show a link between homelessness, victimisation, and the chance of contracting HIV. In addition to its connection to individual risky sexual practices, residential volatility appears to be linked to women's HIV risk. Almost one out of every four sex workers (24%) had been trafficked into the industry.

Almost half of those surveyed (50.2%) were forced or pressured into sex labour before they became 18 (41.7%). FSWs who initially were victims of child sexual abuse had more unprotected transactional intercourse compared to adults (Adjusted Odds Ratio (AOR) = 2.06); however, being forced or coerced into sex work was associated with a lower risk of HIV transmission (AOR = 0.45). Participants were on average, 32 years old, 22% were married. They experienced physical (22%) and sexual (21%) assaults from their customers and spouses. Adjusted logistic regression analysis models suggested FSWs who had experienced client violence were more common among those accepting extra money for unprotected sex (AOR = 1.7; 95% CI;1.4 to 2.2), less likely to be consistent in condom use (AOR = 0.6; 95% CI;0.5 to 0.7), and more likely to report STI symptoms (AOR = 3.5; 95% CI; 2.6 to 4.6) [41].

Reference	Research aim	Study setting/location	Sample size	Study design	Key findings	Limitations
Reed et al. [22]	The current study investigates the relationship between FSW's reported residential instability—defined as a high frequency of reported evictions—and their experiences of violence and sexual risk factors for HIV.	Rajahmundry, within the East Godavari District of Andhra Pradesh, India.	673 female sex workers	Cross-sectional study	Residential instability remained strongly related to STIs independent of the effects of either violence or unprotected sex with clients. Violence associated with residential instability was a contributor to reported STIs. The findings highlight the connection between HIV risk, violence, and residential instability. In addition to its association with collective risky sexual activities, residential instability appears to be linked to women's HIV risk.	The cross-sectional design did not allow for prospective FSW follow-up, a difficulty in research with hard-to-reach populations
Reed et al. [23]	This study explores violence encountered in work and personal contexts and relation to HIV risk factors in these contexts among female sex workers (FSW) in Andhra Pradesh, India.	Andhra Pradesh, India	2335 FSW	Cross-sectional survey	According to models of adjusted logistic regression, FSWs with client violence were less likely to consistently use condoms with clients, more likely to report experiencing STI symptoms, and more likely to report accepting more money for unprotected sex trades. Women who reported spousal violence were also more likely to report STI symptoms, less likely to report consistently using condoms with clients.	Stigma frequently causes sensitive topics or socially unacceptable behaviour to go unreported.

Reference	Research aim	Study setting/location	Sample size	Study design	Key findings	Limitations
Swain et al. [24]	The purpose of this study is to comprehend the relationships between violence, risk factors for HIV infection, and reproductive health among a group of mobile FSWs in India.	22 districts from four high HIV prevalence states (Andhra Pradesh, Karnataka, Maharashtra, Tamil Nadu) in India	5498 FSWs	Cross-sectional behavioural survey	Thirty-five percent of all mobile FSWs said they had been the victim of violence at least once in the previous year; 11% said it had been physical and 19.5% said it had been sexual. The findings show that FSWs who had ever been the victim of physical or sexual abuse were much more likely to be at risk for HIV infection as well as dangers to their reproductive health. FSWs who had suffered sexual violence were more likely to report inconsistent condom usage and develop STI symptoms than those who had experienced physical violence.	First self-reports are very susceptible to underreporting and social desirability biases. Self-reported symptoms of STI may be underestimated. Second, because analyses are cross-sectional, causality cannot be inferred from relationships between violence victimisation and reproductive health measures. Finally, results cannot be applied to other FSWs in India and are particular to mobile FSWs from four states with high prevalence.
Ramesh et al. [25]	This study evaluated the individual and combined relationships between sexual risk behaviours, mobility, and violence, as well as the prevalence of HIV and STIs among female sex workers (FSWs) in India.	eight high HIV prevalence districts of Andhra Pradesh state, India	2042 FSWs	A cross-sectional survey	One fifth of FSWs (19%) reported encountering violence; 68% said they had visited elsewhere in the past year at least once and engaged in sexual activity here. Compared to their peers, mobile FSWs were more likely to report violence (23% vs. 10%, $p < 0.001$). One in five people had an HIV positive test result. In adjusted models, FSWs who reported both mobility and violence	The limitations of self-reported data are widely acknowledged, and this study's primary independent variables were based on self-reported responses.

Reference	Research aim	Study setting/location	Sample size	Study design	Key findings	Limitations
					compared to their counterparts were more likely to report unprotected sex with occasional (adjusted OR: 2.86, 95% CI: 1.76–4.65) and regular clients (adjusted OR: 2.07, 95% CI: 1.40–3.06) and to report HIV infection.	
Blanchard et al. [26]	The authors of this research present an "integrated empowerment framework" based on theoretical and programmatic literature and then employ it to empirically analyse the relationships between empowerment and social transformation and HIV risk reduction among FSWs in south India.	Belgaum, Gulbarga, Gadag and Dharwad districts in Karnataka, and Solapur in Maharashtra.	1750 FSWs	Cross-sectional behavioural tracking surveys	More programme contact was positively correlated with both power within and power with ($p < 0.01$ and $p < 0.001$, respectively). In terms of self-efficacy for condom and health care usage, these empowerment measures were likewise linked to "personal transformation" results ($p < 0.001$). The "social change" factors, such as increased autonomy and decreased aggression and coercion, were most strongly associated with collective empowerment (power with others), especially in districts with longer-running programmes ($p < 0.05$). Power with others was linked to condom use with customers ($p < 0.001$), but power within was linked to more frequent use of condoms with regular partners ($p < 0.01$) and higher service utilisation ($p < 0.05$).	First, because the surveys were cross-sectional, we are unable to determine the causal chain's direction. Second, there could be participation bias. Third, even for variables measuring communal processes of empowerment, the responses were self-reported individually. If the community participation process results in social desirability in each FSW's responses to empowerment questions, the resultant misclassification bias may become even more severe.

Reference	Research aim	Study setting/location	Sample size	Study design	Key findings	Limitations
Travasso et al. [27]	The purpose of this study is to investigate the relationships between FSWs' non-paying partner status, including cohabitation, and their exposure to HIV prevention programmes, involvement in social groups and activities, and use of health care services in three Indian states.	Maharashtra, Andhra Pradesh and Tamil Nadu	8107 FSWs	Cross-sectional survey	Analysis showed that FSWs reporting a non-cohabiting non-paying partner were more likely to be exposed to HIV prevention programmes, attend meetings, and visit a sexually transmitted infections clinic at least twice in the previous 6 months as compared to those reporting no non-paying partner. However, FSWs with a non-paying partner tended to use condoms consistently and were more susceptible to contracting HIV because they lived on the streets ($p < 0.001$) and were in debt ($p < 0.001$).	First, recall and social desirability biases were present. Second, cross-sectional data cannot be used to show causal links between partner status and the use of HIV prevention programmes. Third, only three vulnerability metrics were used to produce the vulnerability score. A further limitation of any studies on women's experiences of violence is that experiences are often measured using questions like those in the IBBA.
Saggurti et al. [28]	The association between mobility indicators, socioeconomic vulnerabilities, and HIV risk behaviours among 5498 mobile female sex workers (FSWs) residing in India's four states with high HIV incidence is examined in this study.	Andhra Pradesh, Karnataka, Tamil Nadu and Maharashtra, India	5498 FSWs	Cross-sectional behavioural survey	Even after adjusting for a number of demographic factors and socioeconomic vulnerabilities like experiences of violence, FSWs with higher levels of mobility reported inconsistent condom use in intercourse with clients considerably more frequently than FSWs with lower levels of mobility. Additionally, it was discovered that brief visits and attendance at Jatra (religious fairs) locations were significantly associated with	First, only mobile FSWs were included in the study population; no non-mobile FSWs were. Second, this study shows that each of the variables analysed, including socio-demographic traits and associated vulnerabilities, raises the risk of HIV infection among mobile FSWs. Thirdly, because the replies to the analysis's questions were self-reported, they were prone to social desirability and memory bias.

Reference	Research aim	Study setting/location	Sample size	Study design	Key findings	Limitations
					the users' inconsistent use of condoms during client interactions, as well as their continued use of sex despite the presence of STI symptoms.	
Javalkar et al. [19].	This study looks at the characteristics of relationships between female sex workers and their intimate partners and how those factors affect IPV.	47 villages in Bagalkot district, north Karnataka.	620 FSWs	Cross-sectional baseline survey	Even though most partnerships started after a sex work encounter, 84% of IPs claimed they were unaware of their current sex work activities. In the past 6 months, 49% FSWs reported experiencing emotional, 33% physical, and 7% sexual violence, whereas 24% FSWs reported experiencing recent severe physical and/or sexual violence from IPs. In the past 6 months, their clients had used physical and/or sexual violence against them, they had engaged in sexual activity with their IP while under the influence of alcohol, and they had provided financial support to their IP.	Researchers are unable to determine if there are temporal or causal relationships between factors and intimate partner violence because the data was cross-sectional. Additionally, there were several discrepancies in the time ranges employed, which could have improved reporting accuracy. There may be underreporting of behaviours.
Blanchard et al. [21]	The goal was to investigate the experiences and understandings of intimate partner violence and HIV/AIDS among Bagalkot sex workers and their intimate partners in order to inform both theories and practice.	Bagalkot district, Karnataka state, India.	38 participants	A community-based, interpretive qualitative methodology	The findings demonstrated that several interrelated, multi-level factors contributed to the broad acceptance of violence and its continued usage in participants' intimate relationships. This included stigma, societal gender norms,	Their goal was to ensure the purposive sample was as representative as possible. However, bias could have developed if people who agreed to participate shared milder examples or were less reluctant to talk about

Reference	Research aim	Study setting/location	Sample size	Study design	Key findings	Limitations
					and restrictions on sex work and personal expectations that justified violence and reflected them.	violence. Particularly with regard to the level of conflict and condom use, there was probably some social desirability bias or non-disclosure in the stories.
Patel et al. [29]	The aims of this study are to identify major depressive symptoms among FSWs in southern India and evaluate the separate and combined relationships between mobility and violence and major depressive symptoms.	Six districts (Ananthapur, Chittoor, Karimnagar, Khammam, Nalgonda and Warangal)	2400 participants	Cross-sectional survey	Major depression was detected in 29% of FSWs, more than one-fourth of the population. In contrast to those who reported neither, FSWs who were both mobile for sex work outside of their district of residence and had encountered any violence (combined association) within the previous year were six times more likely to screen positive for major depression (62% vs. 19%). According to the individual association data, FSWs were three times more likely to screen positive for serious depression if they reported being mobile outside the district and if they had been physically or sexually assaulted within the previous year.	This study's characteristics were based on self-reported responses, and it is well known that self-reported data has certain drawbacks. The FSW populations in this study are a part of the Avahan programme, which aims to empower and engage the community, they might not be representative of all FSW populations. This study only included a small sample of FSWs who were CBO members, its conclusions cannot be applied to all FSWs in India.
Sarkar et al. [30]	To comprehend HIV infection, violence, negotiating skills, and sex trafficking among sex	West Bengal, Eastern India	580 sex workers	Cross-sectional study	In contrast to Bangladeshis (7%) and Indians (9%), Nepalese (43%) had a higher seroprevalence of HIV.	Important research limitations included convenient sampling, self-reported behaviour, the absence of minor girls in

DOI: http://dx.doi.org/10.5772/intechopen.115109

Reference	Research aim	Study setting/location	Sample size	Study design	Key findings	Limitations
	workers in brothels in West Bengal, eastern India.				Twenty-four percent of sex workers entered the industry through being trafficked. When this profession first began, victims of trafficking, including those sold by family members, experienced more violence (57%) than those who entered the field voluntarily (15%). With the most recent two clients, the overall condom negotiating rate was 38%. HIV was found to be substantially linked with sexual violence by multivariate analysis.	brothels as study subjects, interviewing participants in brothels where privacy and appropriate spaces were not always available, the fear of disclosing private information about the brothel owner, lost business hours, and recall bias in some instances.
Erausquin et al. [31]	In this study, researchers investigate the potential links between five police-related incidents and indicators of HIV risk and violence among a sample of female sex workers (FSWs) in Andhra Pradesh, India, and we discuss the implications for HIV prevention.	Andhra Pradesh, India	835 FSWs	Cross-sectional survey	The findings showed that sexually transmitted infection symptoms, inconsistent condom use, accepting more money for sex without a condom, and being arrested were associated with having sex with police to avoid trouble, giving gifts to police to avoid trouble, having police take away condoms, experiencing a workplace raid, and being arrested.	The data analysis was cross-sectional, which limited the capacity to determine causality. Additionally, they only examined the experiences of adult FSWs; no inferences can be made about those of younger FSWs. Furthermore, it is questionable whether FSW self-reports of either HIV risk behaviours or experiences with police in this situation are accurate and reliable.
George et al. [32]	This study looks at connections between the types of sex work done and the prevalence of recent victimisation due to physical and sexual violence	Three districts of Andhra Pradesh state	1138 FSWs	Cross-sectional survey	A significant frequency of sexual and physical violence at work; 77% of FSWs reported sexual violence and 50% of FSWs reported physical	The sampling approach employed in the current investigation restricts the ability to extrapolate and might have created bias if

Reference	Research aim	Study setting/location	Sample size	Study design	Key findings	Limitations
	among a large sample of young FSWs.				violence. Comparatively to women who participate in sex work in their home districts.	individuals were chosen based on an unidentified factor that was pertinent to the findings of the study.
Wirth et al. [33]	Researchers looked into the possibility of both forced and early introduction into sex work as potential explanations for the link between sex trafficking and HIV. They also tested if each of these connections had been altered by sexual violence.	Four districts (Bangalore, Bellary, Belgaum, and Shimoga) in Karnataka, India	1814 adult FSWs	Cross-sectional	Overall, 372 (21%) women fulfilled either one of the two sex trafficking definitional criteria: 278 (16%) people started doing sex work before turning 18, and 107 (5%) people said they were forced into sex work. 13 people (or 0.7%) met both requirements. Regardless of age at entry into sex work, women forced into the sector had a higher likelihood of HIV than women who did so voluntarily (odds ratio = 2.30, 95% confidence interval: 1.08, 4.90). When sexual violence was present, there was a more significant correlation between forced sex work and HIV infection (odds ratio = 11.13, 95% confidence interval: 2.41, 51.40).	Data on sexual assault was only collected for the prior year. Authors will have underestimated the impact of sexual violence. Next, because information on sex work admission was gathered at the same time as HIV status evaluation, they could not confirm that participation in the sex trade preceded HIV infection. The survey did not cover women who were involved in all types of sex work, despite the use of a probability-based sampling framework.
Gupta et al. [34]	The current study's goals were to determine the prevalence of trafficking as a means of entering the sex industry among a sample of FSWs in Andhra Pradesh, India, as well as to look at potential	Coastal Andhra Pradesh, India	812 FSWs	Cross-sectional study	The UN criteria of sex trafficking were met by 1 in 5 (19.3%) FSWs. Women who were trafficked into sex work were more likely than other FSWs to report recent violent experiences, have more clients	The cross-sectional data could not be used to evaluate the temporality of associations. The reliance on self-report may also have caused underreporting of the mode and/or age of entry; however,

Reference	Research aim	Study setting/location	Sample size	Study design	Key findings	Limitations
	differences in HIV risk factors (such as the use or non-use of services targeted towards FSWs) between women who entered the sex work through trafficking and those who did not.				per week, and have more days of sex work per week. Regarding condom use or knowledge of HIV, there were no appreciable variations.	this may mean that the findings understate the HIV-related vulnerabilities of FSWs who enter sex work through trafficking. Lastly, the results are particularly relevant to FSWs whose demographic data are represented in the current study because they are not reflective of a valid probability sample.
Heylen et al. [35]	The current article intends to fill the gap by examining patterns of physical abuse from various partners and alcohol consumption by both the FSWs and abusive partners using data from a quantitative survey among a diverse set of FSWs who solicit and work in different venues in Chirala, Andhra Pradesh.	Andhra Pradesh, India	589 FSWs	Cross-sectional study	Eighty-four percent of FSWs admitted to drinking, and 65% said they had ever been physically abused by a partner. Most abused women experienced abuse from several partners, frequently brought on by intoxication or FSW's defiance. The frequency of alcohol use by the FSW was linked to abuse by clients and the primary partner in multivariate logistic regressions. Still, the primary partner's abuse was the only one for which the partner's alcohol use was significant.	This study was cross-sectional. Hence we were unable to establish causality. Second, it's uncertain how well the study group represented the area's population of more concealed FSWs.
Mahapatra et al. [36]	This study aims to examine the rate of non-disclosure of violence among FSWs in India and exposure to HIV prevention programmes.	Andhra Pradesh, Karnataka, Maharashtra and Tamil Nadu.	1341 FSWs	Cross-sectional survey	With significant variations in the pattern of disclosure between states, about 54% of FSWs did not reveal their experience of violence to	First, answers to the victimisation of violence, non-disclosure, and information about the violent offenders are based on self-reports, and

Reference	Research aim	Study setting/location	Sample size	Study design	Key findings	Limitations
					anybody. 36% more FSWs discussed their experience with an NGO employee or colleague. Violence committed by non-paying partners was twice as likely to be reported as non-disclosure as violence committed by paying partners or a stranger. Similarly, FSWs who were not registered with an NGO/sex worker collective were 40% more likely to report non-disclosure of violence against those noted (58% vs. 53%).	there may be underreporting. Second, there were various ways to answer the question about the person who committed the act of violence. Third, the study did not collect information on the type, extent, cause, or actions in response to the experience of violence.
Prakash et al. [37]	This study intends to investigate the overall (real) impact of violence on FSWs' self-reported STI rates and treatment-seeking behaviour in the Thane district.	Thane district, Maharashtra	2785 FSWs	Cross-sectional behavioural study	At the time of the survey, almost 18% of the sampled FSWs reported experiencing physical abuse. FSWs, who solicited clients in public locations, worked jobs other than sex work, had funds and reported having a high client volume each week had a considerably increased likelihood of experiencing such assault. The average adjusted effect of violence definitely showed a decrease in treatment-seeking (10%, $p < 0.05$) and an increase in the probability of any STI (11%, $p < 0.05$) and many STIs (8%, $p < 0.10$).	Physical abuse, particularly those committed by regular partners, might be unreported. Other than this, the survey did not gather data on sexual violence. There was no quantifiable data in the survey to assess how empowered FSWs were in the study area. Lastly, the results of STI are based on self-reported symptoms rather than cases that have undergone clinical testing.

Reference	Research aim	Study setting/location	Sample size	Study design	Key findings	Limitations
Reed et al. [38]	This study investigates the relationship between the difficulties of motherhood and sexual risk factors for HIV among female sex workers (FSW).	Rajahmundry, within the East Godavari District of Andhra Pradesh, India.	850 FSWs	Cross-sectional survey	FSW who reported having three or more children in the home or currently having child health concerns were considerably less likely to report consistent condom use and more likely to accept more money for sex without a condom. Women who indicated current child health problems were also more likely to report a STI symptom in the previous 6 months. Findings imply that increased vulnerability to HIV risk among FSWs is connected to burdensome caregiving obligations for children.	The cross-sectional design does not allow for prospective FSW follow-up and does not establish the temporality of these associations. Additionally, the analyses' items rely on respondents' self-reported responses. Stigma can frequently lead to underreporting of delicate subjects or socially unwelcome actions, as the sexual risk factors examined in the current study. Additionally, the results of the current study may not be generalizable to other populations of sex workers.
Patra et al. [39]	This study aims to understand more about the factors that influence anal sex behaviours among female sex workers (FSWs) and to look into the relationship between anal sex and HIV-related sexual risk factors in Andhra Pradesh, India.	Andhra Pradesh, India	795 FSWs	Cross-sectional behavioural survey	Anal sex was used by one-fourth (23%) of FSWs in the previous year. The likelihood of engaging in anal sex was higher among FSWs 35 years of age or older than it was among those under 25, among those who had been married in the past as opposed to those who are still married, as well as among those who reported heavy alcohol use as opposed to those who did not and those who had experienced violence as opposed to those who had	First, cross-sectional survey data were gathered, proving a cause-and-effect relationship is challenging. As the information was self-reported and acknowledged that there is a stigma attached to sharing such sensitive experiences, the prevalence of anal sex may be under-reported. Third, no biological samples were taken throughout the survey; rather, self-reported STI symptoms served as a marker for HIV risk.

Reference	Research aim	Study setting/location	Sample size	Study design	Key findings	Limitations
					not. STI-related symptoms were more prevalent among FSWs who engaged in anal intercourse than those solely involved in vaginal sex. There was no connection between using condoms and anal intercourse.	
Deering et al. [40]	This study explored the association between violence and inconsistent condom usage while characterising the nature and frequency of violence against female sex workers (FSWs) committed by their clients and their primary intimate or other non-paying partner (NPP). Additionally, the risk factors for client violence were evaluated.	Karnataka state, India	1219 FSWs	Cross-sectional survey	9.6 and 3.7% of 1219 FSWs reported suffering violence at the hands of clients and the NPP, respectively. Repeat customers produced similar outcomes. The NPP found no statistically significant association between ICU and non-paying partner violence. Only being recently arrested remained substantially linked with experiencing client aggression after multivariable analysis.	This analysis relied on self-reported responses to potentially sensitive topics, and as a result, the questions are prone to social desirability bias. This study may underestimate reports of violence in particular. Although the surveys utilised a relatively broad definition of physical violence, the purpose of sexual violence was more limited and might not have included all forms of violence.

Table 5.
Data extraction table.

Women who reported IPV were more likely to accept more money for unprotected sex trades (AOR = 2.1; 95% CI;1.2 to 3.7), less likely to use condoms consistently with clients (AOR = 0.5; 95% CI;0.3 to 0.8), and more likely to report STI symptoms (AOR = 2.6; 95% CI;1.6 to 4.1). The findings show a significant frequency of work-related physical and sexual violence, with 50% of FSWs reporting physical violence [34] and 77% reporting sexual violence.

When compared to women involved in sex work in their home districts, FSWs undertaking contract labour were at a higher risk of physical and sexual violence during work. Individual association findings suggest that FSWs who reported travelling outside of their area of residence and FSWs who had been beaten or raped in the previous year were three times more likely to screen positive for severe depression. There were no significant variations in HIV awareness or condom usage consistency.

4.3 Female sex workers and sexual violence

Around 54% of FSWs did not inform anybody about their violent experiences, with state-by-state variances. A further 36% of FSWs told an NGO worker or a peer about their experience. Non-paying partners were twice as likely to report non-disclosure as paid partners/strangers (53% vs. 68%, AOR = 1.8, 95%CI; 1.3–2.4).

Physical violence was reported by 18% of the FSWs polled at the time of the study. FSWs who recruited clients in public locations, engaged in other economic activities than sex work, possessed funds and reported a high client volume per week had a much-increased risk of encountering such assault. While engaging in sex with frequent partners and customers, FSWs suffering violence were likewise inconsistent condom users. The most recent two clients' overall condom negotiating rate was 38%. HIV was shown to be substantially linked with sexual violence in multivariate analysis (odds ratio = 2.3; 95% confidence range 1.2–4.5) [27]. The study found that trafficked victims [24] were subjected to more violence, including sexual assault, and that sexual violence was linked to HIV infection.

The average adjusted impact of violence showed an increased probability of any STI (including AIDS). FSWs with three or more children in their home or current child health issues were considerably less likely to report safe sex practices (AORs ranged from 0.5 to 0.6) and more likely to pay more money for sex without a condom (AORs: 2.5). Women with current child health issues were more likely to have experienced a STI symptom in the last 6 months (AOR = 1.6; 95%CI:1.1–2.3).

Overall, 372 women (21%) satisfied one or all of the criteria used to define sex trafficking: 278 (16%) started sex work before the age of 18, and 107 (5%) were forced into sex work. Thirteen people (0.7%) satisfied both requirements [31]. Women who were forced into sex work were more likely to be HIV-positive than women who entered freely (odds ratio = 2.30, 95%CI: 1.08, 4.90).

Anal sex was more common among FSWs aged ≥35 years than those aged less than 25 years (AOR: 2.05, P = 0.05), in those who were previously married compared to those who are currently married (AOR: 1.88, P = 0.01), in those who had an income solely from sex work compared with those who had other sources of income (AOR: 1.54, P 0.05), in those who reported heavy alcohol consumption compared to those who had not (AOR: 2.80, $P < 0.01$).

About 34.9% of FSWs reported that they had been the victim of recent physical or sexual violence. Domestic (27.1%), workplace (11.1%), and community (4.2%) perpetrators were all involved in recent violence, with 6.2% of participants reporting both domestic and non-domestic (workplace/community) perpetrators. According to an adjusted study, workplace/community perpetrators' experience of violence is more relevant than household violence in raising HIV/STI risk during sex work (lack of safe sex practices with clients; client or FSW under the influence of alcohol during last intercourse). When compared to FSWs who only reported violence by domestic or workplace/community perpetrators, women who reported recent violence by domestic and workplace/community perpetrators had the highest odds of high titre syphilis infection, current STI symptoms, and condom breakage at last sex, as well as the lowest odds of condom use at last sex with regular clients.

5. Discussion

The issue of sex work is multifaceted. On one hand, there is a challenge with some communities' moral values and appear to be insupportable, on the other hand, it appears to be an unavoidable reality of life [2].

In India, female sex workers struggle in a violent atmosphere. FSWs who recruited clients in public locations, engaged in other economic activities than sex work, possessed funds and reported a high weekly client volume had a more significant chance of encountering such assault. While engaging in sex with frequent partners and customers, FSWs suffer violence and inconsistent condom users. Almost half (41.7%) of the female sex workers were forced or pressured into sex labour under a malicious ground called sexual slavery before turning 18 years old [42]. FSWs entering as a child had more unprotected transactional intercourse in the previous 90 days than those entering as an adult; nevertheless, being forced or coerced into sex work was associated with a higher risk of HIV transmission. Women were abused by several partners, typically because of intoxication or disobedience on the side of the FSW. This community's other public health challenges include a high HIV prevalence, mental health difficulties, and violence [10–12]. Cutting or stabbing with knives, acid assaults, sexual harassment, and beatings are all examples of violence [12, 18]. Some have even died because of the violence [19].

According to a WHO report, violence against FSWs is common and admitted by many [3].

Law on sex work and its law enforcement regularly have failed to safeguard FSWs and therefore the risk of violence has increased. WHO report on India's sex work indicated that sex workers were beaten by police (70%) and arrested (80%) without acceptable evidence [43].

The violence was fuelled by physical torture, rape, and insistent and forced unsafe sex, which harms the cognitive behaviour of female sex workers. In addition to its link to individual hazardous sexual practices, residential instability appears to be linked to women's HIV risk. Compared to their peers, mobile FSWs were more likely to report violence (23% vs. 10%).

FSWs who were a non-paying spouses were more likely to be exposed to HIV prevention tools [41] and use them than those who did not. According to the findings, FSWs who were not supported financially by their partners and non-cohabiting partners were more likely to use the HIV prevention programmes.

Even after adjusting for many demographic variables and socio-economic vulnerabilities, including experiences of violence, FSWs with more mobility reported inconsistent condom usage in intercourse with clients considerably more frequently than FSWs with reduced mobility. Partner violence is always vulgar and crucial from the perspective of more propensity of spreading HIV infections among female sex workers.

Another important thing is the consumption of alcohol and other recreational drugs by FSWs to alleviate depressive moods. Domestic, workplace, and community perpetrators were the sources of violence, with 6.2% of participants reporting recent abuse from domestic and non-domestic (workplace/community) perpetrators. The widespread acceptability and continuance of violence, as well as the absence of safe sex practices in participants' relationships, were caused by several interconnected, multi-level causes.

Individual expectations that justified violence and mirrored society's gender norms were among them, and they were exacerbated by stigma and economic constraints associated with sex work. In India, there have been significantly high-rate incidents that reported to be work-related physical and sexual assault. FSW alcohol usage was linked to abuse by both the client and primary partner; however, abuse was seen with alcohol usage by only primary partner, not client. Inconsistent condom users were also violent while having sex with regular partners and customers. The average adjusted impact of the violence showed an increase in the probability of any STI including HIV infection. Violence compromises Sexual and Reproductive Health (SRH), with mounting chances of incidents like unplanned pregnancies, STI and in particular AIDS [43].

FSW in India hesitated to indicate if they had Unprotected Receptive Anal Intercourse (URAI) with a client in the previous 30 days as in Face-to-Face Interviews (FTFIs) compared with the anonymous Polling Booth Survey (PBS) that was 18.8% vs. 36.2% [44, 45]. FSWs who had anal intercourse were more likely than those who solely used vaginal sex to have HIV infection sexually transmitted infection (STI) symptoms. Baggaley et al. [46] has reported that the HIV transmission risk from Unprotected Receptive Anal Intercourse (URAI) is up to 18 times higher than from receptive vaginal intercourse (URVI). This is mainly explained by the fact that rectal mucosa lacks the protective immune barrier compared with cervico-vaginal secretions and also is more susceptible to traumatic abrasions that enable transmission [44, 45]. There was no link found between anal intercourse and the usage of safe sex practices.

While engaging in sex with frequent partners and customers, FSWs suffering violence were likewise inconsistent in adhering to safe sex practices The average adjusted effect of violence [47] showed a considerable increase in the probability of any STI (11%) and multiple STIs (8%), as well as a decrease in seeking treatment (10%). The extremity of partner violence and the helpless attitudes of women seemed to extend their harassment at work. There are different prospective studies in South India depicting a bit of diminution in HIV incidence in the last 5 years which could be possible by intensifying condoms among men. Moreover, client violence in sex work and constant harassment by an intimate partner have accelerated the suffering of female workers.

A "harm reduction approach" to complex problems like sex work would not deny that reality, but in contrast, aims to ensure safer and more equitable circumstances for sex workers. FSWs experience very complex, but potential risks including infection with HIV, violence, stigma, personal debt, criminalisation, trafficking, etc. Nevertheless, considering comprehensive governmental agencies strategies such as education, empowerment, prevention, care, occupational health and safety, and decriminalisation, have been proven to be highly effective and supportive for FSWs [2, 48]. But despite these initiatives, problems still exist, such as inequalities in access to treatment and support services and gaps in the healthcare system, especially for marginalised communities.

Generally speaking, as a population health preventive measure if the HIV infection epidemic in India needs to be managed, as one of the main sources of transmission, FSWs should be included in planning for the HIV prevention interventions/programmes [49].

5.1 Recognition of legal

On 19 May 2022, the Supreme Court of India announced sex work as a profession, like any other professionals, and sex workers are subject to dignity and constitutional rights, protective arrangements [50].

The recognition of sex work as a profession by the Supreme Court of India may have a potential positive impact as a kind of protection against the FSWs vulnerability, e.g., physical violence and some kind of social support. FSW must be regulated given that it has been recognised as a profession, and the safety of sex workers should be the primary consideration. This will lead to less harm being done to sex workers and a stronger system for protecting them from abuse and exploitation. Therefore, sex workers including FSWs are less exposed to sexually transmitted diseases like HIV and AIDS, and more likely to be protected from police violence, low pay, and harassment [1].

Nonetheless, the stigmatisation practised by the Indian diverse community for faith and cultural norms remains as barrier to the new legal arrangement being implemented fully. Additionally, to some extent, HIV and other infectious disease risk reduction remain heavily dependent on the behavioural patterns of both FSWs and their clients that would need more compliance to the health protection informed by health education and promotion under this category. Legislative actions and regulations have been attempted to address these challenges in recent years. For instance, discrimination in the workplace and hospital settings is prohibited under legislation in India that safeguards the rights of individuals living with HIV/AIDS. These regulations seek to advance equality and guarantee AIDS/HIV patients' access to necessary care. National policy makers should realise that reduction in violence was proven to be another effective factor in HIV transmission and needs to be part of the joint policies for both public health interventions and social protection initiatives.

Legalisation of sex work in India offers a path to decriminalising the sex work and status as a profession that may ensure a better quality of life and socio-economic living status for the sex workers [50]. Following professional recognition, there is clearly an indication for authorities to establish a mandated health screening programme (especially AIDS) for the FSWs as part of the strict industry regulations [1].

6. Strengths and limitations

To the best of authors knowledge, this study is the first scoping review on HIV and violence among female sex workers in India. To reduce bias, the critical appraisal was conducted twice, with a one-week gap between the first and second appraisals, and the two assessments for each study were then compared. Only peer-reviewed articles were included in the study, both a strength and a weakness. Only papers published in English are included in the review, which adds bias due to location and language. Furthermore, omitting articles that are not available in full text may result in the omission of current articles.

7. Conclusion

In India, female sex workers are a severely stigmatised community. The increased HIV infections associated with sexual harassment has become a crucial issue. Findings suggest that women's entry into sex work are primarily due to financial hardship. Even though female sex workers are acquainted with the violent and risky behaviour of their partner, they cannot negotiate with free consent due to their vulnerability (e.g., physical and financial). The prevalence of violence and its link to reproductive health and HIV risk demonstrates that abuse, in general, is a key driver of reproductive health hazards, and sexual harassment is strongly linked to HIV risk among people who have been victims of violence. FSWs unsafe sex practices, negligence about using condoms, job insecurity, and economic crisis all play crucial roles in enhancing sexual violence and HIV infections among female sex workers. Domestic violence is associated with physical injuries, homicide, suicide, emotional distress as well as spreading of sexually transmitted diseases among female sex workers. The violence rate should be highlighted along with the HIV intervention program. The importance of addressing violence as a significant part of the HIV reduction programme should be clarified to the policy makers. Appropriate measures can reduce the vulnerability of female sex workers, ensure their fundamental rights, and provide a violence-free healthy work environment.

Author details

Russell Kabir[1*], Divya Vinnakota[2], Leila Dehghani[3], Brijesh Sathian[4], Bijaya Kumar Padhi[5], Md Rakibul Hasan[6], Sheikh Shamim Hasnain[7], Ilias Mahmud[8] and Ali Davod Parsa[1]

1 Faculty of Health, Medicine and Social Care, Anglia Ruskin University, Chelmsford, UK

2 Department of Allied Health Professions, Sports and Exercise, University of Huddersfield, Huddersfield, UK

3 Cambridge University Hospitals NHS Foundation Trust, Cambridge, UK

4 Hamad Medical Corporation, Doha, Qatar

5 Department of Community Medicine and Postgraduate Institute of Medical Education and Research (PGIMER), Chandigarh, India

6 Health Promotion and Behavioral Sciences, University of Louisville, United States of America

7 British University in Egypt, Cairo, Egipat

8 London Churchill College, London, UK

*Address all correspondence to: russell.kabir@aru.ac.uk

References

[1] Dave A, Ramnarayan T. Prostitution is legal in India, according to a ruling by the supreme court. Indian Journal of Integrated Research in Law. 2023;**3**:1

[2] Gore MN, Patwardhan AR. Disparities in the cost of living adjusted earnings of female sex Workers in India, Thailand, and the USA: A need to create an equitable economic survival of female sex workers. Journal of Primary Care and Community Health. 2022;**13**: 21501319221101857. DOI: 10.1177/21501319221101857

[3] World Health Organisation. Violence against Women and HIV/AIDS: Critical Intersections. Violence against Sex Workers and HIV Prevention. Information Bulletin Series, Number 3; 2005

[4] Rao A, Mamulwar M, Panda S, Pachuau HZ, Vanlalvenzuali H, Lalruatsanga RT, et al. Finding a way forward with the community: Qualitative inquiry in the generalized HIV epidemic in Mizoram, India. Frontiers in Public Health. 2023;**11**: 1217628. DOI: 0.3389/fpubh.2023.1217628

[5] Godwin J. Sex Work and the Law in Asia and the Pacific. UNAIDS, UNFPA, UNDP; 2012

[6] Lubin G. There are 42 million prostitutes in the world, and here's where they live. Business Insider. 2012. Available from: https://www.businessinsider.com/ [Accessed: September 25, 2023]

[7] Shahmanesh M, Wayal S, Cowan F, Mabey D, Copas A, Patel V. Suicidal behavior among female sex workers in Goa, India: The silent epidemic. American Journal of Public Health. 2009;**99**(7):1239-1246

[8] Pai A, Seshu M, Gupte M, VAMP. Status of Sex Workers in India. Centre for Advocacy on Stigma and Marginalisation, SANGRAM, MASUM, VAMP, CEDAW; 2014. Available from: https://www.ecoi.net/en/document/1353310 [Accessed: September 20, 2023]

[9] Dandona R, Dandona L, Kumar GA, Gutierrez JP, McPherson S, Samuels F, et al. Demography and sex work characteristics of female sex workers in India. BMC International Health and Human Rights. 2006;**6**(1):1-10

[10] Chattopadhyay A, McKaig RG. Social development of commercial sex workers in India: An essential step in HIV/AIDS prevention. AIDS Patient Care and STDs. 2004;**18**(3):159-168

[11] Iaisuklang MG, Ali A. Psychiatric morbidity among female commercial sex workers. Indian Journal of Psychiatry. 2017;**59**(4):465

[12] Jayasree AK. Searching for justice for body and self in a coercive environment: Sex work in Kerala, India. Reproductive Health Matters. 2004;**12**(23):58-67

[13] Mamulwar M, Godbole S, Bembalkar S, Kamble P, Dulhani N, Yadav R, et al. Differing HIV vulnerability among female sex workers in a high HIV burden Indian state. PLoS One. 2018;**13**(2): e0192130. DOI: 10.1371/journal.pone.0192130

[14] Ministry of Health and Family Welfare. HIV Estimations Report: Technical Report. (2019). National AIDS Control Organization & ICMR-National Institute of Medical Statistics. New Delhi: Ministry of Health and Family Welfare Government of India; 2020

[15] NACO India HIV Estimations; Fact sheet NACO. 2021. Available from: http://naco.gov.in/sites/default/files/India%20HIV%20Estimates%202021%20_Fact%20Sheets__Final_Shared_24_08_2022.pdf [Accessed: September 24, 2023]

[16] UN Women and Social Development Direct (UN WSD). Avahan, RESPECT Preventing Violence against Women Programme Summary. 2020. Available from: https://www.unwomen.org/sites/default/files/Headquarters/Attachments/Sections/Library/Publications/2020/RESPECT-implementation-guide-Programme-summary-Avahan-en.pdf [Accessed: September 25, 2023]

[17] National AIDS Control Organization (NACO). Annual Report 2018–2019. 2019. Available from: https://main.mohfw.gov.in/sites/default/files/24%20Chapter%20496AN2018-19.pdf [Accessed September 25, 2023]

[18] Asthana S, Oostvogels R. Community participation in HIV prevention: Problems and prospects for community-based strategies among female sex workers in Madras. Social Science & Medicine. 1996;**43**(2):133-148

[19] Javalkar P, Platt L, Prakash R, Beattie T, Bhattacharjee P, Thalinja R, et al. What determines violence among female sex workers in an intimate partner relationship? Findings from North Karnataka, South India. BMC Public Health. 2019;**19**(1):1-14

[20] Challacombe SJ. Global oral inequalities in HIV infection. Oral Diseases. 2016;**22**:35-41

[21] Blanchard AK, Nair SG, Bruce SG, Ramanaik S, Thalinja R, Murthy S, et al. A community-based qualitative study on the experience and understandings of intimate partner violence and HIV vulnerability from the perspectives of female sex workers and male intimate partners in North Karnataka state, India. BMC Women's Health. 2018;**18**(1):1-12

[22] Reed E, Gupta J, Biradavolu M, Devireddy V, Blankenship KM. The role of housing in determining HIV risk among female sex workers in Andhra Pradesh, India: Considering women's life contexts. Social Science & Medicine. 2011;**72**(5):710-716

[23] Reed E, Erausquin JT, Groves AK, Salazar M, Biradavolu M, Blankenship KM. Client-perpetrated and husband-perpetrated violence among female sex workers in Andhra Pradesh, India: HIV/STI risk across personal and work contexts. Sexually Transmitted Infections. 2016;**92**(6):424-429

[24] Swain SN, Saggurti N, Battala M, Verma RK, Jain AK. Experience of violence and adverse reproductive health outcomes, HIV risks among mobile female sex workers in India. BMC Public Health. 2011;**11**(1):1-10

[25] Ramesh S, Ganju D, Mahapatra B, Mishra RM, Saggurti N. Relationship between mobility, violence and HIV/STI among female sex workers in Andhra Pradesh, India. BMC Public Health. 2012;**12**(1):1-8

[26] Blanchard AK, Mohan HL, Shahmanesh M, Prakash R, Isac S, Ramesh BM, et al. Community mobilization, empowerment and HIV prevention among female sex workers in South India. BMC Public Health. 2013;**13**(1):1-13

[27] Travasso SM, Mahapatra B, Saggurti N, Krishnan S. Non-paying partnerships and its association with HIV risk behavior, program exposure and service utilization among female sex workers in

India. BMC Public Health. 2014; **14**(1):1-9

[28] Saggurti N, Jain AK, Sebastian MP, Singh R, Modugu HR, Halli SS, et al. Indicators of mobility, socio-economic vulnerabilities and HIV risk behaviours among mobile female sex workers in India. AIDS and Behavior. 2012;**16**(4): 952-959

[29] Patel SK, Ganju D, Prabhakar P, Adhikary R. Relationship between mobility, violence and major depression among female sex workers: A cross-sectional study in southern India. BMJ Open. 2016;**6**(9):e011439

[30] Sarkar K, Bal B, Mukherjee R, Chakraborty S, Saha S, Ghosh A, et al. Sex-trafficking, violence, negotiating skill, and HIV infection in brothel-based sex workers of eastern India, adjoining Nepal, Bhutan, and Bangladesh. Journal of Health, Population, and Nutrition. 2008;**26**(2):223

[31] Erausquin JT, Reed E, Blankenship KM. Police-related experiences and HIV risk among female sex workers in Andhra Pradesh, India. Journal of Infectious Diseases. 2011;**204**(suppl_5): S1223-S1228

[32] George A, Sabarwal S, Martin P. Violence in contract work among female sex workers in Andhra Pradesh, India. Journal of Infectious Diseases. 2011;**204** (suppl_5):S1235-S1240

[33] Wirth KE, Tchetgen Tchetgen EJ, Silverman JG, Murray MB. How does sex trafficking increase the risk of HIV infection? An observational study from southern India. American Journal of Epidemiology. 2013;**177**(3):232-241

[34] Gupta J, Reed E, Kershaw T, Blankenship KM. History of sex trafficking, recent experiences of violence, and HIV vulnerability among female sex workers in coastal Andhra Pradesh, India. International Journal of Gynecology & Obstetrics. 2011;**114**(2): 101-105

[35] Heylen E, Shamban E, Steward WT, Krishnan G, Solomon R, Srikrishnan AK, et al. Alcohol use and experiences of partner violence among female sex workers in coastal Andhra Pradesh, India. Violence Against Women. 2019; **25**(3):251-273

[36] Mahapatra B, Battala M, Porwal A, Saggurti N. Non-disclosure of violence among female sex workers: Evidence from a large-scale cross-sectional survey in India. PLoS One. 2014;**9**(5):e98321

[37] Prakash R, Manthri S, Tayyaba S, Joy A, Raj SS, Singh D, et al. Effect of physical violence on sexually transmitted infections and treatment seeking behaviour among female sex workers in Thane District, Maharashtra, India. PLoS One. 2016;**11**(3):e0150347

[38] Reed E, Silverman JG, Stein B, Erausquin JT, Biradavolu M, Rosenberg A, et al. Motherhood and HIV risk among female sex workers in Andhra Pradesh, India: The need to consider women's life contexts. AIDS and Behavior. 2013;**17**(2):543-550

[39] Patra RK, Mahapatra B, Kovvali D, Proddutoor L, Saggurti N. Anal sex and associated HIV-related sexual risk factors among female sex workers in Andhra Pradesh, India. Sexual Health. 2012;**9**(5):430-437

[40] Deering KN, Bhattacharjee P, Mohan HL, Bradley J, Shannon K, Boily MC, et al. Violence and HIV risk among female sex workers in southern India. Sexually Transmitted Diseases. 2013; **40**(2):168-174

[41] George A, Sabarwal S. Sex trafficking, physical and sexual violence, and HIV risk among young female sex workers in Andhra Pradesh, India. International Journal of Gynecology & Obstetrics. 2013;**120**(2):119-123

[42] Panchanadeswaran S, Johnson SC, Sivaram S, Srikrishnan AK, Latkin C, Bentley ME, et al. Intimate partner violence is as important as client violence in increasing street-based female sex workers' vulnerability to HIV in India. International Journal of Drug Policy. 2008;**19**(2):106-112

[43] Mazumder N. Violence against Sex Workers, a Violation of their Rights. Alliance India. Available from: https://allianceindia.org/violence-sex-workers-violation-rights/: Sexual & Reproductive Health office; 2016 [Accessed: September 28, 2023]

[44] Belec L, Dupre T, Prazuck T, Tevi-Benissan C, Kanga JM, Pathey O, et al. Cervicovaginal overproduction of specific IgG to human immunodeficiency virus (HIV) contrasts with normal or impaired IgA local response in HIV infection. The Journal of Infectious Diseases. 1995;**172**:691-697

[45] Levy JA. The transmission of AIDS: The case of the infected cell. Journal of the American Medical Association. 1988; **259**:3037-3038

[46] Baggaley RF, Nazareth J, Divall P, Pan D, Martin CA, Volik M, et al. National policies for delivering tuberculosis, HIV and hepatitis B and C virus infection services for refugees and migrants among Member States of the WHO European Region. Journal of Travel Medicine. 2023;**30**(1):taac136

[47] Beattie TS, Bhattacharjee P, Ramesh BM, Gurnani V, Anthony J, Isac S, et al. Violence against female sex workers in Karnataka state, South India: Impact on health, and reductions in violence following an intervention program. BMC Public Health. 2010;**10**(1):1-11

[48] Open Society Foundation. Public Health Programs, Harm Reductions, Health and Human Rights and Sex Work. 2022. Available from: www.opensocietyfoundations.org [Accessed: September 29, 2023]

[49] Mahapatra B, Bhattacharya R, Atmavilas Y, Saggurti N. Measuring vulnerability among female sex workers in India using a multidimensional framework. PLoS One. 2018;**13**(9): e0204055. DOI: 10.1371/journal.pone.0204055

[50] Amritha VS, Babu J, Ashifa KM. Legalization of sex work in India: Perspectives on changes in socio-economic and living conditions of female sex workers. Journal of Survey in Fisheries Sciences. 2023;**10**(4S):409-418

Chapter 2

Transnational Marriage in Malaysia: Case Study and a Critical Review Based on Convention on the Elimination of All Forms of Discrimination against Women (CEDAW) and Narrative Analysis of Topical Stories

Nor Jana Saim, Norulhuda Sarnon, Ali Abbas, Nur Saadah Mohamad Aun and Afifah Idris

Abstract

This chapter examines child citizenship in transnational marriages involving Malaysian women and foreign spouses. The discussion is based on the critical reviews of the Malaysian laws in regard to transnational marriages and its adherence to the Convention on the Elimination of All Forms Discrimination against Women (CEDAW). In Malaysia, most marriages are endogamous (within the same ethnic group), but mixed marriages between diverse backgrounds are on the rise. The federal constitution shows differing citizenship provisions for children of transnational marriages based on the gender of the Malaysian spouse, indicating potential gender inequality in the legislation. Therefore, this chapter discusses the importance of addressing transnational marriage issues in line with the ratified CEDAW, which Malaysia adopted in August 1995. The review focuses on Malaysian mothers with non-Malaysian citizen children and identifies five themes from the data: divorce-related emotional distress, lack of awareness of child citizenship status, unresponsiveness from authorities, prioritizing child welfare, and uncertainty about the future. Gender inequality in legislative provisions impacting mothers and children with different nationalities is highlighted. The review urges the government to take decisive action to comply with the convention and ensure justice for affected mothers and their children.

Keywords: transnational family, mixed marriage, gender inequality, CEDAW, Malaysia

1. Introduction

In this review, we discuss the issue of transnational marriage in the context of determination of child citizenship as a result of the marriage of a Malaysian woman with a foreign spouse. The discussion is based on the critical reviews of the Malaysian laws in regard to transnational marriage and its adherence to the Convention on the Elimination of All Forms Discrimination against Women (CEDAW) as well as the narrative analysis of topical stories from the affected mothers. It is important to discuss the topic as it affects the future of the discriminated children.

The definition of transnational marriage can be defined as a nuclear family; be it a spouse, father, mother, or child; sometimes also includes grandparents who have different nationalities [1]. Studies show that transnational family members always ensure mutual well-being and unity despite being geographically separated [2]. One of the earliest transnational marriage took place in 1511 involving Spaniards: Gonzalo Guerrero and the daughter of King Mayan. According to Jones [3], the story begins when Gonzalo Guerrero was on a journey from Panama to Santo Domingo when his ship was broken. As a result, he and his friends have been stranded in Mexico. They were then captured by the Mayans and made as slaves. For their safety, Gonzalo Guerrero had to learn the Mayan language and taught the Mayan how to fight. He was later accepted by the Mayan people and considered a god. He also later married the daughter of the King Mayan, Zazil HA. They were blessed with three children from this transnational marriage. According to Jones [3], the marriage between Gonzalo Guerrero and King Mayan's daughter was probably the first transnational marriage in the Latin American regions.

While the earliest transnational marriage in Asia took place in India in 1800. The transnational marriage took place among British diplomats; Colonel James Achilles Kirkpatrick with the princess of the King Mogul; Khair un-Nissa [4]. Although Colonel James Achilles Kirkpatrick was then a British Ambassador in Hyderabad, this marriage led to his dismissal. In Malaysia, a transnational marriage took place when the Ming Dynasty sent Admirals Zheng He and Princess Hang Li Po with 500 escorts to Malacca. Princess Hang Li Po later wed Sultan Mansor Shah and bore a child who was given the title Paduka [5]. The escorts who accompanied Princess Hang Li Po lived in Bukit Cina and married locals, resulting in the birth of descendants who came to be known as Baba and Nyonya. This information shows that transnational marriage is not something new in societies from ancient times and received various reactions.

In 1958, a mixed marriage in modern history; the couple Richard and Mildred Loving were arrested by police at their home for being found guilty of interracial marriage. They were later sentenced to several days in prison. At that time, 24 states in the United States banned interracial marriage until the law was repealed in 1967 [6]. Marriages in most communities are usually "endogamous," which is that marriage takes place between members of the same ethnic group. Hence, when there is mixed marriage, interracial marriage, or transnational marriage, all is seen as a diversion from the norm of marriage.

Most countries are not rigid in regard to transnational marriage such as marriages between Russian-Turkish [7] and Swedes and binational partners [8]. According to Jones and Shen [9], the statistics of international marriages in East and Southeast Asia in 2005 are about 0.1 to 32%. The lowest statistic was in China and the highest was in Taiwan. In Singapore, the statistic was about 17%. The Prime Minister of Singapore, Lee Hsien Loong gave a favorable comment on the trend saying that it was natural as more Singaporeans now live and work abroad and many foreigners live and work in Singapore [9].

However, there are about 27 countries in the world that limit automatic citizenship transfer from women to their children. Most of these countries are in Middle East and North Africa such as Saudi, Jordan, Burundi, Liberia, and Togo. Malaysia is among four countries (other than Brunei, Iran, and Nepal) in Asia that limit mother's equal rights as father's in regards to conferring their nationality to their children [10].

Many other countries such as Indonesia and Singapore are providing equal rights for their citizens to confer their nationality to their children either from men or women. For example, according to Indonesian Law No. 12 of 2006, it is noted that a child born from a legal marriage from an Indonesian citizen father or mother with foreign citizen spouse is considered an Indonesian citizen [11]. Similarly in Japan, according to Article 2, Law No.147 of 2004 and Law No.88 of 2008, a child will be a Japanese national when, at the time of its birth, the father or the mother is a Japanese national [12, 13].

Studies found that transnational families typically have language barriers, differences in traditions, different parenting approaches, and legal constraints [14, 15] as well as financial constraints [16]. This critical review paper is an attempt to shed light on the transnational marriage of Malaysian women and foreign men from the perspective of Malaysian law enforcement and the Convention on the Elimination of All Forms of Discrimination Against Women (CEDAW).

According to Tedong et al. [17] foreign spouses who are married to Malaysians face social marginalization in Malaysia due to discriminatory policies that enforce them to rely on their Malaysian partners either for obtaining a visa or job opportunities.

It is also possible for the transnational family having issues with conferring child citizenship that will affect education, health services, and future of their children such as in Malaysia. This situation can happen such as a child from a transnational marriage who does not have Malaysian citizenship might have difficulty to be registered in a government school. A student visa or long-term social visit pass is required for the child, which needs to be renewed annually or after a specific period set by the Immigration Department of Malaysia. In some cases, the widow or widower of a Malaysian citizen may be required to return to their home country if their long-term social visit pass is not renewed due to reasons such as the absence of a Malaysian citizen child, or the lack of an eligible sponsor who must be a Malaysian citizen [18]. Failing to address this issue could result in the loss of talent and human capital, as well as jeopardizing one's life. Therefore, this review paper aims to advocate for the idea that there is a gender bias in the Malaysian Federal Constitution [19, 20] that impacts the transnational marriages of Malaysian women with foreign spouses. This chapter also aims to examine and address the circumstances surrounding Malaysian women who are having children with foreign nationality due to being born outside of Malaysia.

2. Transnational marriages in Malaysia

In Malaysia, it is estimated that in 2005, 14.3% (8733) of transnational marriages for non-Muslim couples were registered [21]. The number of transnational marriages keeps increasing by more than threefold. According to the Registration Department of Malaysia, there were about 29,698 transnational marriages among non-Muslim couples registered from 2018 until November 2022 [22]. The same statistic also noted that about 20,273 registered marriages are between Malaysian men and foreign women. Whilst about 9425 marriages are between Malaysian women with foreign men. The Kedah Islamic Religious Affairs Department (JHEIK) data estimates that, in 2018, there was a 12.3% increase in transnational marriages compared to 2017 [23]. Statistic from the Malaysian Immigration Department (2016 in Todeng et al. [17] reported that the numbers of transnational marriages were 55,88 in 2012 and increased to 118,581 marriages in 2015. In addition, transnational marriage statistics can be viewed based on proxies such as the increasing number of members or followers of a Facebook account. For example, the Foreign Spouses Support Group Facebook page, which has around 16,000 people, even though it just started in 2019. The same trend can be seen on Facebook page; Love is Not Tourism Malaysia, Malaysian Mixed Marriages, which has members of around 11,000 (started in 2020 or 2021) and 1600 members, respectively. While, the Facebook page Family Frontier Malaysia has approximately 2800 members and followers. Based on these observations, the number of transnational marriages is increasing, and many people are planning for international marriages.

3. Convention on the elimination of all forms of discrimination against women (CEDAW) and Malaysia Federal Constitution Laws in regards of transnational marriages

Malaysia has ratified the Convention on the Elimination of All Forms of Discrimination Against Women (CEDAW) since 1995. As a state party that has ratified the convention, Malaysia is expected to adhere to and respect the articles within the convention. The convention consists of 30 articles, including equality, stereotypes and prejudices, smuggling and prostitution, politics, education, employment, and the economy (UN [24]). However, the discussion in this chapter focuses only on Articles 2, 9, 15, and 16 as shown in **Table 1**:

3.1 Article 2: Government responsibility

Based on Article 2, the Convention on the Elimination of All Forms of Discrimination Against Women (CEDAW) states that after ratifying, the government is responsible for the immediate implementation of the content of the convention. This is to demonstrate the commitment of the ratified convention. In addition, it is a legislative bond between the government and the convention. The government is then responsible for reporting every four years to the convention. The responsibilities of the government in implementing the convention are as follows:

Article 2 Government responsibilities	Article 9 Citizenship
Article 15 Equality in law Women have the same right to contact, selection of property and residence	Article 16 Marriage and family life

Table 1.
Articles 2, 9, 15, and 16 CEDAW.

3.2 Respect

The government is responsible for enacting laws that do not discriminate against women as well as implementing practices that do not discriminate against women. In addition, the government needs to be sensitive to laws that discriminate against women and repeal the law.

3.3 Protect

In order to protect women's rights, the government should look into complaints and provide mechanisms for dealing with such complaints. For the purpose of protection, the government should establish regulation for institutions and individual. These regulations should aim to prevent any form of discrimination against women and prohibit discriminatory practices.

3.4 Promote

The government should also promote public awareness of women's rights. This is to ensure that the community is aware of gender equality and gender discrimination.

3.5 Fulfilling

The government must strive to develop women's capacity to prevent gender discrimination. Thus, the government is also able to ensure that the legal and reality of gender equality can be achieved.

3.6 Article 9: determination of child citizenship

Article 9 in CEDAW states that:

1. "States Parties shall grant women equal rights with men to acquire, change or retain their nationality. They shall ensure in particular that neither marriage to an alien nor change of nationality by the husband during marriage shall automatically change the nationality of the wife, render her stateless or force upon her the nationality of the husband.

2. States Parties shall grant women equal rights with men with respect to the nationality of their children."

For many transnational marriage couples, the determination of child citizenship is among the main issues. **Table 2** is the translation of Summary Information on Determining Citizenship by Operation of Law [Ringkasan Kaedah Penentuan Kewarganegaraan Secara Kuat Kuasa Undang-undang] released on the official Facebook account of the Malaysia National Registration Department on January 17, 2019 [25].

The Malaysian Embassy in Santiago also published the same table on their official website on January 25, 2021 [26], which may serve as a reference for transnational marriage couples residing abroad. Although, the statement "This table does not apply to specific cases" is included with the table, it was without further explanation of what those specific cases may entail. The table suggests that all children born from a legal

Citizenship status		Marital status	Citizenship of the child
Father	**Mother**		
Citizen	Citizen	✓/×	Citizen
Non-citizen	Non-citizen	✓/×	Non-citizen
Non-citizen	Citizen	✓/×	Citizen
Citizen	Non-citizen	×	Non-citizen
Citizen	Non-citizen	✓	Citizen
Permanent resident	Permanent resident	✓/×	Citizen
Non-citizen	Permanent resident	✓/×	Citizen
Permanent resident	Non-citizen	×	Non-citizen
Permanent resident	Non-citizen	✓	Citizen

Adapted from summary information on determining citizenship by operation of law [25].

Table 2.
Child citizenship determination by operation of law.

marriage between Malaysian citizens and a foreign national, regardless of the gender of the Malaysian citizen, will acquire Malaysian citizenship status. The National Registration Department has issued a schedule stating that children born from a legal marriage between Malaysian citizens and a foreign national, whether male or female, will obtain Malaysian citizenship status. However, an issue arises when Malaysian women marry foreigners and give birth abroad.

According to the Malaysia Federal Constitution:

Article 14 (1)(b)(1) – (b) and (c) [19] stated as follows:

(b) every person born outside the Malaysia whose father at the time of birth is a citizen and whether born in the Federation or at the time of such birth is in federal service or service a State; and

(c) every person born outside the Federation whose father at the time of birth is a citizen and within 1 year after the birth occurs or within such further period as may be authorized by the Federal Government, the birth is registered in a Federal consulate.

Clearly Article 14 (1)(b)(1) – (b) and (c) specifically only refer to the term "father." Due to that, a child born overseas from the transnational marriages of Malaysian women with foreign spouses is unable to acquire Malaysian citizenship by operation of law. On the other hand, a child born overseas from the transnational marriages of Malaysian men with foreign spouses have the privilege to register their children in any Malaysian embassy or consulate in order to obtain Malaysian citizenship status. In many cases, in order to ensure that a child obtains Malaysian citizenship status, Malaysian women are forced to travel long distances either by land or air while they are pregnant to return to Malaysia to give birth. Surely, this situation will endanger the safety of the women and the baby. There are also Malaysian women who are unable to return to Malaysia to give birth on the advice of medical officers due to the high risk to their health as well as to the babies. Although, despite having supporting medical documents, a child born overseas from Malaysian mothers is still unable to obtain Malaysian citizen status.

Under the provision of Article 15(1) of the Malaysia Federal Constitution [19], it is stated that a child overseas-born could apply for citizenship. However, the percentage of citizenship approval is very small. According to Singh [27], the citizenship applications from 2018 to October 2021 recorded 2352 applications. Yet, the number approved is only about 21 applications, which is less than 0.89%. In addition, the Malaysian mother of a child born overseas also could not submit an application for resident pass or permanent resident. This is because those applications can only be submitted after the citizenship application is rejected. But the decision on the application for citizenship often waits for years for an approval with the possibility of rejection without explanation [28]. There are also applications that have no result until the child is over 18 years old and is not eligible to apply for citizenship due to having surpassed the age limit. This gender discrimination might lead to the increasing number of statelessness in Malaysia [28].

In April 2010, the Minister of Home Affairs announced that Malaysian women married to foreigners have the opportunity to apply for citizenship for their children born overseas. This can be done by submitting their applications at Malaysian embassies or high commissions located in the respective foreign country [29]. However, in 2020, a group of six Malaysian mothers through an NGO, Family Frontier Malaysia, made an application to the court and was decided in September 2021. On September 23, 2021, the High Court sided with Family Frontier Malaysia to allow citizenship status to be granted to children born overseas by Malaysian women. Sadly, two days later, on September 25, 2021, the Malaysia Government submitted an application to suspend the decision on citizenship rights and take the case to the Court of Appeal. On November 15, 2021, the High Court rejected the application to suspend the decision on citizenship rights (further details in Suriani Kempe and six others and Government of Malaysia in [28]). The case still keeps going until now.

It is also worth noting that children with non-Malaysian citizenship will be discriminated against in terms of getting education in government schools, have to pay high medical fees, have no Malaysian passport, as well as no welfare aid from the Welfare Department, and not eligible for a funding for educational purpose such as from National Higher Education Fund Corporation [Perbadanan Tabung Pendidikan Tinggi Nasional, abbreviated PTPTN] [30] or zakat (Islamic funding for Muslims) [31]. A summary of this citizenship discrimination against children as a result of the marriage of Malaysian women with foreigners can be described in **Figure 1**.

3.7 Article 15 equality in law

Article 15 is on the basis that women have the same legal rights on signing contracts, property selection, and choosing a place to live. However, due to the constraints set out in Article 14 (in Federal Constitution), it has denied the women's right to choose their place of residence. This is because Article 14 (Federal Constitution) has made it clear that the children of Malaysian women who are married to foreigners must be born in Malaysia in order to obtain citizenship. This has denied women's right to be in their chosen place of residence and environment during childbirth.

As a result, Malaysian women who marry foreigners and live abroad are forced to go through long-distance journeys either by land or air and possibly endanger themselves and their pregnancies just for giving birth in Malaysia. This situation can be life-threatening not only to the baby but also to Malaysian women.

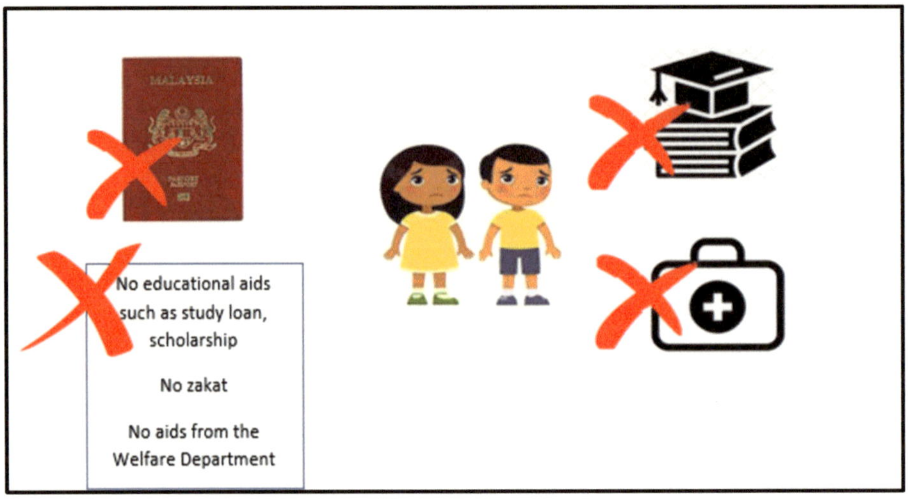
MALAYSIA
No educational aids such as study loan, scholarship
No zakat
No aids from the Welfare Department

Figure 1.
Summary discrimination on children overseas-born with no-Malaysian citizenship status as a result of the marriage of Malaysian women with foreigners.

Due to the restriction in Article 14 (Malaysia Federal Constitution), it also resulted Malaysian women being forced to stay away from their families during the confinement period after giving birth; at least two (2) or three (3) months; due to financial constraints if they plan to bring all their family members back to Malaysia. Not only the journeys are harmful to themselves and their pregnancies but they also might need to go through the confinement period on their own if there is no immediate family who wants to help them. This discrimination makes the life of Malaysian women and their families, especially the children, seem worthless and become second-class citizens based on Article 14 (Malaysia Federal Constitution).

3.8 Article 16: marriage and family life

The Articles 19 (1) and (3) of Malaysia Federal Constitution of states as follows:

i. he has been resident in the Federation for a period of not less than 10 years in 12 years

   a. that he is of good character; and

   b. that he has an adequate knowledge of the Malay language.

The Article 15 of Malaysia Federal Constitution states as follows:
Citizenship through registration (wife and child of citizens)

a. that she has been resident in the Federation for a period of 2 years prior to the date of the application and intends to do so on a permanent basis; And

b. that she is of good character.

Article 19 of Federal Constitution pertains to transnational marriages involving Malaysian women and foreigners, specifically in terms of citizenship status and the naturalization process [20]. According to Article 15 of the Malaysian Constitution, foreign spouses of Malaysian women are required to undergo a naturalization period that is five times longer than those of foreign spouses of Malaysian men. Additionally, male spouses of Malaysian women are subject to have knowledge of Malay language, which is not applicable to female spouses of Malaysian citizens (**Figure 2**).

3.9 Long-term social visit pass

Normally, the spouse of a Malaysian citizen would apply for a long-term social visit pass in order to continue residing with their spouse in Malaysia [32]. This application would include the couple's information, accompanied by a statement stating that "*Any form of employment is strictly prohibited*" although transnational couples may apply to the Immigration Department for permission to work in the event of a job opportunity, however, the fact is many employers are hesitant to offer employment due to the presence of this statement. It is due to the misleading statement that makes Malaysian companies hesitant. A study by Tedong et al. [17] noted that numerous Malaysian companies are not in favor to employ foreign spouses as they did not have permanent resident or citizenship status.

Thus, many foreign spouses with qualifications and the ability to work remain unemployed, resulting in a loss of valuable human resources in the job market. As a result, many transnational couples rely on a single breadwinner. While this may not pose a significant challenge for Malaysian men in such marriages, it can be burdensome for Malaysian women, who are typically expected to assume the role of the primary provider. This can create a role conflict that may result in divorce. Furthermore, due to this policy, transnational marriages involving Malaysian women are more likely to fall below the poverty line compared to those involving Malaysian men. **Figure 2** illustrates the discrimination in transnational marriages between a Malaysian woman and her foreign husband compared to a Malaysian man and his foreign wife.

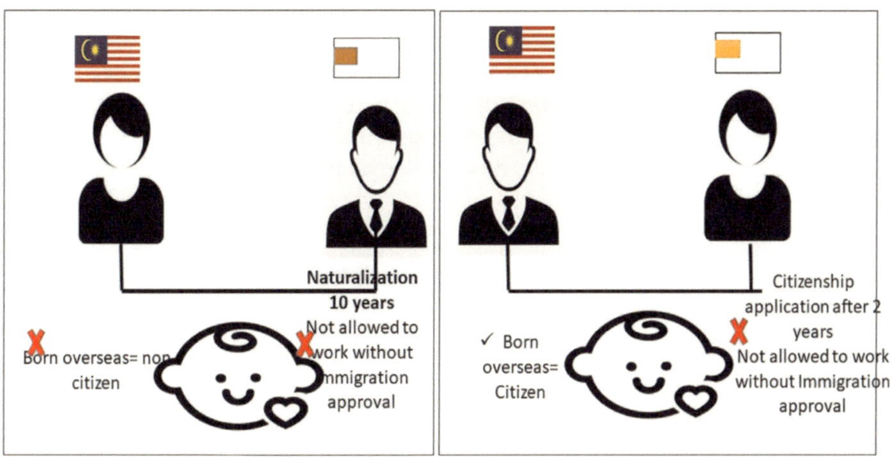
Naturalization
10 years
Born overseas= non citizen
Not allowed to work without Immigration approval
Citizenship application after 2 years
✓ Born overseas= Citizen
Not allowed to work without Immigration approval

Figure 2.
The discrimination between transnational marriages between Malaysian woman and foreign husband vs. Malaysian man and foreign wife.

4. Method

In order to understand the circumstances surrounding Malaysian women who are having children with foreign nationality, the researchers have obtained information related to this matter. The main researcher contacted informants who were part of the Facebook page "Foreign Spouse Support Group." After getting to know them, the main researcher reached out to them through email and WhatsApp group. In the beginning, there were four informants who agreed to participate in the study and gave their consent *via* WhatsApp group. However, one informant who initially agreed to participate later declined due to an ongoing divorce court case. Subsequently, the researchers added an additional informant who shared her experience through a sharing session on a Facebook page. She was later contacted by the main researcher and gave her consent via Facebook messenger. All the informants, except for Informant 4, sent their stories *via* email to the main researcher. The main researcher verbatim transcribed the sharing session of Informant 4. The letters and the verbatim were then analyzed using narrative analysis [33].

5. Findings

5.1 Informants' background

Table 3 provides an illustration of the background of the informants. It has been observed that the informants have between one to three children. All of them were born outside Malaysia and aged below 18 years old. Another notable fact is that among the four informants, only one is married, whereas the remaining three have been through a divorce. It is interesting to note that all of the individuals who underwent the divorce process did it outside of Malaysia, except for one who had their divorce proceedings within the country. Additionally, two of the informants are living in Malaysia, one is living in Italy and one living in Saudi Arabia.

5.2 Emotional distress caused by divorce

The informants that were going through the divorce process experienced emotional distress. It is most probably because the divorce happened outside Malaysia, and it makes them feel "lonelier" and without close family members to support them.

P, Informant 1, narrated her divorce situation as below:

	Nickname/place of living	Marital status	Number of children	Number of children with Malaysian citizenship	Number of children with foreign citizenship
Informant 1	P/Malaysia	Divorced	2	-	2
Informant 2	L/Italy	Divorced	1	-	1
Informant 3	R/Malaysia	Divorced	3	1	2
Informant 4	A/Saudi Arabia	Married	2	1	1

Table 3.
Informants' background.

> *My basic goal was to start from the bottom like any other woman after divorce. Before leaving France with my two babies, I had to do it nicely; and amicable. I signed away proper basic monthly support which can help for monthly living expenses, and schooling or their basic needs to be able to have full child custody like they were under French law. We shared the lawyer but the lawyer seemed to be on his side. I will sign anything as long as I have my daughters with me in Malaysia. … ..I had been through a divorce, and it was traumatic back then. My entire five years of my life packed in three (3) luggage under 30 kg and 70 euro in my wallet. I traveled two flights from Lyon - Amsterdam - Kuala Lumpur on economy flight with one toddler; 5 years old and one infant; 3 years old with no help. When I reached Kuala Lumpur International Airport, I cried buckets.*

> *Marriage is not always guaranteed to be smooth sailing as in my case. Because of disloyalty, I live as a single mother, raising my girl. It was a stressful and traumatic experience going through the divorce, even though I got full custody of my child. It is not easy as a single mother in a foreign country without any support systems. I also know from the experiences of other mothers that I will have a hard time if I bring her back to Malaysia. It will be a huge struggle for both options* (L, Informant 2).

However, for L, Informant 2, although she has no support after her divorce, she decided to remain in Italy due to her daughter's citizenship status. In her opinion, because her daughter is considered a foreigner in Malaysia then there is no difference either staying in a foreign country or her homeland. Despite having gone through a divorce and having no support, she was compelled to face the challenges of raising her child abroad because of her citizenship status, leaving them with no other choice.

Whilst R, Informant 3, has had a different story. She, her husband, and three children moved back to live in Malaysia after years in the UK. They decided to move back to Malaysia because lack of family support while they were staying there. They hope to be close to her family as all her family members living in Malaysia. However, her marriage was shattered after 5 years of their moving to Malaysia.

> *My marriage broke down towards the end of 2020. My husband and I decided to part ways. We signed the divorce paper in April 2021, with me having full custody of both our children. Now that I'm a single mother, my elder child's citizenship is even more important to me than ever before* (R, Informant 3).

5.3 Uninformed about the child citizenship status by Malaysian constitution

The analysis revealed that the informants exhibited a lack of knowledge about the citizenship status operation by law. Consequently, due to that reason, informants were full of hope to get the citizenship for their children. One of informants signed away her rights to get financial support from her ex-husband in order to gain full custody of her children and brought them to Malaysia. She was unaware that her children were unable to get Malaysian citizenship by law.

> *After returning to Malaysia not knowing at all they cannot get citizenship. My basic goal was to start from the bottom like any other woman after divorce. Before leaving France with my two babies, I had to do it nicely; and amicable. I signed away proper basic monthly support which can help for monthly living expenses, and schooling or their basic needs to be able to have full child custody like they were under French law.*

> *We shared the lawyer but the lawyer seemed to be on his side. I will sign anything as long as I have my daughters with me in Malaysia* (P, Informant 1).

P, Informant 1, further stated her frustration as follows:

> *In 2015, at the Department of Registration in Malacca State, I will never forget that eerie, sad feeling that almost felt like death when they said "Can't get [citizenship] for your kids". I returned to Malaysia not knowing at all they cannot get citizenship. I felt cornered and an end of the world feeling* (P, Informant 1).

Another informant received misleading advice from the Malaysian Embassy in Italy that she could register her child's citizenship there and it would take only a year. However, despite waiting for 7 years, until now her child has still not been granted Malaysian citizenship.

> *I delivered my baby in Italy where I was living. The reason I chose to deliver my baby in Italy was I had a miscarriage during my first pregnancy in 2015 and was advised by doctors to not travel and take rest. -Prior to my delivery, I checked with the Malaysian Embassy in Italy and was told that I could register my child's citizenship at the embassy. The Embassy told me that the application process will take about a year. I still keep that email until now. Once assured there would be no legal complications, I remained in Italy for the remainder of my pregnancy..* (L, Informant 2).

R, Informant 3, illustrated that she faced a difficult battle for her children's citizenship after getting married in the UK.

> *I moved to the United Kingdom (UK). I found love and got married to an Irish citizen in March 2012. Honestly, I was naïve at that time, and did not think much of what would become one of the greatest, saddest and most tiring battles of my life – my children's citizenship and she is becoming a Permanent Residence in Malaysia.* (R, Informant 3).

On the other hand, M, Informant 4, was informed by the officer at the Malaysian Consulate in Jeddah to give birth in Malaysia.

> *Alhamdulillah (Praise to Allah), Malaysian Consulate in Jeddah was very nice, giving advice and help at their level best. I asked their advice. And their advice was always the same – 'Madam, please go back to Malaysia'. 'Madam, if you can. Please go back to Malaysia'. 'Madam, please go back to Malaysia'. The same answer, the same tone and their faces look ashamed. Because they cannot help me for more. Limited. Because it is not under their capacity. The Constitution stopped them.*

However, although she was informed about the laws of Malaysia regarding children born overseas, but she had no other option during her second pregnancy where she gave birth in Saudi Arabia due to time and financial constraints. Her second daughter was registered as a refugee as her husband.

> *Meanwhile, my second daughter, Maryam was born in Saudi Arabia due to some reasons. For that, Maryam is a refugee, having no country, having no passport. She has no place to go for help if anything happened to her* (A, Informant 4).

5.4 The struggles of raising children with foreign citizenship

All informants expressed their struggles raising children with foreign citizenship. Most of the informants were worried about the short-term visa or the non-permanent document that their children need to apply for residing in Malaysia. For instance, L, Informant 2, was worried about her daughter's visa if they choose to back to Malaysia. She described her feeling as below:

> *Early 2020 when the COVID-19 pandemic brought disaster to Italy, I was of course affected like everyone else. I got to know that Malaysians were being repatriated free of charge, but I could not and was scared to take up the offer to return. As I was informed that my daughter would only be given a short-term visa. And where I am supposed to go for a visa run (exit the country and return to get a visa) when her visa expired during the pandemic?*
>
> *I was desperate to avoid the rampant of Covid-19 situation in Italy, however I was unsure of my daughter's visa status upon our return. One government source told me that my daughter would be able to acquire a one-month visa. However, to be honest, I felt our legal status in a third country, Italy, is more secure where both my daughter and I have Permanent Residence permits. Compared to the uncertainty of her visa in Malaysia; even obtaining a long-term visit visa is a question mark, let alone to apply for Malaysian citizenship which for now remains a distant dream* (L, Informant 2).

P, informant 1, also narrated her struggles with visa renewal after coming back to Malaysia. It was because her 5- and 3-year-old daughters were unable to get any other visa other than tourist visa. For that reason, they need to go out of Malaysia every 90 days to make it eligible for visa renewal.

> *I have been struggling so much since coming back to Malaysia in 2015 after my divorce from France. After returning I had to go in and out 90 days either in Singapore or Thailand for two years plus, with my 5 and 3 year old which affected their kindergarten and my career. My daughters were under tourist visa as I cannot get any other visa for them. Immigration did not help or aid my girls with a visa from a Malaysian mother* (P, Informant 1).

A, Informant 4, depicted that there is no word that can describe her feeling when her daughter with refugee status was not allowed to be in Malaysia for more than 30 days.

> *Emm..I cannot be in my own country more than 30 days without requested visa. It was because Maryam is not allowed to be in Malaysia more than 30 days. I feel sad.. No words can express my feeling. ... The first time I felt like I was hit on my head was when I arrived in Malaysia, the Malaysian Immigration Department stamped on Maryam's passport with a validity 30 days. Only 30 days we allowed to stay in my own country, 'tempat tumpahnya darah ku'. It was like we staying in Malaysia and started to count 30, 29, 28... That how it was to me, my kids, Sarah and Maryam. If they stamped on Maryam's passport validity only 30 days, it goes the same to me. I cannot just put it alone to Maryam and say; "Ok. Goodbye Maryam. I am going back to Malaysia to enjoy my life"* (A, Informant 4).

During her sharing session, she mentioned that "Tempat tumpahnya darahku" is a line from Malaysian National anthem, which literally means "the place where my blood will be spilled." Her expression conveys a sense of betrayal by her own county, the place where she should rightfully belong and receive protection. However, instead of receiving support, she feels let down as her country denied her opportunity to confer citizenship by operation by law to her daughter, simply because she is a woman who married a foreigner and gave birth to her baby outside the country.

R, Informant 3, voices her disappointment as follows:

> *My first born? Still unwelcomed in Malaysia. This year my eldest turns 17 years old, which strips it away from being eligible for a Long-Term Social Visit Pass. The only way for it to continue staying in Malaysia is through a student visa* (R, Informant 3).

> *Now that I'm a single mother, my elder child's citizenship is even more important to me than ever before. To me, he is my flesh and blood, and he has spent more of his time in Malaysia than in his birth country. He is learning the culture and language here, building relationships with his extended family and friends here. He barely has any memory or association with his birthplace – and yet, he is being seen as a foreigner in this country. Not a 'he', but still an 'it'.* (R, Informant 3).

Some informants also described their difficulties in regard to health and education.

> *Not only he has limited options when it comes to education, he also must pay double the cost on medical, insurance or even local attractions, just because the government refused to recognize the rights of a mother.* (R, Informant 3).

> *Currently, every year I have to pay for my kids' schooling expenses: the visa renewal is a huge headache. Every 12 months they require more and more difficult documents. I need to pay RM1000 for the kids' student visa and RM1600 for the medical insurance (AIA). This medical insurance is a must to have otherwise the student visa will not be approved* (P, Informant 1).

Since their children are not Malaysian citizens, they incur higher expenses as they have to bear the costs of education, health insurance, and visa renewals. They typically have to pay a higher cost when they go on vacation since their children are charged based on tourist rates instead of local rates. They are also not entitled to receive financial assistance meant for children such as *Bantuan Awal Sekolah* (Early School Aid) or PTPTN; education loan for higher education. In addition, they also do not qualify to apply for zakat assistance even if they are Muslims.

5.5 Absence of a response to their application

All informants were aware of their children's citizenship status, and they promptly applied to the appropriate authority to obtain citizenship status under Article 15 (Malaysia Federal Constitution). However, they have not received any response from the authority despite their efforts to make calls and emails. Their applications are either pending or unanswered.

In February 2015, I registered our marriage at High Commission of Malaysia in London, and submitted my child's Malaysian citizenship application through the same place. I was told by the officer that the whole process would take two years. I was right to make that choice. One year has passed. my husband fell ill, and we had no family support in London. We decided to move back to Malaysia, where there will be support to raise our child, and where there will be help to let my husband focus on his recovery. We have not left the country [Malaysia] since that day. Upon returning home to Malaysia, I contacted the High Commission of Malaysia in London to inform them that I had moved, so they could update the contact address of my application. I have lost count of how many times I called JPN Putrajaya, time and time again, to get a status update. Each time I called; I would always receive the same, short answer: "Pending". When I asked how long it would take, I was told on the phone that it would take up to 6 years, contrary to the 2-year timeframe I was given in London (R, Informant 3).

Now, my daughter is four years old, and I have applied for her citizenship since the time she was born, but I have yet to receive any response from the government. What hope is there for my child to get Malaysian citizenship and for me to return to Malaysia? I always write to JPN and the Embassy to check the status of my citizenship in the last four years. I really need help!! (L, Informant 2).

According to A, Informant 4, although the staff that she was dealing with at the Malaysia Consulate in Jeddah were nice and tried to help her, however, they were unable to do much as it is not in their capacity to make decisions. For her, it was Malaysia Federal Constitution that limits the staff for further processing her application, and yet she has not received answer although she applied since last 3 years.

Throughout my application, I never met any rude or questioning my decision to marry a foreigner. All of them tried their level best. I have never felt offended because all of them understand my situation. They also wanted the best for me and my daughter, but the Constitution stopped them. May Allah rewards their kindness. I had been applying Maryam's citizenship since last 3 years. So far, there is no news about my application. I tried to call from time to time. But I am making calls from overseas. Sometime due to different time zone, some time Malaysia still on public holiday [so I did not manage to talk to them] (A, Informant 4).

The lack of communication from the authority has left them in limbo and unable to proceed to the next stage.

5.6 Uncertainty and apprehension of the future

As mentioned in the previous section, their applications for their children's citizenship are still pending or unanswered. Consequently, the informants feel uncertainty and apprehension about their future. Most of the informants have this fear that they will be separated from their children once they turn 18 years old if they are not granted Malaysian citizenship status.

I am imagining when they are over 17 years old, their school is over, I have to say 'bye bye' to them at KLIA and that is it if I cannot get them Malaysian citizenship. They will be aliens in France as they cannot even speak one word in French. They are 100% more Malaysian. I have no problem with the French Embassy or my ex-husband

> *because we still need his signature for the passport renewal but my kids get Malaysian citizenship, then we do not need to worry any more* (P, Informant 1).

> *To me, he is my flesh and blood, and he has spent more of his time in Malaysia than in his birth country. He is learning the culture and language here, building relationships with his extended family and friends here. He barely has any memory or association with his birthplace – and yet, he is being seen as a foreigner in this country. Not a 'he', but still an 'it'* (R, Informant 3).

The informants are concerned about how their children will cope if they were compelled to relocate to an unfamiliar country.

> *Maryam knew that she is not a Malaysian citizen based on different colors on her passport compared to her sister. The color of Sarah's passport is red, and her passport is blue. Mama's passport is red and Dad's passport is blue. She keeps asking 'Why I am not Malizie?' Malizie is Arabic word for Malaysia. Help me to explain this to a 3 year old girl. Sometime she said; 'I will follow Dad, isn't? and you will take Kakak [her sister; Sarah]. The day when the High Court was siding on our side, I hugged her and said, 'Maryam, you are a Malaysian now'. She was happy and she was dancing. She said, 'Can I call Teta (her Palestinian grandmother)? She called her and said, 'Teta, I am Malaysian now!' She keeps repeating, 'I am Malaysian now. Kakak [her sister, Sarah], I am the same as you! After three days, the bad news comes when the government withdraw the decision of the High Court* (A, Informant 4).

A, Informant 4, further expressed that if something happened between her and her husband, they somehow knew that her refugee daughter will go to her husband and her Malaysian daughter will go to her. For her, it is almost impossible to have both daughters due to vast adversities because of their citizenship status.

6. Discussion and conclusion

The provisions of the law should be equal without any discrimination or second-class citizens being denied their rights. It should be in line with Article 8 (1) and (2), which states the right to equality before the law. Therefore this study urges the Government of Malaysia and all parties involved to uphold the law so that there is no discrimination against citizens solely on the grounds of religion, race, place of birth, or gender in any law.

Therefore, it is time for stakeholders to raise the issue of gender inequality so that Malaysian legislation is seen as standing in the eyes of the world equally with the other countries in accordance with Article 9 of the Convention on the Elimination of All Forms of Discrimination Against Women [34]. For the elimination of gender inequality, it is proposed to amend Part II of the Second Schedule of the Federal Constitution by substituting the word "father" for "parent" so that the children from transnational marriages are not discriminated against simply because they have a Malaysian mother who married a foreign husband. With the amendment, it will be in line with the aspirations of Article 8 (2) of the Federal Constitution, there is no gender-based discrimination. Improvements from the discussion in this review are taking the same stance as Nik Salida Suhaila, Syahirah, and Wan Abdul Fattah's articles [35].

The same goes for the granting of citizenship status. Investigations need to be refined to ensure that transnational marriages actually take place regardless of whether it is a transnational marriage of a Malaysian man or a Malaysian woman. Granting citizenship status should be based on the ability of the spouse to be a Malaysian citizen in understanding and appreciating citizenship as a Malaysian and not based on gender as a mere partner.

Based on the analysis of the topical stories from the affected mothers who have children with foreign citizenship, regardless of their marital status, the child citizenship is still weighty issue for the mothers. In some situations, the mothers are informed about the citizenship status of the baby being born out of Malaysia. However, due to health, financial, and other reasons, they have no other option other than to give birth to their babies out of Malaysia. We strongly urge the government and related authorities to take serious action to adhere to the ratified Convention on the Elimination of All Forms of Discrimination against Women (CEDAW). The failure to address these gender-bias discriminations has resulted in denying all affected individuals to enjoy the rights that they rightfully deserve. As saying goes, justice delayed is justice denied.

Author details

Nor Jana Saim[1*], Norulhuda Sarnon[1], Ali Abbas[2], Nur Saadah Mohamad Aun[1] and Afifah Idris[1]

1 Social Work Program, Faculty of Social and Human Sciences, National University of Malaysia, Bangi, Selangor, Malaysia

2 School of Distance Education, Science University of Malaysia, Penang, Malaysia

*Address all correspondence to: janasaim@ukm.edu.my

References

[1] Mazzucato V. Child well-being and transnational families. In: Michalos AC, editor. Encyclopedia of Quality of Life and Well-Being Research. Dordrecht: Springer; 2014. DOI: 10.1007/978-94-10 007-0753-5_3870

[2] Bryceson D, Vuorela U. Transnational families in the twenty-first century. In: Suhakam CEDAW, Bryceson D, Vuorela U, editors. The Transnational Family: New European Frontiers and Global Networks. Oxford: Berg; 2002

[3] Jones GD. The Conquest of the Last Maya Kingdom. California: Stanford University Press; 1998

[4] Dalrymple W. White Mughals: Love and Betrayal in Eighteenth-Century India. India: Penguin Publishing Group; 2004

[5] Kong Y. Zheng He and the Malay World Cruise. Bangi: Penerbit University National Malaysia; 2000

[6] Sue DW, Rasheed MN, Rasheed JW. Multicultural Social Work Practice: A Competency-Based Approach to Diversity and Social Justice. 2nd ed. New Jersey: John Wiley; 2016

[7] Deniz A, Özgür EM. Mixed marriage and transnational marriage migration in the grip of political economy: Russian-Turkish case. Turkish Studies. 2021;**22**(3):437-461

[8] Haandrikman K. Binational marriages in Sweden: Is there an EU effect? Population, Space and Place. 2014;**20**(2): 177-199

[9] Jones GW, Shen H. International marriage in East and Southeast Asia: Trends and research emphases. Citizenship Studies. 2008;**25**(1): 9-25

[10] UNHCR. Background Note on Gender Equality, Nationality Laws and Statelessness 2014. Geneva: UNHCR; 2014

[11] Susi Dwi Harijanti. Report on Citizenship Law: Indonesia. Global Citizenship, Observatory (GLOBALCIT) Robert Schuman Centre for Advanced Studies. Badia Fiesolana: European University Institute; 2017

[12] Ministry of Justice. Law.No. 147 of 2004: The Nationality Law. 2023a. Available from: https://www.moj.go.jp/ENGLISH/information/tnl-01.htmlE Nationality Law

[13] Ministry of Justice. Law No. 88 of 2008: The Nationality Law. 2023b. Available from: https://www.moj.go.jp/ENGLISH/information/tnl-01.htmlE Nationality Law

[14] Bryceson D, Vuorela U, editors. The Transnational Family: New European Frontiers and Global Networks. New York: Routledge; 2020

[15] Jørgensen MB. 4 Danish regulations on marriage migration: Policy understandings of transnational marriages. In: Transnational Marriage. London: Routledge; 2013. pp. 60-78

[16] Tschirhart N, Diaz E, Ottersen T. Accessing public healthcare in Oslo, Norway: The experiences of Thai immigrant masseuses. BMC Health Services Research. 2019;**2019**(19):1-10

[17] Tedong PA, Roslan K, Abdul Kadir AR. Marriage migration: Lived experience of foreign spouses married to Malaysian citizens. Pertanika Journal of Social Sciences & Humanities. 2018;**26**(2):945-960

[18] Wahid AS. Adik jaga kakak cerebral palsy selepas ibu ditahan Imigeren [Younger brother taking care of cerebral palsy sister after their mother been detained by the Immigration]. Sinar Harian. 2021. Available from: https://m.sinarharian.com.my/mobile-article?articleid=169015

[19] Federal Legislation. Federal Constitution. 2020. Available from: https://lom.agc.gov.my/federal-constitution.php

[20] Law of Malaysia Federal Constitution. National Printing. Kuala Lumpur: Malaysia Berhad; 2009

[21] Chee HL. International marriages in Malaysia: Issues arising from state policies and processes. In: Jones WJ, Terrence HH, Mohamad M, editors. Changing Marriage Patterns in Southeast Asia: Economic and Socio-Cultural Dimensions. London: Routledge Contemporary Southeast Asia Series; 2011

[22] Abd Halim NH. Ramai Lelaki Tempatan Kahwin Wanita Vietnam [Most Local Men Married to Vietnamese Women]. Kuala Lumpur: Utusan Malaysia Online; 2023

[23] Nur Amirah Abdullah. More and more people choose foreigners. 2019. Available from: http:www//sintoknews.com/marriage-citizen-local-together-citizen-foreigner-kian-increased/

[24] UN Women. Convention on the Elimination of All Forms of Discrimination against Women. 2009. Available from: https://www.un.org/womenwatch/daw/cedaw/

[25] National Registration Department. Summary on Determining Citizenship by Law. 2019. Avaialble from: https://www.facebook.com/ModeratorJPN/posts/ringkasan-kaedah-penentuan-kewarganegaraan-secara-kuat-kuasa-undang-undangtaraf-/2042018939177478/

[26] Malaysian Embassy in Santiago. Summary on Determining Citizenship by Law. 2021. Available from: https://www.kln.gov.my/web/chl_santiago/news-from-mission/-/blogs/ringkasan-kaedah-penentuan-kewarganegar

[27] Singh R. Question of mother's rights. November 13, 2021. Penang Women's Development Corporation-PWDC. 2021. Available from: https://www.facebook.com/PWDCMalaysia/videos/659830105019251/

[28] Rahman SAKBA, Sharifuddin SBA, Hafidz MBBM. Citizenship rights in Malaysia: A constitutional reform. Current Legal Issues. 2021;**3**:41-49

[29] Malaysian Women Can Register Children Born Abroad. The Star Online. 12 April 2010. Available at: https://www.thestar.com.my/news/nation/2010/04/12/malaysian-women-can-register-children-born-abroad/

[30] UKMShape. Maklumat umum & Tatacara Memohon Perbadanan Tabung Pendidikan Tinggi Nasional (PTPTN) [General information & Application Procedures for the National Higher Education Fund (PTPTN)]. 2018. Available from: https://www.ukm.my/ukmshape/ptptn-maklumat-umum-tatacara-memohon/

[31] Lembaga Zakat Selangor. 2015. Mesyuarat Pertama Pengggal Ketiga Dewan Negeri Selangor tahun 2015 [The First Meeting of the Third Term of the Selangor State Assembly for 2015]. Available from: http://dewan.selangor.gov.my/question/lembaga-zakat-selangor-2/

[32] Immigration Department of Malaysia. Long Term Social Visit. 2021.

Available from: https://www.imi.gov.my/index.php/en/main-services/pass/visitor-pass/social-visit-pass/long-term-social-visit-pass/

[33] Smith B. Narrative analysis. In: Lyons E, Coyle A, editors. Analysing Qualitative Data in Psychology. 2nd ed. London: Sage; 2016

[34] Human Rights Commission of Malaysia. Convention on the Elimination of all Forms of Discrimination against Women. Kuala Lumpur: SUHAKAM; 2009

[35] Saleh NSSN, Shukor SA, Ismail WAFW. Equality and citizenship for women in Malaysia: Where and when? Malaysian Journal of Syariah and Law| بمالءيزيا والقانون الشريعة مجلة|. 2021;**9**(1):103-113

Chapter 3

Gender-Based Violence is a Never to be Forgotten Social Determinant of Health: A Narrative Literature Review

Anna Maria Giammarioli, Eloise Longo and Raffaella Bucciardini

Abstract

Gender-based violence (GBV) has been internationally recognized as a serious and pervasive phenomenon affecting women's lives and health. The World Health Organization (WHO) reports that about 30% of women have experienced worldwide some form of violence. GBV (in addition to clearly visible immediate effects) induces long-term effects, including an increased incidence of many noncommunicable diseases such as diabetes or cancer. In the last few years, it has also been demonstrated that the signs of violence interfere with genome plasticity and gene expression through epigenetic mechanisms. The underestimation of the problem does not allow us to put in place preventive health mechanisms that could cushion the damage (prevent post-traumatic stress disorders—PTSDs—and the evaluation of epigenetic changes) to avoid the onset of the diseases. Appropriate interventions could reduce many of these long-term health effects while failure to intervene could be a significant source of health inequalities. The aim of this narrative review is to summarize the available evidence on the relationship between GBV, its long-term effects on health, and as victims' living conditions, and socioeconomic position of determining both.

Keywords: equal rights, health disparities, social determinants of health, gender-based violence, intimate partner violence

1. Introduction

Gender-based violence (GBV) refers to harmful acts directed against a person based on their gender, sexual orientation, or gender identity. GBV is a severe violation of human rights and a life-threatening health that include physical, sexual, psychological, and socioeconomic violence, including sexual harassment and stalking [1].

Both women and men, as well as people who do not fit within the narrow parameters of the assigned societal gender-based roles, may experience GBV but worldwide the majority of victims of GBV are women and girls. Even in the case of lesbian, gay,

IntechOpen

bisexual, and transgender (LGBT) people, violence is predominantly suffered by women (LGBT women and transgender men), who the assailants perceive as a challenge to socially constructed norms. For this reason, although this is incorrect, GBV and violence against women and girls (VAWG) are used interchangeably [1]. Both VAWG and GBV are based on hierarchical and unequal structural power relations that are rooted in norms, roles, and relationships between socioeconomic groups as well as in socially constructed characteristics of women and men, which in turn influence violence and abuse [2, 3]. In the last few decades, GBV has increasingly been recognized as a public health problem affecting almost all health outcomes throughout life (including mental health and noncommunicable diseases such as diabetes or cancer). In many countries, violence against LGBT women and its health effects are not adequately investigated and are certainly underreported, so the available data for LGBT women are further much more limited than those for non-LGBT women. In this chapter we focused on the health effects produced by violence against non-LGBT women, assuming that they are similar for LGBT women (hereinafter both referred to as women).

Our aim is to summarize the available evidence on the relationship between GBV and its long-term health effects, arguing that many of these health effects could be avoided by helping victims of violence with recovery interventions. We would also like to point out that women living in environments with limited social, educational, and economic opportunities (in addition to being at increased risk of multiple forms of violence) have fewer opportunities to access GBV recovery interventions. GBV turns out to be a key indicator of health inequalities and we suggest that it should start to be considered a social determinant of health.

2. Materials and methods

A narrative literature review was conducted to seek to examine a collection of qualitative and quantitative studies. A narrative literature review is particularly useful as a means of linking together studies from different fields and methodologies in order to develop a more comprehensive, intersecting, and overarching synthesis. There are some possible limitations in this analysis and some articles that talk about GBV may not be covered in this narrative review.

For the purpose of this study, we used a search on the following online databases: PubMed/MEDLINE and Google Scholar. In PubMed/MEDLINE, we used the Boolean operators, "AND" and OR, to link keywords and MeSH headers as shown below: i) (Gender-based violence OR intimate partner violence OR domestic violence) AND (post-traumatic stress disorder OR psychological stress OR stress-related disorders OR mental health OR trauma, nervous system OR disease OR illness); ii) (Gender-based violence OR intimate partner violence OR domestic violence) AND (health veterans OR women veterans OR veterans OR military sexual trauma); iii) (Gender-based violence OR intimate partner violence OR domestic violence) AND (epigenomics OR epigenesis, Genetic OR epigenetic); iv) (Gender-based Violence OR intimate partner violence OR domestic violence) AND (health service accessibility OR health personnel OR health personnel education); v) (gender-based violence OR intimate partner violence OR domestic violence) AND (social determinant of health OR health disparities OR health equity). In Google Scholar we searched articles not indexed in PubMed/MEDLINE. The terms used and their combinations were similar to those utilized in the PubMed/MEDLINE research. We focused all searches from January 2000 to January 2023. Some references were not identified using the online databases but were obtained through reference lists of other articles. Reports from World Health Organization (WHO) and United Nations were downloaded from the official websites, and web addresses have been reported in the references. The criteria for inclusion in the research are the following: scientific articles and/or papers written in English and/or Italian and with human subjects. We excluded expert opinions, case reports, studies on abused children, and studies addressing the effects of violence on LGBT communities. Two authors were involved in the search and screening process of scientific articles and/or papers.

3. Patriarchal culture and international conventions to tackle gender-based violence

GBV is not a private matter, but it concerns the whole of society. It is a phenomenon that has deep roots entrenched in a social context that feeds on prejudice and stereotypes and is not limited to the dramatic cases of femicide. Secular patriarchal structures and attitudes make lasting progress difficult. Most societies have been shaped by religious doctrine whereby attitudes and systems that promote male dominance have become the norm. This doctrine has distorted sacred scriptures by selecting texts where women are subordinate and inferior to men. Alongside these patriarchal systems, violence in society has also been normalized, and factors of social poverty have amplified violence. GBV is accepted in many spheres of social life [4].

According to WHO, sex-gender inequalities are deeply rooted in society [5] and are both cause and consequence of violence, so social prevention measures aim to achieve cultural change in attitudes and behaviors of men and women and eradicate prejudices, attitudes, and habits based on negative gender stereotypes [6].

Over the past decades, international institutions and organizations have focused on promoting women's rights, complaining, and warring against GBV. As a result, essential declarations and resolutions have been issued, and the most significant ones are listed below in chronological order:

- The international Convention on the Elimination of All Forms of Discrimination against Women (CEDAW), adopted in 1979 by the United Nations General Assembly, defines discrimination against women as.

  "...any distinction, exclusion or restriction made based on sex which has the effect or purpose of impairing or nullifying the recognition, enjoyment or exercise by women, irrespective of their marital status, based on equality between men and women, of human rights and fundamental freedoms in the political, economic, social, cultural, civil or any other field" [7].

- The Council of Europe Convention is the first international treaty that specifically addresses violence from a gender perspective. "Preventing and combating violence against women and domestic violence (also known as The Istanbul Convention) "*.... any act of violence based on sex, or the threat of such acts, which produces or is likely to produce physical, sexual, or psychological harm or suffering, coercion or arbitrary deprivation of liberty, whether in the public or private lives of women*" [6];

- The Beijing World Conference on Women and its Platform for Action specify that "*... violence against women is the manifestation of the historical difference in* *power within gender relations such inequality has resulted and results in systematic discrimination against them, we call upon, therefore, governments to make greater efforts regarding the quantification and evaluation of its consequences on women's health*" [8];

- The World Health Organization (WHO) report on violence is defined as "*a huge, global health problem" and urges health services to make more significant efforts "to provide comfort to women who experience acts of physical violence and sexual abuse*" [9];

- The WHO World Report on Violence and Health presents the first comprehensive global-scale analysis of the problem of violence [10].

Prevention of GBV has been included as a target in the 2030 United Nations Agenda for Sustainable Development (Goal 5), and many countries are working in this direction. However, we all still have a long way to go [11].

Human rights conventions and declarations obligate countries that have ratified them to treat GBV as a human rights violation and to define laws and actions to tackle the phenomenon. Regrettably, much more often than desired, this applicability has been undermined by social conditioning and structural and organizational barriers in many countries. The tradition of a patriarchal culture that still feeds the practice of possession in the affective relationship prevents one from reading the imbalance of man/woman relationships that is at the root of violence. It is, therefore, important to recognize the signs of mistreatment and abuse in its various forms: psychological, physical, economic, social, and cultural.

4. Different forms of gender-based violence

Although violence disproportionately affects women living in low- and lower-middle-income countries, GBV runs across all cultures, social classes, and ethnicities everywhere in the world.

As previously described, it is an expression of unequal power relations, underpinned by social norms and beliefs linked to dominance, power, and abuse of authority, and formalized through social institutions' laws, policies, and regulations [12, 13]. GBV can take many forms, including physical, psychological, and sexual violence; social violence, which cuts survivors off from their communities or social groups, and economic violence, which results in economic deprivation [1].

Depending on the types of relationship between the victim and the perpetrator of violence (e.g., known versus unknown, intimate versus acquaintance), women have experienced intimate partner violence (IPV) and non-intimate partner violence (NPV). The Centers for Disease Control and Prevention (CDC) defines IPV as physical violence or psychological aggression perpetrated by a current or former partner [14]. At the same time, NPV is violence perpetrated by a person with whom the victim has only a passing acquaintance. As many studies show, IPV fits into a broader spectrum of possible violence that occurs within the home and involves not only spouses or partners but also the father with respect to the daughter or other relatives and family members who may perpetrate acts of violence on female relatives [15].

The World Health Organization (WHO) reports that about 30% of women worldwide (1 in 3 women) have experienced some form of physical and sexual violence by an intimate partner or non-partner sexual violence or both, with severe consequences on physical and psychological health [16]. Data are even more alarming in poorer countries where women who have experienced physical and/or sexual violence in their lifetime account for around 37%, with some of these countries having a prevalence of up to one in two. In addition, the information regarding violence is often not collected or under-reported due to the women's reluctance to declare violence, given that the victims are often blamed for what happened to them and the phenomenon is undoubtedly underestimated worldwide. In many countries, the situation is even worse concerning violence against LGBT women, which is not adequately investigated and is certainly under-reported.

Differently from what one is prepared to believe, the World Health Organization (WHO) reports that globally IPV is the most common type of GBV, as on average 27% of women worldwide have experienced physical and/or sexual violence from their intimate partner [16]. The prevalence estimates of intimate partner violence range from 20% in the Western Pacific, 22% in high-income countries and Europe, 25% in the WHO regions of the Americas to 33% in the WHO African region, 31% in the WHO Eastern Mediterranean region, and 33% in the WHO South-East Asia region [16]. The variations in prevalence can be explained by the fact that different multilevel factors (including individual, relational, community, and social aspects) may interact with each other to increase or reduce the risk of being a victim of IPV [12, 13, 17]. IPV is also characterized by systematic underreporting due to the tendency of victims not to verbalize or report the abuse they have suffered, which makes it extremely difficult to estimate the burden of disease associated with incidents of IPV.

An understudied and underestimated phenomenon is also violence in pregnancy. Widespread is the stereotype that pregnancy has a protective function with respect to violence [18–20]. The data, however, contradict this reality. According to the WHO, worldwide one in four women has been victim of some form of violence during pregnancy [10]. The underestimation is probably due to women's reluctance to report violence suffered by their partners during the period of expecting a son/daughter. Nevertheless, several studies highlight how episodes of violence and sexual abuse suffered in the past and not sufficiently and psychologically treated are reactualized in pregnancy or during childbirth, a phenomenon so-called "surviving women," that is still little studied [21]. Domestic partner violence during pregnancy is associated with adverse health outcomes—fatal and nonfatal—for the pregnant woman and her baby because of direct physical trauma as well as the physiological effects of current or past abuse-related stress on the growth and development of the fetus [22, 23].

Data show that every type of emergency and crisis may exacerbate existing violence against women. This also happened during the COVID-19 pandemic where the lockdown and its social and economic impacts have increased the exposure of women to abusive partners and known risk factors [24, 25]. Before the pandemic, the Human Development Office for the United Nations Development Program (UNDP) reported that only 107 of 195 countries had data available on IPV [26]. Today, despite the huge efforts made to monitor the increase of IPV due to the pandemic, research has yet to establish exactly the estimates of IPV during the lockdown and in periods other than the pandemic outbreak.

5. Gender-based violence has long-term as well as immediate health effects

GBV has immediate and long-term health effects and different levels of severity, where fatal outcomes such as femicide are the most severe form. Among victims of violence, many women often report immediate physical injuries such as bruises, lacerations, and burns to the head, neck, or face but also fractures and broken bones or teeth. Until a few years ago, the connection between long-term health effects and GBV was often lost and only in the last few years, attention has been paid to this aspect. Among the long-term effects, in addition to those concerning sexual and reproductive spheres (sexual infections and gynecological problems, pregnancy complications, and unintended pregnancy), we would like to emphasize that victims of violence are at high risk of many physical diseases, such as asthma, irritable bowel syndrome, frequent headaches, chronic pain, diabetes, and mental health problems [16, 27]. Among mental health consequences, victims can manifest chronic mental illness, post-traumatic stress disorder (PTSD), depression, and anxiety [28, 29]. PTSD symptoms may include severe anxiety, flashbacks, nightmares, symptoms of increased arousal, such as irritability or anger, or symptoms of persistent avoidance of trauma-related situations [30]. Sexual abuse and victimization from multiple forms of violence have also been associated with greater odds of cervical cancer diagnoses, as victims have an increased risk of acquiring a sexually transmitted infection such as human papilloma virus [31, 32]. Experiencing violence has also been associated with harmful use of alcohol and drug abuse, smoking, and eating disorders, which in turn predispose individuals to a higher risk of noncommunicable diseases [33].

5.1 The body's adaptive response to trauma

The human body can cope or maintain stability during changes and excessive exposure to stress and/or traumatic events such as GBV. This body's adaptive response can occur through complex neuronal, neuroendocrine, and immune responses [see [34] for a comprehensive review]. It is nonspecific as, whatever the nature of the stressor, the mechanism triggered is always the same. Although discussing the body's adaptive response mechanisms is not the focus of this chapter, some notions can be briefly summarized. The threat evokes a physical and emotional reaction (also known as fight or flight); the sympathetic nervous system (SNS), the hypothalamic–pituitary–adrenal (HPA) axis, and the cardiovascular system are activated and these, in turn, affect the immune system [29]. When the danger is perceived as overcome, the parasympathetic nervous system (PSNS) acts to return to a state of normal basal equilibrium. Prolonged exposure to trauma, such as violence or painful memories, can prevent the body's adaptive response from switching off.

When the trauma pain is deep and its impact persists, increased production of stress hormones can wear down the body, keeping it in an unstable or weakened state. When this happens, the body is more susceptible to adverse health conditions such as cardiovascular disease, chronic pain, pregnancy complications, PTSD, and anxiety. The inability to minimize or stop adaptive response activity can lead to serious long-term health consequences. This is well known and it is recommended to assist trauma survivors (e.g. due to natural disasters such as tornadoes, hurricanes, fires, and floods or abused children, holocaust survivors, or stressors faced by members of military service in war, etc...) in an ongoing process of healing and recovery.

5.2 Gender-based violence, post-traumatic stress disorders, and epigenetic modifications

Several studies have shown that violent experiences affect genome regulation and expression by epigenetic modification as response to trauma [35–37].

Over the past two decades, a body of research has expanded rapidly and provided good evidence about the underlying biological mechanisms regulating the relationship between the risk of developing PTSD and epigenetic modifications consistent with perturbations with the HPA axis [38]. Epigenetics refers to changes in gene expression (active versus inactive genes) that do not involve changes to the underlying DNA sequence. Epigenetic changes include DNA methylation, modifications of histone proteins, and small RNA-mediated gene silencing (miRNAs), affecting gene expression. Epigenetics is an important part of biology as it regulates development and adaptations during the life of an organism as the epigenome dynamically responds to the environmental influences. In the last few years, several studies have demonstrated that stressors, incorrect lifestyles, and/or adverse psychosocial environments may influence epigenetic mechanisms by altering the epigenetic pattern of DNA methylation and/or chromatin structure. As previously mentioned, the remarkable growth in understanding epigenetic mechanisms and the impact of epigenetics on contemporary biology has added insight into the molecular processes that connect the brain with behavior, neuroendocrine responsiveness, and immune outcome [39]. Scientific studies have also highlighted the relationship between PTSD and the presence of epigenetic marks in genes regulating the HPA axis [37, 40, 41]. A starting point for understanding better the correlation between GBV, epigenetics, and PTSD was the finding that abused women veterans' health is poorer than that of their active duty military and non-abused civilian counterparts. In some countries, great attention has been given to the GBV suffered by the women veterans and this has created a critical priority for clinicians, researchers, and policymakers to better understand the impact of violence on women's health. Studies on war veterans have widely demonstrated that violence can impact women's health by inducing molecular modifications at the epigenetic level, which in turn can contribute to the onset of mental, physical, and chronic diseases [42, 43]. Until now, few studies have examined the relationship between PTSD, epigenetic changes, and GBV in nonveteran women.

Although few studies have examined the relationship between PTSD, epigenetic changes, and GBV beyond those on veteran women, nevertheless some exciting considerations can be drawn. Studies on nonveteran women have confirmed correlations between PTSD symptoms and epigenetic signatures (differential hyper-methylation) of trauma/stress-related genes [37]. Past and present violence and trauma can remain imprinted in the genome through epigenetic modifications, increasing the risk to women's health [35, 36]. Epigenetic changes due to parental experience of violence can be transferred to offspring through prenatal and postnatal epigenetic modifications indicating that epigenetic changes, although theoretically reversible, are heritable [35, 36, 44]. Importantly, the potentially reversible nature of epigenetic modifications suggests that trauma-induced epigenetic effects could be not necessarily permanent and that specific interventions could reduce the high prevalence of poor health among victims of violence and their children.

Nevertheless, this field of research is relatively young and there are still many questions that need to be elucidated concerning violence-induced epigenetic effects and their impact on women's health and/or health of their offspring. Currently, it is hard to find longitudinal studies or research studies for any of the health associations with GBV and epigenetic modifications in civilian women.

6. The social context and social determinant of health

Currently, many countries show reluctance to define specific recovery interventions for GBV victims or interventions to prevent GBV. People who grow up and live in environments with limited social, educational, and economic opportunities, in addition to being at greater risk of multiple forms of violence, have fewer opportunities to access the process of healing and recovery [45]. Evidence-based research shows that PTSD onset appears to be influenced by the type, duration, and severity of violence and the processes put in place to recover and heal the kind of trauma suffered [38, 45]. GBV has immediate and long-term health effects, but socioeconomic factors can influence (and in some cases worsen) the health outcomes of specific groups of people based on their social position. Social and economic factors between countries and within the same country, in addition to put women at greater risk of multiple forms of violence, can determine the unequal treatment of women victims of violence where women belonging to less advantaged people may not have adequate psychological and health support for the recovery and/or treatment of trauma. Health is the result of multiple factors or determinants of health that significantly influence health, whether positive or negative. In addition to biological characteristics, social factors are just as important to health outcomes and the likelihood of generating diseases. WHO defines social determinants of health (SDH) as "the conditions in which people are born, grow, live, work, and age [46]. SDH perspective is based on all factors that can make people healthy or not healthy, including education, income, labor market position, ethnicity, and gender bias.

Extensive research has shown that people who are less advantaged in terms of socioeconomic position have worse health (and shorter lives) than those who are more advantaged. Disparities in social, educational, and economic opportunities are the fundamental cause of health inequalities [46]. Health inequalities are widely recognized as a public health problem as they determine a significant share of potentially avoidable mortality and morbidity. The 2008 report of the WHO Commission on Social Determinants of Health (CSDH) "*Closing the gap in a generation*" provided a comprehensive synthesis of knowledge and evidence on health inequalities and a set of recommendations to develop comprehensive and integrated policies to contrast them [47].

The Service for Sexual and Domestic violence (when present) has long denounced this. Women who are less advantaged in terms of socioeconomic position and/or living in contexts where GBV victims are not supported by recovery interventions often face GBV trauma by using drugs, drinking alcohol, smoking, or overeating, further worsening their health condition. Research studies show that about 90% of women with substance use disorders have experienced physical or sexual violence [48]. The effects of violence on health have been underestimated and there is still a reluctance to consider violence as a problem to be addressed at a social, economic, and health level. In other words, it is a problem to consider GBV as a social determinant of health.

7. Network approach to cope with health effects of gender-based violence

The prevention of, and response to GBV, requires coordinated action across multiple sectors, including psychologists, social workers, lawyers, territorial associations, and other professionals but in this subsection, we focus our attention on healthcare professionals.

The WHO encourages the development of prevention and awareness programs to help reduce the prevalence of GBV, as well as establishing health services for GBV victims' care (particularly on mental health) and educating communities to take advantage of available care. In 2013, to address the issue of women's reluctance to declare violence, WHO published the clinical and policy guidelines "Responding to Intimate Partner Violence and Sexual Violence against Women" [49]. Guidelines recommended that healthcare professionals should ask about GBV, whenever there is an identified risk or health condition that GBV may have caused. Healthcare professionals play a unique role in coping health effects of GBV as they are often the first contact for abused women in healthcare services [50]. Victims of violence approach service providers in different institutional settings, with varying levels of awareness. Victims often do not find the words to tell what is happening to them, or they can be in hospital for other needs, and operators should be able to decode narratives and understand latent needs, which in turn have linked to the identification of GBV survivors. Healthcare professionals are ideally placed to identify and provide support to GBV victims and help prevent the long-term health consequences associated with violence. As evidenced by several studies worldwide, many barriers can prevent healthcare professionals from identifying and responding adequately to women who suffer violence. The first of all is the lack of adequate training, which makes healthcare professionals insecure in taking any initiative to ask for information about GBV [51, 52]. Healthcare professionals with insufficient training to respond to the victim of GBV may be miscommunicating and cause harm, such as arguing that women should leave an abusive relationship without providing survivors with a safety plan or considering the survivor's point of view [51, 52]. Other common barriers are lack of time, privacy, and resources. Some healthcare professionals had reported fear of offending women when they asked about violence. Another essential aspect of breaking down these barriers is creating a multidisciplinary network, including lawyers, psychologists, social workers, territorial associations, and other professionals to identify and support victims of GBV correctly [53].

8. Conclusion

GBV is based on prejudices and stereotypes handed down over centuries that require slow and very long times to be changed and geographically diversified interventions (both socioeconomic and cultural). Thus, GBV prevention can be promoted by considering individual, relationship, community, and societal risk and protective factors. In the last few years, sociocultural interventions have increased awareness of the various forms of violence that can occur (physical, sexual, psychological, and socioeconomic) and have activated processes of critical reflection on gender bias and stereotypes still rooted in society. Unfortunately, this is still not enough and an equity lens should be applied to all processes to prevent GBV and to remove all systemic barriers that prevent people from accessing adequate health care (after violence) due to their social, economic, gender, or cultural characteristics. The prevention of, and response to GBV, requires coordinated action across multiple sectors, in which health is one of the most relevant. All women who have been exposed to violence have increased risks of getting sick, indicating that violence can be considered a social determinant of health. All women who have been exposed to violence should be able to obtain comprehensive and gender-sensitive health services. All women should be able to address the physical and mental health consequences of their experience and all women should be helped in their recovery from the traumatic event. GBV is a multicausal problem influenced by social, economic, cultural, psychological, legal, and biological factors. Particular attention should be given to interventions for the assistance of GBV victims within each country to avoid that the unequal distribution of economic, social, and environmental conditions could penalize less advantaged women in society.

At the same time, we know that cases of GBV are significantly underreported, and new strategies should be evaluated to help GBV victims make reporting easier, safer, and more confidential. In this context, interesting results have been obtained by providing specific training to healthcare professionals.

Finally, they are essential for both the existence of international protocols and guidelines with clear procedures and the creation of a network of experts involved in the issue of violence both locally and nationally for bringing out the phenomenon—mostly underreported and underestimated—and guaranteeing support, listening, acceptance, and protection to women. GBV is widespread worldwide, and its resulting health problems are preventable issues that must pose serious challenges to public health and policy.

Conflict of interest

The authors declare no conflict of interest.

Author details

Anna Maria Giammarioli[1]*, Eloise Longo[2] and Raffaella Bucciardini[1]

1 Center of Global Health, National Institute of Health, Rome, Italy

2 Department of Neuroscience, National Institute of Health, Rome, Italy

*Address all correspondence to: anna.giammarioli@iss.it

References

[1] European Institute for Gender Equality–EIGE. What is Gender-Based Violence? Available from: https://eige.europa.eu/gender-based-violence/what-is-gender-based-violence

[2] Montesanti SR, Thurston WE. Mapping the role of structural and interpersonal violence in the lives of women: Implications for public health interventions and policy. BMC Women's Health. 2015;**15**:100. DOI: 10.1186/s12905-015-0256-4

[3] Semahegn A, Torpey K, Manu A, Assefa N, Tesfaye G, Ankomah A. Are interventions focused on gender-norms effective in preventing domestic violence against women in low and lower-middle income countries? A systematic review and meta-analysis. Reproductive Health. 2019;**16**(1):93. DOI: 10.1186/s12978-019-0726-5

[4] Curter J. Patriarchy and violence against women and girls. Lancet. 2014;**385**:e40-e41. DOI: 10.1016/S0140-6736(14)62217-0

[5] World Health Organization-WHO. The Global Plan of Action to Strengthen the Role of the Health System within a National Multisectoral Response to Address Interpersonal Violence, in Particular against Women and Girls, and against Children. Geneva: WHO; 2016

[6] Council of Europe Convention on preventing and combating violence against women and domestic violence, Istanbul, 11.V.2011; Available from: https://rm.coe.int/168008482e

[7] Convention on the Elimination of All Forms of Discrimination against Women–CEDAW, ONU, December 18, 1979; Available from: https://www.ohchr.org/en/instruments mechanisms/instruments/convention-elimination-all-forms-discrimination-against-women

[8] The Beijing World Conference on Women and its Platform for Action: Available from: https://www.unwomen.org/en/how-we-work/intergovernmental-support/world-conferences-on-women#beijing

[9] United Nations (UN) Economic and Social Council –1996- "Further Promotion And Encouragement Of Human Rights And Fundamental Freedoms, Including The Question Of The Programme And Methods Of Work Of The Commission Alternative Approaches And Ways And Means Within The United Nations System For Improving The Effective Enjoyment Of Human Rights And Fundamental Freedom." Available from: http://hrlibrary.umn.edu/commission/thematic52/53-wom.htm

[10] World Health Organization-WHO-2002. Uurges Governments to take action to reduce violence against women. Available from: https://www.who.int/news/item/22-11-2002-who-urges-governments-to-take-action-to-reduce-violence-against-women

[11] United Nations (UN) General Assembly: The 2030 Agenda for Sustainable Development. Available from: The Sustainable Development Agenda - United Nations Sustainable Development

[12] Kabir R, Khan HTA. A cross-sectional study to explore intimate partner violence and barriers to empowerment of women in Armenia. BioMed Research International.

2019;**16**(2019):6939684. DOI: 10.1155/2019/6939684

[13] Kabir R, Harish H, Alradie-Mohamed A, Afework S, Mohammadnezhad M, Arafat SY. Experience of intimate partner violence of women at reproductive age group in India and their decision-making power. Advances in Human Biology. 2021;**11**(1):89

[14] Centers for Disease Control and Prevention. Intimate Partner Violence. 2021. Available from: https://www.cdc.gov/violenceprevention/intimatepartnerviolence/

[15] Santambrogio J, Colmegna F, Trotta G, Cavalleri PR, Clerici M. Intimate partner violence (IPV) e fattori associati: una panoramica sulle evidenze epidemiologiche e qualitative in letteratura. Riv Psichiatr. 2019;**54**(3):97-108. DOI: 10.1708/3181.31598

[16] World Health Organization - WHO. Global, regional and national prevalence estimates for intimate partner violence against women and global and regional prevalence estimates for non-partner sexual violence against women. In: Violence against Women Prevalence Estimates, 2018. Geneva: WHO; 2021

[17] Vinnakota D, Arafat SMY, Kar SK, et al. Pornography and sexual violence against women in India: A scoping review. Journal of Psychosexual Health. 2021;**3**(3):216-221. DOI: 10.1177/26318318211023935

[18] Dubini V, Cruriel P. La violenza come fattore di rischio in gravidanza. AOGOI Risveglio ostetrico. 2004; **anno I**(1/2):1-11

[19] Kabir R, Chakraborty R, Vinnakota D, Siddika N. Intimate partner violence constrains timely utilisation of antenatal care services among Armenian women: Results from a nationally representative sample. International Journal of Critical Illness and Injury Science. 2021;**11**(4):209-214. DOI: 10.4103/IJCIIS.IJCIIS_199_20 Epub 2021 Dec 18

[20] Vinnakota D, Parsa AD, Sivasubramanian M, Mahmud I, Sathian B, Kabir R. Intimate partner violence and pregnancy termination among Tajikistan women: Evidence from nationally representative data. Women. 2022;**2**(2):102-114. DOI: 10.3390/women2020012

[21] Simkin P, Klaus P. When Survivors Give Birth: Understanding and Healing the Effects of Early Sexual Abuse on Childbearing Women. 1st edition Classic Day Publishing; 2004. p. 450. ISBN-10: 1594040222

[22] Garcia-Moreno C, Jansen HA, Ellsberg M, Heise L, Watts CH. WHO multi-country study on Women's health and domestic violence against women study team. Prevalence of intimate partner violence: Findings from the WHO multi-country study on women's health and domestic violence. Lancet. 2006;**368**(9543):1260-1269. DOI: 10.1016/S0140-6736(06)69523-8

[23] Longo E, Ghirini S. "Violenza domestica nella perinatalità" in Camoni L, Palumbo G, Gigantesco A (a cura di) La salute mentale nel periodo perinatale. Uno sguardo tra diverse discipline; Il pensiero scientifico Ed., Roma, 2022

[24] Gupta J. What Does Coronavirus Mean for Violence against Women? [Internet]. 19 March 2020. Available from: https://womensmediacenter.com/news-features/what-does-coronavirus-mean-for-violence-against-women

[25] Women's Aid UK. The Impact of COVID-19 on Women and Children

Experiencing Domestic Abuse, and the Life-Saving Services That Support Them. UK: Women's Aid UK; 2020

[26] United Nation Development Programme (UNDP). Annual Report 2018. Available from: https://www.undp.org/publications/undp-annual-report-2018

[27] Rivara F, Adhia A, Lyons V, Massey A, Mills B, Morgan E, et al. The effects of violence on health. Health Affairs. 2019;**38**(10):1622-1629. DOI: 10.1377/hlthaff.2019.00480

[28] Santaularia J, Johnson M, Hart L, Haskett L, Welsh E, Faseru B. Relationships between sexual violence and chronic disease: A cross-sectional study. BMC Public Health. 2014;**14**:1286. DOI: 10.1186/1471-2458-14-1286

[29] Silove D, Ventevogel P, Rees S. The contemporary refugee crisis: An overview of mental health challenges. World Psychiatry. 2017;**16**:130-139. DOI: 10.1002/wps.20438

[30] Castro-Vale I, Carvalho D. The pathways between cortisol-related regulation genes and PTSD psychotherapy. Healthcare (Basel). 2020;**8**(4):37. DOI: 10.3390/healthcare8040376

[31] Leite FMC, Amorim MHC, Primo CC, Gigante DP. Violence against women and cervical cancer screening: A systematic review. Journal of Clinical Nursing. 2016;**26**:2126-2136. DOI: 10.1111/jocn.13328

[32] Reingle Gonzalez JM, Jetelina KK, Olague S, Wondrack JG. Violence against women increases cancer diagnoses: Results from a meta-analytic review. Preventive Medicine. 2018;**114**:168-179. DOI: 10.1016/j.ypmed.2018.07.008. Epub 2018 Jul 6

[33] World Health Organization - WHO. Global and Regional Estimates of Violence against Women: Prevalence and Health Impacts of Intimate Partner Violence and Non-partner Sexual Violence. Geneva: WHO; 2013

[34] Djuric Z, Bird CE, Furumoto-Dawson A, Rauscher GH, Ruffin MT 4th, Stowe RP, et al. Biomarkers of psychological stress in health disparities research. The Open Biomarkers Journal. 2008;**1**:7-19. DOI: 10.2174/1875318300801010007

[35] Conching AKS, Thayer Z. Biological pathways for historical trauma to affect health: A conceptual model focusing on epigenetic modifications. Social Science & Medicine. 2019;**230**:74-82. DOI: 10.1016/j.socscimed.2019.04.001

[36] Serpeloni F, Nätt D, Assis S, Wieling E, Elbert T. Experiencing community and domestic violence is associated with epigenetic changes in DNA methylation of BDNF and CLPX in adolescents. Psychophysiology. 2020;**57**(1):e13382

[37] Piccinini A, Bailo P, Barbara G, Miozzo M, Tabano S, Colapietro P, et al. Violence against women and stress-related disorders: Seeking for associated epigenetic signatures, a pilot study. Healthcare (Basel). 2023;**11**(2):173. DOI: 10.3390/healthcare11020173

[38] Cao-Lei L, Saumier D, Fortin J, Brunet A. A narrative review of the epigenetics of post-traumatic stress disorder and post-traumatic stress disorder treatment. Front Psychiatry. 2022;**13**:857087. DOI: 10.3389/fpsyt.2022.857087

[39] Mathews HL, Janusek LW. Epigenetics and psychoneuroimmunology: Mechanisms and models. Brain Behav

Immun. 2011;**25**(1):25-39. DOI: 10.1016/j.bbi.2010.08.009. Epub 2010 Sep 9

[40] Gudsnuk K, Champagne FA. Epigenetic influence of stress and the social environment. ILAR Journal. 2012;**53**(3-4):279-288. DOI: 10.1093/ilar.53.3-4.279

[41] Dick A, Provencal N. Central Neuroepigenetic regulation of the hypothalamic-pituitary-adrenal Axis. Progress in Molecular Biology and Translational Science. 2018;**158**:105-127. DOI: 10.1016/bs.pmbts.2018.04.006. Epub 2018 Jun 6

[42] Gerber MR, Iverson KM, Dichter ME, Klap R, Latta RE. Women veterans and intimate partner violence: Current state of knowledge and future directions. Journal of Womens Health. 2014;**23**(4):302-309. DOI: 10.1089/jwh.2013.4513

[43] Schmidt EM, Magruder K, Kilbourne AM, Stock EM, Cypel Y, El Burai Félix S, et al. Four decades after war: Incident diabetes among women Vietnam-era veterans in the health ViEWS study. Women's Health Issues. 2019;**29**(6):471-479. DOI: 10.1016/j.whi.2019.08.002

[44] Yehuda R, Lehrner A. Intergenerational transmission of trauma effects: Putative role of epigenetic mechanisms. World Psychiatry. 2018;**17**(3):243-257. DOI: 10.1002/wps.20568

[45] St John L, Walmsley R. The latest treatment interventions improving mental health outcomes for women, following gender-based violence in low-and-middle-income countries: A mini review. Frontiers in Global Women's Health. 2021;**2**:792399. DOI: 10.3389/fgwh.2021.792399

[46] Wilkinson R, Marmot M. Social determinant of health: the solid facts. 2nd Ed. World Health Organization. Regional Office for Europe; 2003. Available from: https://apps.who.int/iris/handle/10665/326568

[47] World Health Organization. Closing the gap in a generation: health equity through action on the social determinants of health. Final Report of the Commission on Social Determinants of Health. 2008. Available from: https://apps.who.int/iris/bitstream/handle/10665/43943/9789241563703_eng.pdf?sequence=1

[48] Beijer U, Scheffel Birath C, DeMartinis V, Af KB. Facets of male violence against women with substance abuse problems: Women with a residence and homeless women. Journal of Interpersonal Violence. 2015;**33**(9):1391-1411

[49] World Health Organization. Responding to Intimate partner violence and sexual violence against women. 2013. ISBN: 978 92 4 154859 5. Available from: https://apps.who.int/iris/bitstream/handle/10665/85240/9789241548595_eng.pdf

[50] Alshammari K, McGarry J, Higgingbottom G. Nurse education and understanding related to domestic violence and abuse against women: An integrative review of the literature. Nursing Open. 2018;**5**(3):237-253. DOI: 10.1002/nop2.133

[51] World Health Organization. Global Plan of Action: Health systems address violence against women and girls. 2016. Available from: https://www.who.int/publications/i/item/WHO-RHR-16.13

[52] Kirk L, Bezzant K. What barriers prevent health professionals screening

women for domestic abuse? A literature review. The British Journal of Nursing. 2020;**29**(13):754-760. DOI: 10.12968/bjon.2020.29.13.7

[53] Colucci A, Luzi AM, Fanales Belasio E, Barbina D, Mazzaccara A, Farchi S, et al. A blended training programme for healthcare professionals aimed at strengthening territorial networks for the prevention and contrast of gender-based violence. Epidemiologia e prevenzione. 2019;**43**(2-3):177-184. DOI: 10.19191/EP19.2-3.P177.057

Section 2

Maternal Health and Menstrual Issues

Chapter 4

The Premenstrual Assessment Form: Short Form (PAF-SF) – Additional Psychometric Analyses of a Brief Measure of Premenstrual Symptoms

Kayla M. Joyce and Sherry H. Stewart

Abstract

The Premenstrual Assessment Form–Short Form (PAF-SF) is a 10-item measure that assesses premenstrual symptom severity. There is little research assessing the PAF-SF's psychometrics and proposed subscales (affect/water retention/pain). This chapter aims to assess the 10-item PAF-SF's psychometric properties (i.e., internal consistency, and structural/criterion-related/known groups validity). Eighty-seven naturally cycling females (M_{age} = 28.86 years, *SD* = 6.11) participated. Participants completed the 10-item PAF-SF; the State-Trait Anxiety Inventory–Trait subscale (STAI-T); and the Structured Clinical Interview for DSM-5 (SCID-5) premenstrual dysphoric disorder (PMDD) module. With principal components analysis, we extracted and compared three-factor (affect/water retention/pain) and two-factor (psychological/physiological) solutions for the PAF-SF. The two-factor solution was selected for its greater interpretability, simple structure, internal consistencies, and parsimony. Participants with versus without a provisional PMDD diagnosis had higher psychological subscale scores; unexpectedly, PMDD group differences were not observed on the physiological subscale. Psychological, but not physiological, subscale scores were positively correlated with trait anxiety and PMDD affective symptom count. Scores on the physiological subscale were positively correlated with the PMDD somatic symptom count. Psychological subscale scores were also positively correlated with the PMDD somatic symptom count. The 10-item PAF-SF appears to be a reliable and valid measure of premenstrual symptom severity and comprises psychological and physiological symptom domains.

Keywords: premenstrual assessment form – short form, premenstrual, psychometric, reliability, validity, factor analysis

1. Introduction

Menstrual cycle-related fluctuations in mood, behavior, and physical symptoms have been well-documented (e.g., [1–4]). The menstrual cycle can be broken down

IntechOpen

into five phases, consisting of the menstrual (days 1–5), follicular (days 6–12), ovulatory (days 13–14), luteal (days 17 – premenstrual phase), and premenstrual phases (five days prior to menstrual bleeding; [5–7]). Although all five menstrual cycle phases have been linked to changes in females' mood, behavior, and physical symptoms [1–4], the premenstrual phase is of particular interest given considerable evidence for increases in depressed mood, risky behaviors (e.g., substance use), and pain during this phase [1–4, 8–10].

There are, however, marked individual differences in the degree of changes in mood, behaviors, and/or physical symptoms experienced in the five days prior to menstruation [1–4, 8–10]. For those females experiencing more substantial changes during the premenstrual phase, there are two diagnoses that can be considered – premenstrual syndrome (PMS; prevalence rate of 47.8%; [11]) and premenstrual dysphoric disorder (PMDD; prevalence rate of 3–8%; [12, 13]). PMS and PMDD are two classifications along a spectrum of premenstrual symptoms. PMS is defined as moderate emotional, physical, and behavioral symptoms that occur premenstrually [14]. In contrast, PMDD is an affective disorder recognized in the *Diagnostic and Statistical Manual of Mental Disorder, 5th Edition* (DSM-5; [15]) that is associated with severe increases in emotional, physical, and behavioral symptoms premenstrually that impair the affected individual's daily functioning. Given the high prevalence of PMS and the impairing nature of the symptoms comprising PMDD, it is critical that clinicians and researchers have access to measures that accurately assess individual differences in premenstrual symptoms.

Several self-report measures have been developed to assess premenstrual symptoms, such as the Premenstrual Assessment Form (PAF; [13]), the Menstrual Distress Questionnaire (MDQ; [16]), and the Premenstrual Symptoms Screening Tool (PSST; [17]). Many of these measures are shown to be both reliable and valid (e.g., [18]); however, they commonly pose two main issues in clinical and research settings which limits their usability. First, these measures are onerous for respondents given their length. For instance, the PAF has 95 items [13], the MDQ has 47 items [16], and the PSST has 19 items [17]. Second, scoring measures with many items can be problematic for researchers and clinicians given time-intensive requirements for scoring and/or the financial burden of purchasing expensive scoring software. For these reasons, brief measures are viewed as advantageous in both clinical and research settings because they provide informative data in a timely fashion while also enabling researchers and clinicians to simultaneously utilize additional measures to gather other pertinent information. While there is clearly a need for brief questionnaires to assess premenstrual symptom severity since PMDD has been in the *Diagnostic and Statistical Manual* for a decade, we must ensure the strong psychometric properties of brief questionnaires to guarantee they have not sacrificed good measurement in the search for brevity and usability.

To address the above limitations of existing premenstrual symptom measures, Allen et al. [19] developed a shortened 10-item version of the PAF, i.e., the Premenstrual Assessment Form – Short Form (PAF-SF). The PAF-SF assesses severity of premenstrual affective and somatic changes on a 6-point scale. Items are summed for a total PAF-SF (all 10 items) and three subscale scores (i.e., affect [four items], water retention [three items], and pain [three items]), making the PAF-SF a measure with broad coverage of premenstrual symptomatology, yet with few items, helping to reduce burden on respondents, researchers, and clinicians alike.

To develop this measure, Allen et al. [19] selected the 20 items from the original PAF [13] that were most frequently reported to change in the week prior to menstruation. These 20 items were administered to a sample of 217 females with regular menstruation in a smoking cessation trial at two time points: baseline and 6-month follow-up. The 20 items were subject to principal component analysis (PCA) with Varimax rotation which identified three factors: affective, water retention, and pain premenstrual symptoms. Allen et al. [19] trimmed items that did not show salient loadings in this PCA or that did not contribute to internal consistency to produce their final 10-item measure. They conducted preliminary analyses to establish the good psychometric properties of the 10-item total scale and its three subscales (i.e., internal consistencies, test-retest reliability, and criterion-related validity in relation to a measure of nicotine withdrawal symptoms). However, Allen et al. [19] did not conduct a PCA on the final 10-item version of the scale, and specific internal consistency values for the resultant subscales were not reported. Given its brevity and broad symptom coverage, Allen et al.'s [19] preliminary analyses suggest that the PAF-SF might be a good brief measure to administer in clinical and research settings to assess premenstrual symptom severity.

However, beyond the original measure development and preliminary validation study [19], there is a dearth of research examining the psychometric properties of the PAF-SF. Further psychometric analyses in an independent sample are required to determine whether the three PAF-SF subscales suggested by Allen et al. [19] – affect, water retention, and pain – are structurally valid, internally consistent, and show validity in relation to other theoretically-related criterion variables. To achieve this, the current study: (1) identified empirically derived subscales on the PAF-SF using PCA; (2) assessed the internal consistency of the identified subscales; (3) assessed concurrent criterion-related validity of the identified subscales in relation to trait anxiety and specific dimensions of PMDD symptoms as assessed through a gold-standard structured clinical interview; and (4) assessed a form of validity called known groups validity, that measured each identified subscale's ability to distinguish among groups of females with and without a provisional diagnosis of PMDD based on a gold-standard clinical interview.

We hypothesized [H1] that our exploratory factor analysis of the PAF-SF would reveal a three-factor solution with a good simple structure and factors reflecting affective, water retention, and pain symptoms, respectively [19]. We also hypothesized [H2] that subscales derived from the chosen factor structure would each show acceptable to excellent internal consistency. We further hypothesized that the factorially-derived subscales would show good concurrent criterion-related validity in terms of differential associations with our chosen criterion measures. Specifically, we expected [H3] only the PAF-SF affective subscale would be positively correlated with scores on a validated measure of dispositional anxiety. Given affective symptoms from the PAF-SF include anxiety symptoms [19], we reasoned there should be a strong overlap with a measure tapping the tendency to experience anxiety across situations. We also expected [H4] only the PAF-SF affective subscale would be positively correlated with a symptom count of affective PMDD symptoms endorsed on a gold-standard clinical interview for PMDD (i.e., the Structured Clinical Interview for DSM-5 Disorders; SCID-5; [20]). In contrast, we predicted [H5] only the PAF-SF water retention and pain subscales would be positively correlated with a symptom count of somatic PMDD symptoms endorsed on the SCID-5. Finally, we hypothesized that the factorially-derived PAF-SF subscales would show known group validity.

More specifically, we expected [H6] females with a provisional PMDD diagnosis on the SCID-5 would show elevations on all PAF-SF subscales relative to those females without a provisional PMDD diagnosis.

2. Methods

2.1 Participants

Eighty-seven female cannabis users were originally recruited for a study on cannabis use across the menstrual cycle [21]. Eligibility criteria for the original study were as follows: (1) being between 19 and 45 years old, (2) owning/having access to a smartphone (with a data/texting plan), (3) having no known interference with their menstrual cycle (i.e., past six months or current pregnancy, use of hormonal contraceptives, immediate plans of conceiving, breastfeeding, hysterectomy, amenorrhea, or perimenopausal/postmenopausal), (4) having an average length menstrual cycle (i.e., 25–32 days), (5) not having a pain disorder diagnosis, (6) not prescribed medicinal cannabis, (7) not stopping hormonal contraceptive use within the three months prior to study participation, (8) using cannabis >4 times in the month prior to study involvement, and (9) not abstaining from, trying to abstain from, or in treatment for cannabis use. See **Table 1** for sample demographics and clinical characteristics.

2.2 Procedure

The study protocol was approved by an institutional research ethics board at Dalhousie University (REB #: 2017–4249) and is a secondary analysis of data collected by Joyce et al. [21]. Recruitment was done *via* advertisements in the community, on social media, in the local newspaper, and on the radio. The larger study was divided into five sessions; further information on the larger study protocol can be found in Joyce et al. [21]. Only sessions relevant to the current study are described here.

2.2.1 Telephone screening

Participants completed a telephone screening with K.M.J. to determine eligibility (see the above inclusion/exclusion criteria). If deemed eligible, they were scheduled for a baseline assessment where all data relevant to the present study were collected in person.

2.2.2 Baseline assessment

During the baseline assessment, participants provided informed consent, completed three self-report questionnaires (i.e., Demographics, 10-item PAF-SF [19], and State-Trait Anxiety Inventory – Trait Subscale [22]), and took part in a clinical interview, namely the PMDD module of the SCID-5 [20]. The SCID-5 interviews were conducted by K.M.J, a graduate student in psychiatry research at the time of data collection, who was trained and supervised by S.H.S., a licensed clinical psychologist[1].

[1] Data from the SCID-5 was missing for one participant. As such, they were excluded from all analyses including SCID-5 data.

Demographic/Clinical Variable	Mean (Standard Deviation) / Percentage (%)
Age (in years)	28.86 (6.11)
Ethnicity	
Caucasian	72.4%
Other[a]	27.6%
Education Level	
College/University Graduate or More[b]	69.0%
Some Colleges/Universities or Less[c]	31.0%
Menstrual Cycle Length (in days)[d]	27.70 (4.91)
Trait Anxiety[e]	45.50 (7.25)
Number of Affective PMDD Symptoms[f]	2.37 (1.53)
Number of Somatic PMDD Symptoms[f]	2.21 (1.46)
Premenstrual Dysphoric Disorder[g]	27.5%
Premenstrual Assessment Form – Short Form	32.32 (9.24)
PAF-SF Three-Factor Solution	
Affect Subscale	13.97 (4.79)
Water Retention Subscale	8.14 (3.77)
Pain Subscale	10.22 (3.06)
PAF-SF Two-Factor Solution	
Psychological Subscale	13.97 (4.79)
Physiological Subscale	18.36 (5.91)

[a]*Categories are too small to report individually; however, this category consisted of: South East Asians, Blacks, South Asians, Arab/West Asians, Latin Americans, Native Canadians, and others.*
[b]*Includes: college/university graduates, some post-graduate, and post-graduate degree.*
[c]*Includes: some college/university, high school graduates, and some high school.*
[d]*Self-reported menstrual cycle length.*
[e]*Determined by the State-Trait Anxiety Inventory – Trait Subscale [22].*
[f]*Determined by symptom count of affective and somatic premenstrual dysphoric disorder symptoms, respectively, endorsed on the Structured Clinical Interview for DSM-5 Disorders [20].*
[g]*Percentage of the sample meeting DSM-5 diagnostic criteria for the premenstrual dysphoric disorder (PMDD) on the Structured Clinical Interview for DSM-5 Disorders [20].*

Table 1.
Demographic and clinical descriptives for the full sample (N = 87).

2.3 Materials

2.3.1 Premenstrual assessment form: Short form (PAF-SF)

The PAF-SF contains 10 items pertaining to physiological and psychological changes experienced premenstrually (e.g., feeling bloated) [19]. For each item, the intensity of change experienced premenstrually was rated from 1 ("*Not present at all or no change from usual level*") to 6 ("*Extreme change – the degree of change in severity is so different from your usual state that it is very apparent to you OR even people who do not know you well might notice*"). The PAF-SF total score has excellent internal consistency (α = .95), the total score and three proposed subscales (affect, water retention, pain)

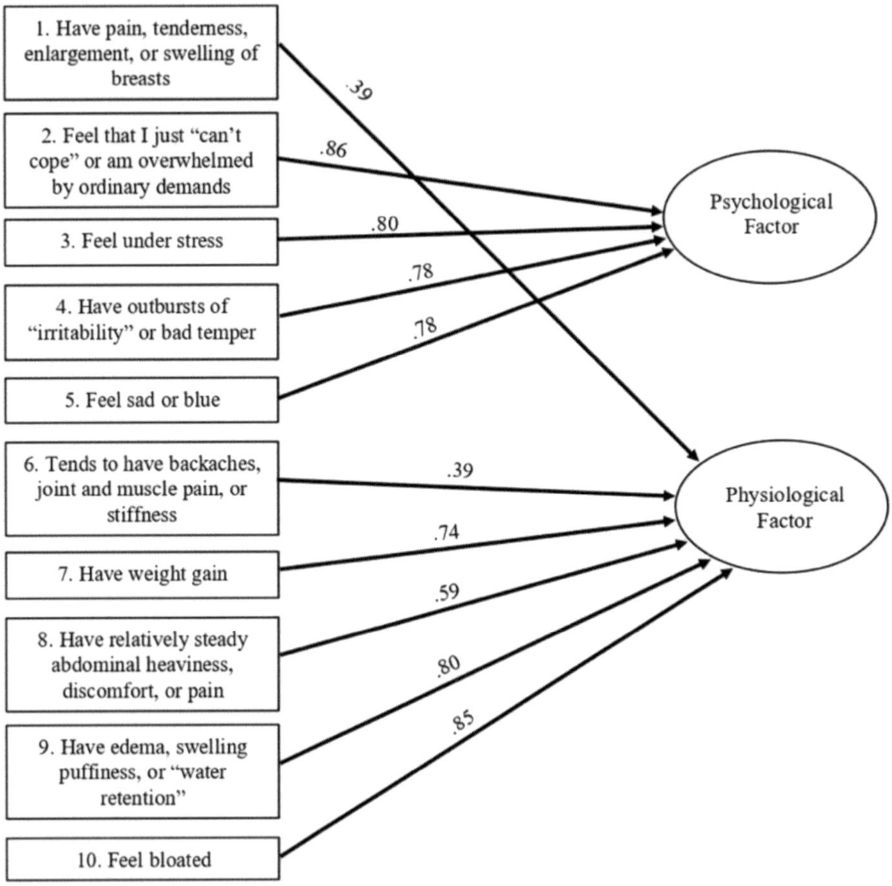

Figure 1.
Depiction of the two factors, that is, psychological and physiological symptoms, and items from the Premenstrual Assessment Form – Short Form [19] showing salient loadings (≥ .30) on each factor.

show acceptable test-retest reliability across a 6-month follow-up (*r*'s = .60–.70), and the total score shows criterion-related validity against a measure of nicotine withdrawal symptoms in a sample of smokers undergoing smoking cessation (*r*'s ~ .40; [19]). PAF-SF items are provided in **Figure 1**.

2.3.2 State-Trait anxiety inventory: Trait subscale (STAI-T)

The STAI-T [22] was used to examine trait anxiety levels, i.e., the relatively stable aspect of anxiety proneness. The STAI-T consists of 20 items rated on a 4-point scale ranging from 1 ("*Almost never*") to 4 ("*Almost always*"). The STAI-T involves 13 anxiety-present (e.g., "*I feel nervous and restless*") and 7 anxiety-absent items (e.g., "*I feel pleasant*"); the latter are reverse-scored prior to the calculation of the STAI-T total score. Higher total scores on the STAI-T are indicative of elevated trait anxiety. The STAI has demonstrated good-to-excellent internal consistency across studies (α = .86–.95; [22–24]) and test-retest reliabilities have ranged between marginally acceptable-to-good (*r*'s = .69–.89; [23]). The trait subscale of the STAI is considered a valid measure of general negative affect (i.e., anxiety and depression) [25].

2.3.3 Structured clinical interview for DSM-5 disorders: Research version (SCID-5)

The SCID-5 is the gold-standard clinical interview for mood disorder diagnoses in research settings [20]. It was used in the present study for two purposes: (1) to identify the number of DSM-5 affective and somatic premenstrual-related symptoms endorsed, respectively, and (2) to divide participants into those with and without a provisional PMDD diagnosis for our known groups' analysis of construct validity.[2] The affective premenstrual symptom count on the SCID-5 included four questions pertaining to (a) mood swings; (b) irritability; (c) dysphoric mood; and (d) anxious mood (i.e., Criteria B1-B4, respectively, of the DSM-5 PMDD diagnostic criteria; [15]). The somatic premenstrual symptom count on the SCID-5 included four questions on: (a) fatigue; (b) increased appetite; (c) sleep disruptions; and (d) pain/water retention (i.e., Criteria C3-C5 and C7, respectively, on the DSM-5 PMDD diagnostic criteria; [15]). The SCID-5 [20] has good test-retest reliability over one week (r = .76) and very good-to-excellent inter-rater reliability (κ = .62–.82; [26]). While an analysis of the reliability and validity of PMDD diagnoses via the SCID-5 is currently lacking, Accortt et al. [27] have found that structured interviews for PMDD diagnoses have a high inter-rater agreement (ICC = .86–1.00) and reliability (κ = .96).

2.4 Data analysis

Descriptive statistics were used to characterize the sample on sociodemographic and clinical characteristics. We then compared our sample to norms on the clinical measures (i.e., mean PAF-SF total, mean STAI-T, proportion with provisional PMDD diagnoses).

Next, we conducted an exploratory PCA to examine the factor structure underlying the PAF-SF. An exploratory, as opposed to confirmatory, approach was used since the present study represents the first examination of the factor structure of the 10-item version of the PAF-SF. We utilized orthogonal (Varimax with Kaiser normalization) rotation to improve interpretability of the resultant factor solution and for consistency with the approach used by Allen et al. [19] with the 20-item version of the PAF-SF during test development. To determine the number of factors to retain, we considered the results of both the commonly used Kaiser's [28] eigenvalue >1.0 rule and the more stringent parallel analysis criterion. Parallel analysis is a procedure that statistically determines the break in the scree plot [29, 30]. We compared obtained eigenvalues to mean eigenvalues generated using Monte Carlo simulations based on the study's sample size (i.e., N = 87) and the number of variables (i.e., 10 PAF-SF items) [29].

For each factor solution, we calculated sample means and standard deviations (SD) on the associated subscales and examined resultant subscales' inter-correlations and internal consistencies (Coefficient alphas). We considered alphas > .70 as acceptable and > .80 as good [30]. We used all information (i.e., simple structure [31], factor interpretability, internal consistency of subscales, parsimony) to select the most suitable factor solution. Subscale scores associated with the selected solution were used in all subsequent criterion-related and construct validity analyses.

---

[2] Our PMDD diagnoses in the present study were considered 'provisional' as they were based entirely on the SCID-5 interview and were not confirmed by prospective daily ratings during at least two symptomatic cycles as required in Criterion F of the DSM-5 PMDD diagnostic criteria [15].

To determine the criterion-related and construct validity of the factorially-derived PAF-SF subscales, a series of bivariate correlations were conducted to examine relationships between the PAF-SF subscales and (a) STAI-T scores, (b) PMDD affective symptom count from the SCID-5, and (c) PMDD somatic symptom count from the SCID-5. We used Cohen's [32] convention of considering a correlation of $r = .10$ as a small correlation, $r = .30$ a moderate correlation, and $r = .50$ a large correlation. Finally, a pair of between-sample *t*-tests were used to compare those with and without a provisional SCID-5 diagnosis of PMDD on each subscale of the PAF-SF. We calculated effect sizes for these group differences using Cohen's *d* and used Cohen's [32] convention of considering a $d = .20$ as a small effect, $d = .50$ a moderate effect, and $d = .80$ a large effect size.

3. Results

3.1 Sample characteristics

The mean (± *SD*) score on the PAF-SF total score in our sample of 32.3 ± 9.2 (see **Table 1**) was about half of a standard deviation above the sample mean of 27.4 ± 10.9 reported by Allen et al. [19] in the PAF-SF development sample at baseline. Just over one-quarter of the sample met SCID-5 [20] criteria for a provisional PMDD diagnosis (see **Table 1**), which is about three times higher than the rate of PMDD in the general population [12, 13]. The mean (± *SD*) STAI-T score was 45.5 ± 7.3 (see **Table 1**), which is comparable to the mean trait anxiety score in the general population of 44.4 ± 11.3 [33].

3.2 Factorial validity

We conducted a PCA to examine the underlying factor structure of the PAF-SF. We first tested assumptions. Given the Kaiser-Meyer-Olkin (KMO) measure of sampling adequacy was > .60 (i.e., .82) and given the significant Bartlett's test of sphericity ($\chi^2(45) = 321.82, p < .001$), we determined that the PAF-SF data was suitable for PCA.

Kaiser's [29] eigenvalues >1.0 criterion was first used to determine the number of factors to retain. It suggested a three-factor solution; obtained eigenvalues appear at the bottom of **Table 2**. The three factors together accounted for 67.0% of the variance in PAF-SF item scores. **Table 2** shows PAF-SF item loadings on the three extracted factors following orthogonal (Varimax) rotation. Communality values (see **Table 2**) were strong ranging from .56 (item 8) to .78 (item 10) suggesting that the three factors together explained 56–78% of the variance in individual item scores. Salient loadings were considered those ≥ .30 and are shown in bold (see **Table 2**).

Factor 1 was labeled affect, as it showed salient positive loadings from all four intended affect items (**Table 2**). Factor 2 was labeled water retention, as it showed its three strongest positive salient loadings from the three intended water retention items; however, it showed salient positive loadings from all three intended pain items as well (**Table 2**). Factor 3 was labeled pain, as it showed salient loadings from all three intended pain items; however, one of these was a positive loading (Item 1) and the other two were unexpectedly negative loadings (Items 6 and 8; see **Table 2**). The simple structure for the rotated three-factor solution was poor: while there were no hyperplane items (i.e., items showing no salient loadings on any factor), three

PAF-SF Item Content (original subscale)	Factor 1 Affect	Factor 2 Water Retention	Factor 3 Pain	Communality
1. Painful Breasts (Pain)	.11	**.30**	**.71**	.61
2. Overwhelmed (Affect)	**.87**	.02	−.04	.75
3. Feel Under Stress (Affect)	**.80**	.23	.00	.70
4. Irritable Outbursts (Affect)	**.78**	.25	−.01	.68
5. Feel Sad or Blue (Affect)	**.77**	.28	−.01	.68
6. Back/Joint/Muscle Pain (Pain)	.28	**.48**	**−.59**	.66
7. Weight Gain (Water Retention)	.21	**.75**	−.01	.61
8. Abdominal Pain (Pain)	.19	**.64**	**−.34**	.56
9. Water Retention (Water Retention)	.16	**.78**	.21	.68
10. Feel Bloated (Water Retention)	.20	**.85**	.16	.78

Notes: Observed eigenvalues = 4.19, 1.49, 1.02, .87, .60, .46, .43, .38, .29, .27.
Salient loadings ≥ .30 are shown in bold.

Table 2.
Results of the principal component analysis: Loadings of each Premenstrual Assessment Form – Short Form item on the orthogonally-rotated three-factor solution.

	1	2	3	4	5
1. Psychological[a]	—				
2. Physiological[a]	.49*	—			
3. Affect[b]	1.0*	.49*	—		
4. Pain[b]	.40*	.83*	.40*	—	
5. Water Retention[b]	.43*	.89*	.43*	.49*	—

Notes: [a]Two-Factor Solution; [b]Three-Factor Solution.
An asterisk (*) denotes a significant correlation coefficient (p < .001).
The psychological and affect subscales, from the two- and three-factor solutions, respectively, include the same four Premenstrual Assessment Form – Short Form items.

Table 3.
Bivariate correlations between subscales were identified via two-factor and three-factor solutions from the principal component analysis.

of the 10 items showed complex loadings (i.e., a salient loading on more than one factor). All three complex loadings were from the intended pain items which showed salient loadings on both the water retention and pain factors (i.e., Factors 2 and 3, respectively). Given that all items showed salient loadings on (at least) their intended factor, we calculated scores on the original PAF-SF subscales using the scoring suggested by Allen et al. [19]. Bivariate correlations between the three subscales ranged from $r = .40$ (affect – pain) to $r = .49$ (water retention – pain; see **Table 3**). While these were moderate to large inter-subscale correlations [34], they were somewhat lower than the inter-subscale correlations (r's > .60) reported by Allen et al. [19]. Coefficient alpha values were good for the water retention and affect subscales ($\alpha = .83$ and .85, respectively) but unacceptably low for the pain subscale ($\alpha = .45$; [34]), inconsistent with H2. The unacceptably low alpha for the pain subscale was likely due to constituent items having salient loadings of different directions on

Factor 3 (pain). Taken together, these results strongly suggest that the three-factor solution involves factor over-extraction; more specifically, separate pain and water retention factors do not appear to be justified.

A more stringent parallel analysis criterion for determining the number of factors to extract was then utilized. Comparing against mean eigenvalues, parallel analysis suggested two factors should be retained rather than the three suggested by the less stringent Kaiser's [28] eigenvalues >1.0 criterion. The two factors together accounted for 56.8% of the variance in PAF-SF item scores. **Table 4** shows PAF-SF item loadings on the two extracted factors following orthogonal (Varimax) rotation. Salient loadings ≥ .30 are shown in bold (see **Table 4**). There was a good simple structure [31] for the rotated two-factor solution: no hyperplane items, only one complex item, and each factor containing at least five salient loadings.

Factor 1 was labeled psychological premenstrual symptoms, as it showed strong salient positive loadings from all four affect items and an additional moderate loading from one pain item (**Table 4** and **Figure 1**). Factor 2 was labeled physiological premenstrual symptoms, as it showed strong positive salient loadings from all three water retention items as well as moderate positive salient loadings from all three pain items (see **Table 4** and **Figure 1**). Communality values (see **Table 4**) were not as strong overall compared to the three-factor solution given the loss of one factor. They ranged from .15 (Item 1) to .77 (Item 10) suggesting that the two factors together explained 15–77% of the variance in individual item scores. The lowest communality values were for the intended pain items which ranged from .15 (Item 1) to .42 (Item 8); the remaining items all showed high communality values ranging from .61 (Item 7) to .77 (Item 10). The one pain item that showed the complex loadings (i.e., Item 6: back/joint/muscle pain) showed similarly sized moderate salient positive loadings on both the psychological and physiological factors. Since this item conceptually fit best with the physiological factor, it was included with the other Factor 2 items in scoring of the factorially-derived subscales. The two subscales were inter-correlated at

PAF-SF Item Content (original subscale)	Factor 1 Psychological	Factor 2 Physiological	Communality
1. Painful Breasts (Pain)	.01	**.39**	.15
2. Overwhelmed (Affect)	**.86**	.00	.74
3. Feel Under Stress (Affect)	**.80**	.21	.69
4. Irritable Outbursts (Affect)	**.78**	.23	.67
5. Feel Sad or Blue (Affect)	**.78**	.26	.67
6. Back/Joint/Muscle Pain (Pain)	**.40**	**.39**	.31
7. Weight Gain (Water Retention)	.15	**.74**	.61
8. Abdominal Pain (Pain)	.27	**.59**	.42
9. Water Retention (Water Retention)	.15	**.80**	.66
10. Feel Bloated (Water Retention)	.20	**.85**	.77

Notes: Salient loadings ≥ .30 are shown in bold.
While item 6 showed a complex loading on both factors, for subscale scoring purposes, it was included with Factor 2 (Physiological symptoms) given its superior conceptual fit with this factor.

Table 4.
Results of the principal component analysis: Loadings of each Premenstrual Assessment Form – Short Form item on the orthogonally-rotated two-factor solution.

r = .49, a large magnitude correlation (**Table 3**). Consistent with H2, internal consistencies for the resultant subscales ranged from acceptable (physiological subscale; α = .76) to good (psychological subscale; α = .85; [34]). The internal consistency of the physiological subscale remained essentially unchanged if the one cross-loading item (item 6) was removed (α = .75); thus, item 6 was retained in scoring the physiological subscale.

Given its superior simple structure and interpretability, the acceptable to good internal consistencies of the resultant subscales, and based on the principle of parsimony, the two-factor solution was chosen above the three-factor solution as the best representation of the factor structure underlying the PAF-SF. Bivariate correlations between all subscales identified using the PCAs are shown in **Table 3**.

3.3 Criterion-related validity

Bivariate correlations suggested significant convergent/discriminant relationships between the two PAF-SF subscales and various criterion measures. Consistent with H3, the PAF-SF was correlated with the STAI trait anxiety subscale only in the case of the psychological but not the physiological PAF-SF subscale. Specifically, higher scores on the psychological subscale of the PAF-SF were associated with significantly more trait anxiety (r = .47, p < .001) on the STAI trait anxiety subscale; the correlation was large in magnitude supporting the PAF-SF psychological subscale's validity but not so large as to suggest redundancy with trait anxiety. Also consistent with H3, scores on the physiological subscale of the PAF-SF were not significantly related to scores on the trait anxiety subscale of the STAI (r = .14, p = .213; small magnitude correlation). Comparison of dependent-sample correlations revealed that the correlation between STAI-T and the PAF-SF was significantly stronger in the case of the psychological than the physiological PAF-SF subscale (z = 3.23, p = .001).

Consistent with H4, the PAF-SF subscales were also correlated with the affective symptom count on the SCID-5 PMDD module only for the psychological, but not the physiological PAF-SF subscale. A significant large magnitude positive correlation was observed between the number of affective symptoms endorsed on the SCID-5 and scores on the psychological subscale of the PAF-SF (r = .49, p < .001). In contrast, scores on the physiological subscale of the PAF-SF were not significantly related to affective symptom count on the SCID-5 PMDD module (r = .20, p = .062; small magnitude correlation). Comparison of dependent-sample correlations revealed that the correlation between SCID-5 PMDD affective symptom count and the PAF-SF was significantly stronger in the case of the psychological than the physiological PAF-SF subscale (z = 2.89, p = .002).

Partially consistent with H5, a significant positive correlation of moderate magnitude was observed between the number of somatic premenstrual-related symptoms endorsed on the SCID-5 and scores on the physiological subscale of the PAF-SF (r = .29, p = .008). But contrary to H5, scores on the psychological subscale of the PAF-SF were also significantly related to the somatic symptom count on the SCID-5 PMDD module with a correlation coefficient of similar moderate magnitude to that seen with the physiological subscale of the PAF-SF (r = .29, p = .007).

3.4 Construct validity: Known groups validation

Partially consistent with H6, females with a provisional diagnosis of PMDD on the SCID-5 reported higher scores on the psychological subscale of the PAF-SF than those

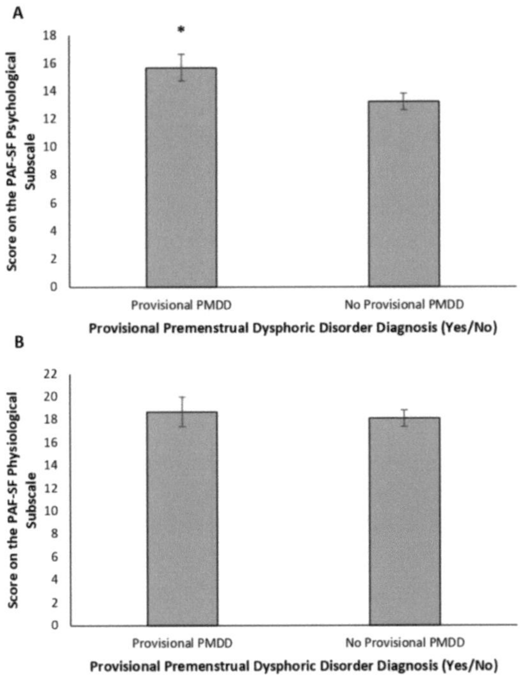

Figure 2.
Mean (A) psychological and (B) physiological subscale scores on the Premenstrual Assessment Form – Short Form (PAF-SF; [19]) in females with (n = 24) and without (n = 63) a provisional premenstrual dysphoric disorder (PMDD) diagnosis. Error bars represent standard errors. An asterisk (*) indicates significantly higher PAF-SF psychological subscale scores in females with a provisional PMDD diagnosis versus those without ($p < .05$).

without a diagnosis ($t_{85} = -2.25, p = .03; d = .52$ [medium effect size]; see **Figure 2A**). However, inconsistent with H6, scores on the physiological subscale of the PAF-SF did not differ between PMDD groups ($t_{85} = -.62, p = .54; d = .15$ [small effect size]; see **Figure 2B**).

4. Discussion

One of the purposes of the present study was to examine the factorial validity of the 10-item PAF-SF since it had never been subject to factor analysis before. While in the initial test development and validation study, Allen et al. [19] did find support for a three-factor solution to an earlier 20-item version of the PAF-SF (i.e., affect, water retention, and pain factors), they further reduced the scale to 10-items but did not confirm the assumed three-factor structure of the reduced scale. In the present study, the traditional Kaiser's [28] eigenvalues >1.0 criterion for determining the number of factors to retain suggested a three-factor solution which, at first glance, resembled the three-factor structure suggested by Allen et al. [19] with Factors 1–3 capturing affect, water retention, and pain symptoms, respectively. However, there were several problems with this solution. First, there were several complex loadings between the water retention and pain factors with all intended pain items showing primary or secondary loadings on Factor 2, water retention. Second, contrary to theory, the three intended pain items showed opposite direction salient loadings on Factor 3 with breast pain showing a positive loading, and abdominal pain and back/joint/muscle pain showing negative loadings, on this factor. Finally, while the affect and water retention subscales [19] showed good internal consistencies (α's > .80), the internal consistency for the pain subscale (i.e., α = .45) was unacceptably low [34]. Taken together, these findings suggested that the three-factor solution represented factor over-extraction and provided little in the way of factorial validity for a pain factor that was distinct from the water retention factor. Indeed, when Allen et al. [19] reduced their 20-item PAF-SF to the current 10-item version, they had to lower the magnitude of acceptable factor loadings for item retention from their intended minimum of .40 to find sufficient items that could be retained for their pain subscale. Each of their retained three pain items had secondary (or primary) salient loadings on the water retention factor in their PCA of the 20-item version of the PAF-SF [19]. Thus, it is perhaps not surprising that there was a lack of stability of a separate pain factor in our replication.

The more stringent parallel analysis criterion (using mean eigenvalues) for determining the number of factors to retain suggested a two-factor solution with factors that we labeled psychological and physiological premenstrual symptoms, respectively. All four items in Allen et al.'s [19] affect subscale comprised the first factor (psychological), and the remaining water retention and pain items all showed salient loadings on the second factor (physiological). This two-factor solution showed a superior simple structure [31] relative to the three-factor solution and both resultant subscales from the two-factor solution showed acceptable to good internal consistencies (α's > .70). Thus, we opted to select the more parsimonious two-factor structure over the three-factor structure. While this runs contrary to the results of Allen et al. [19] and H1, parallel analysis has been found to produce more accurate factor extractions than Kaiser's [29] eigenvalue >1.0 rule [35], providing further impetus for our selecting the two-factor over the three-factor solution. All additional validation tests were conducted using subscale scores derived from the two-factor solution.

We saw strong support for the criterion-related validity of the psychological symptom subscale of the PAF-SF in that this subscale showed theoretically expected significant positive, large magnitude correlations with trait anxiety and with the count of premenstrual affective symptoms endorsed on the SCID-5 PMDD module [20]. This shows that females who are more dispositionally anxious (i.e., showing a tendency to experience greater anxiety across a variety of situations; [22]) are also more likely to self-report changes in negative affect, including anxious affect, in the five days prior to menstruation on the PAF-SF. These criterion-related validity results also show that females who endorse experiencing more affective symptoms on a gold-standard clinical interview for diagnosing PMDD also self-report a greater severity of psychological premenstrual symptoms on the PAF-SF. Moreover, these significant criterion-related validity findings were specific to the psychological symptom subscale of the PAF-SF and were not seen with the PAF-SF physiological symptoms subscale. Additionally, the magnitudes of the correlations of these two criterion measures with the PAF-SF were significantly stronger for the psychological subscale than for the physiological subscale. Overall, this provides strong criterion-validation for the PAF-SF psychological symptoms subscale, consistent with H3.

The test of criterion-related validity of the PAF-SF physiological symptoms subscale produced results that were less definitive. Consistent with H4, this subscale showed a significant positive correlation of moderate magnitude with a symptom count measure of somatic symptoms endorsed on the SCID-5 PMDD module [20]. However, this relation was not unique to the physiological symptom subscale of the PAF-SF; indeed, a similar moderate magnitude correlation with the PMDD somatic symptom count was seen for the PAF-SF psychological symptom subscale. At first glance, this might suggest relatively poor criterion-related validity for the physiological symptom subscale of the PAF-SF. However, certain limitations of the symptom count of PMDD somatic symptoms endorsed on the SCID-5 as the criterion measure against which the PAF-SF physiological symptoms subscale was assessed should be acknowledged. There was substantial content overlap between the PAF-SF psychological scale and the SCID-5 PMDD affective symptom count criterion measure. However, this was less true of the content match between the PAF-SF physiological scale and the SCID-5 PMDD somatic symptom count criterion measure where all six PAF-SF physiological scale items corresponded to only one of four of the PMDD somatic symptoms assessed (i.e., DSM-5 PMDD Criterion C7: pain/water retention). We considered using only endorsement on the SCID-5 of the single symptom, Criterion C7 from the DSM-5, as our criterion-validity check for our test of H5. However, the use of single-item measures as criterion measures are usually advised against in the psychometric literature due to measurement error concerns [36]. Moreover, factor analytic work on the symptoms of PMDD in the DSM-5 [15] has shown that the pain/water retention symptom (Criterion C7) shows a moderate but salient loading on a factor defined by strong salient loadings from the affective symptoms (Criteria B1-B4) rather than loading with the remaining "somatic" symptoms (Criteria C3-C5) on their separate second factor [37, 38]. The lack of clear division of DSM-5 PMDD symptoms into affective versus somatic domains may explain why both the PAF-SF physiological and psychological subscales correlated to the same moderate degree with the PMDD somatic symptom count on the SCID-5. Thus, while the correlation of the PAF-SF physiological subscale with the PMDD somatic symptom count on the SCID-5 provides some preliminary criterion-related validation for this PAF-SF subscale, more work needs to be done to definitively support its validity in the future.

Our known groups validity analysis yielded results partially consistent with H6. Specifically, females with a provisional diagnosis of PMDD on the gold-standard SCID-5 scored significantly higher than those without provisional PMDD on the psychological symptom subscale of the PAF-SF, with the group difference proving moderate magnitude [32]. This provides important evidence of construct validity for this PAF-SF subscale. Unexpectedly, those in the provisional PMDD group did not score significantly higher on the physiological symptom subscale of the PAF-SF (a small magnitude group difference; [32]). While this might at first glance suggest a lack of construct validity for the physiological symptom subscale, it is important to remember that water retention and pain symptoms (tapped by the six items of the PAF-SF physiological symptoms subscale) represent only a single symptom (Criterion C7) of 11 symptoms on the SCID-5 PMDD module. Indeed, factor analytic work on the symptoms of PMDD in the DSM-5 has shown higher importance of the affective symptoms (Criteria B1-B4) as opposed to water retention and pain symptoms (Criterion C7) as core symptoms of PMDD [37].

While the primary purpose of the present study was practical – i.e., further evaluation of the psychometric properties of the 10-item PAF-SF [19] – our findings also contribute to the theoretical understanding of the underlying structure of premenstrual symptoms. Like our PCA supporting two factors underlying the structure of premenstrual symptoms, other recent findings have supported two factors [37, 38]. Where these various findings converge is in identifying a primary factor comprised of affective premenstrual symptoms (e.g., mood swings, anxious mood, dysphoric mood) and a separate second factor comprised of physiological symptoms. However, the specific symptoms loading onto the second factor have varied across studies depending on the premenstrual symptom measure used. With our PCA of the 10-item

PAF-SF, the physiological symptoms loading on Factor 2 were a set of six items comprising water retention and pain (captured with a single item [C7] in the DSM-5). For the other two studies [37, 38], the factor analyses were of the DSM-5 items where Factor 2 included salient loadings from somatic symptoms like sleep disturbance and appetite changes. Interestingly, the DSM-5 water retention/pain item showed a salient loading on the first (affective) factor rather than the second factor in both studies [37, 38]. This suggests that one may need to have a greater weighting of water retention and pain symptoms within the measurement tool than currently represented in the DSM-5 definition of PMDD for a separate water retention/pain factor to emerge. It remains to be determined if, when added to the DSM-5 to replace the current single water retention/pain symptom, the six PAF-SF physiological symptoms would load with the other DSM-5 somatic symptoms or on their own separate factor.

Several potential study limitations should be acknowledged that may affect the interpretation of our results and suggest useful directions for future research. First, our sample size was relatively small for conducting a PCA. While our sample size of $N = 87$ participants exceeds some rules-of-thumb for PCA sample size such as a minimum of five participants per variable ($N = 50$ minimum in our case; [39]) or 20 participants per factor ($N = 60$ minimum in the case of our three-factor solution; [40]), it was just short of the sample size recommended by other rules-of-thumb such as 10 participants per variable ($N = 100$ minimum in our case; [36]) or $N = 100$ participants minimum overall [41]. The biggest risk of having an inadequate sample size for a PCA is a potential lack of replicability of the factorial solution [42]. Thus, it will be important for future studies to replicate our recommended two-factor solution for the PAF-SF using a larger sample and confirmatory factor analytic methods. Second, our sample had several characteristics that may limit generalizability of our results. For example, participants were all regular cannabis users for reasons related to the larger study from which this secondary data was drawn [19]. Like the original measure development sample (female smokers undergoing tobacco cessation; [19]), results obtained with substance-using samples may not generalize to non-substance users. As another example, a relatively large proportion of the sample (over one-quarter) met DSM-5 criteria for a provisional PMDD diagnosis which is substantially higher than the 3–8% of the general female population with PMDD [12, 13]. This high rate may have been due to (a) the original study [21] being advertised as concerning cannabis use across the menstrual cycle which may have preferentially attracted females with PMDD concerns and/or (b) our failure to confirm PMDD diagnoses with prospective daily ratings of symptoms for two symptomatic cycles as required by DSM-5 [15]. Either way, it will be important to examine the psychometric properties of the PAF-SF in a more representative sample of naturally cycling females in the future. Finally, as with the original validation study [19], only a small number of criterion measures were included in the present study to examine the criterion-related validity of the PAF-SF. Thus, future studies should include a broader range of validating tools, particularly those that might theoretically be expected to show unique correlations with the physiological subscale of the PAF-SF.

5. Conclusion

In conclusion, our study provides additional support for the good psychometric properties of the PAF-SF that builds upon the results presented by Allen et al. [19] in their original test development and preliminary validation study. However, contrary to Allen et al.'s [19] recommendations that this self-report measure should be scored on three subscales, our findings suggest that the PAF-SF should be scored according to two subscales – psychological (the equivalent of Allen et al.'s [19] 4-item affect subscale) and physiological symptoms (the equivalent of the sum of Allen et al.'s [19] 3-item water retention subscale and their 3-item pain subscale). Both of our suggested subscales show at least partial evidence of criterion-related validity in relation to theoretically relevant criterion variables, and the psychological subscale shows evidence of known groups validity in relation to PMDD diagnoses. Overall, our findings add to the preliminary results of Allen et al. [19] in supporting the 10-item PAF-SF as a useful brief measure of premenstrual symptom severity for both research and clinical settings, that can overcome the practical limitations of longer measures of premenstrual symptoms.

Acknowledgements

Funding for the larger project was obtained from the Department of Psychiatry Research Fund at Dalhousie University.

At the time of data collection, Kayla Joyce's graduate studies in psychiatry research at Dalhousie University were supported by a Nova Scotia Graduate Scholarship, the Scotia Scholar Award from the Nova Scotia Health Research Foundation, and the Joseph-Armand Bombardier Canada Graduate Scholarship from the Social Sciences and Humanities Research Council of Canada. Kayla Joyce's doctoral degree in clinical psychology at the University of Manitoba, which she was completing at the time of writing this chapter, was supported by a Vanier Canada Graduate Scholarship from the Social Sciences and Humanities Research Council. Sherry Stewart is supported by a Canadian Institutes of Health Research Tier 1 Canada Research Chair in Addictions and Mental Health at Dalhousie University.

Conflicts of interest

The authors declare no conflict of interest.

Author details

Kayla M. Joyce[1*] and Sherry H. Stewart[2]

1 Dalhousie University, Halifax, Canada and University of Manitoba, Winnipeg, Canada

2 Dalhousie University, Halifax, Canada

*Address all correspondence to: joycek1@mymanitoba.ca

References

[1] Joyce KM, Good KP, Tibbo P, Brown J, Stewart SH. Addictive behaviors across the menstrual cycle: A systematic review. Archives of Women's Mental Health. 2021;**24**:529-542. DOI: 10.1007/s00737-020-01094-0

[2] Lorenz TK, Gesselman AN, Vitzthum VJ. Variance in mood symptoms across menstrual cycles: Implications for premenstrual dysphoric disorder. Women's Reproductive Health. 2017;**4**:78-88. DOI: 10.1080/23293691.2017.1326248

[3] Iacovides A, Avidon I, Baker FC. Does pain vary across the menstrual cycle? A review. European Journal of Pain. 2015;**19**:1389-1405. DOI: 10.1002/ejp.714

[4] de Tommaso M. Pain perception during menstrual cycle. Current Pain and Headache Reports. 2011;**15**:400-406. DOI: 10.1007/s11916-011-0207-1

[5] Fehring RJ, Schneider M, Raviele K. Variability in the phases of the menstrual cycle. Journal of Obstetric, Gynecologic, and Neonatal Nursing. 2006;**35**:376-384. DOI: 10.111/j.1552-6909.2006.00051.x

[6] Lenton EA, Landgren B, Sexton L. Normal variation in the length of the luteal phase of the menstrual cycle: Identification of the short luteal phase. BJOG: An International Journal of Obstetrics & Gynaecology. 1984;**91**:685-689. DOI: 10.111/j.1471-0528.1984.tb04831.x

[7] Walsh RN, Budtz-Olsen I, Leader C, Cummins RA. The menstrual cycle, personality, and academic performance. Archives of General Psychiatry. 1981;**38**:219-221. DOI: 10.1001/archpsyc.1981.01780270105015

[8] Collins A, Eneroth P, Landgren BM. Psychoneuroendocrine stress responses and mood as related to the menstrual cycle. Psychosomatic Medicine. 1985;**47**:512-527. DOI: 10.1097/00006842-198511000-00002

[9] Aganoff JA, Boyle GJ. Aerobic exercise, mood states and menstrual cycle symptoms. Journal of Psychosomatic Research. 1994;**38**:183-193. DOI: 10.1016/0022-3999(94)90114-7

[10] Reed SC, Levin FR, Evans SM. Changes in mood, cognitive performance and appetite in the late luteal and follicular phases of the menstrual cycle in women with and without PMDD (premenstrual dysphoric disorder). Hormones and Behavior. 2008;**54**:185-193. DOI: 10.1016/j.yhbeh.2008.02.018

[11] Direkvand-Moghadam A, Sayehmiri K, Delpisheh A, Satar K. Epidemiology of premenstrual syndrome (PMS) - a systematic review and meta-analysis study. Journal of Clinical & Diagnostic Research. 2014;**8**:106-109. DOI: 10.7860/JCDR/2014/8024.4021

[12] Wittchen HU, Becker E, Lieb R, Krause P. Prevalence, incidence and stability of premenstrual dysphoric disorder in the community. Psychological Medicine. 2002;**32**:119-132. DOI: 101017/S0033291701004925

[13] Halbreich U, Borenstein J, Pearlstein T, Kahn LS. The prevalence, impairment, impact, and burden of premenstrual dysphoric disorder (PMS/PMDD). Psychoneuroendocrinology. 2003;**28**:1-23. DOI: 10.1016/S0306-4530(03)00098-2

[14] Dickerson LM, Mazyck PL, Hunter MH. Premenstrual syndrome.

American Family Physician. 2003;**15**:1743-1752

[15] American Psychiatric Association. Diagnostic and Statistical Manual of Mental Disorder. 5th ed. Arlington, VA: APA Press; 2013

[16] Moos RH. The development of a menstrual distress questionnaire. Psychosomatic Medicine. 1968;**30**:852-867. DOI: 10.1097/00006842-196811000-00006

[17] Steiner M, Macdougall M, Brown E. The premenstrual symptom screening tool (PSST) for clinicians. Archives of Women's Mental Health. 2003;**6**:203-209. DOI: 10.1007/s00737-003-0018-4

[18] Halbreich U, Endicott J, Schacht S, Nee J. The diversity of premenstrual changes as reflected in the premenstrual assessment form. Acta Psychiatrica Scandinavica. 1982;**65**:46-65. DOI: 10.1111/j.1600-0447.1982.tb00820.x

[19] Allen SS, McBride CM, Pirie PL. The shortened premenstrual assessment form. Journal of Reproductive Medicine. 1991;**36**:769-772

[20] First MB, Williams JBW, Karg RS, Spitzer RL. Structured Clinical Interview for the DSM-5 – Research Version. Arlington, VA: American Psychiatric Association; 2015

[21] Joyce KM, Thompson K, Good KP, Tibbo PG, O'Leary ME, Perrot TS, et al. The impact of depressed mood and coping motives on cannabis use quantity across the menstrual cycle in those with and without pre-menstrual dysphoric disorder. Addiction. 2021;**116**:2746-2758. DOI: 10.1111/add.15465

[22] Speilberger CD, Gorsuch RL, Lushene R, Vagg PR, Jacobs GA. Manual for the State-Trait Anxiety Inventory. Palo Alto, CA: Consulting Psychologists Press; 1983

[23] American Psychological Association. The State-Trait Anxiety Inventory (STAI) [Internet]. 2011. Available from: https://www.apa/org/pi/about/publications/caregivers/practice-settings/assessment/tools/trait-state

[24] Gustafson LW, Gabel P, Hammer A, Lauridsen HH, Petersen LK, Andersen B, et al. Validity and reliability of state-trait anxiety inventory in Danish women aged 45 years and older with abnormal cervical screening results. BMC Medical Research Methodology. 2020;**20**:89. DOI: 10.1186/s12874-020-00982-4

[25] Balsamo M, Romanelli R, Innamorati M, Ciccarese G, Carlucci L, Saggino A. The state-trait anxiety inventory: Shadows and lights on its construct validity. Journal of Psychopathology and Behavioral Assessment. 2013;**35**:475-486. DOI: 10.1007/s10862-013-9354-5

[26] Tolin DF, Giliam C, Wootton BM, Bowe W, Bragdon LB, Davis E, et al. Psychometric properties of a structured diagnostic interview for DSM-5 anxiety, mood, and obsessive-compulsive and related disorders. Assessment. 2018;**25**:3-13. DOI: 10.1177/1073191116638419

[27] Accortt EE, Bismark A, Schneider TR, Allen JJB. Diagnosis of premenstrual dysphoric disorder: The reliability of a structured clinical interview. Archives of Women's Mental Health. 2011;**14**:265-267. DOI: 10.1007/s00737-011-0209-3

[28] Kaiser HF. The application of electronic computers to factor analysis. Education and Psychological Measurement. 1960;**20**:141-151. DOI: 10.1177/001316446002000116

[29] Longman RS, Cota AA, Holden RR, Fekken GC. A regression equation for the parallel analysis criterion in principal components analysis: Mean and 95th percentile eigenvalues. Multivariate Behavioral Research. 1989;**24**:59-69. DOI: 10.1207/s15327906mbr2401_4

[30] Horn JL. A rationale and test for the number of factors in factor analysis. Psychometrika. 1965;**30**:179-185. DOI: 10.1007/BF02289447

[31] Thurstone LL. Multiple Factor Analysis. Chicago, IL: The University of Chicago Press; 1947

[32] Cohen J. Statistical Power Analysis for the Behavioral Sciences. Hillsdale, NJ: Lawrence Earlbaum Associates; 1988

[33] Asido AN, Teleki SA, Csokasi K, Rozsa S, Bandi SA. Developmental of the short version of the Spielberger state-trait anxiety inventory. Psychiatry Research. 2020;**291**. DOI: 10.1016/j.psychres.2020.113223

[34] Cortina JM. What is coefficient alpha? An examination of theory and applications. Journal of Applied Psychology. 1993;**78**:98-104. DOI: 10.1037/0021-9010.78.1.98

[35] Zwick WR, Velicer WF. Comparison of five rules for determining the number of components to retain. Psychological Bulletin. 1986;**99**:432-442. DOI: 10.1037/0033-2909.99.3.432

[36] Nunally JC, Bernstein IH. Psychometric Theory. 3rd ed. New York: McGraw Hill; 1994

[37] Teng CT, Vieira Filho AH, Artes R, Gorenstein C, Andrade LH, Wand YP. Premenstrual dysphoric symptoms among Brazilian college students: Factor structure and methodological appraisal. European Archives of Psychiatric and Clinical Neuroscience. 2004;**255**:51-56. DOI: 10.1007/s00406-004-0535-9

[38] Wang YP, Teng CY, Vieira Filho AHG, Gorenstein C, Andrade LH. Dimensionality of the premenstrual syndrome: Confirmatory factor analysis of premenstrual dysphoric symptoms among college students. Brazilian Journal of Medical and Biological Research. 2007;**40**:639-647. DOI: 10/1590/s0100-879x2007000500006

[39] Hatcher L. A Step-by-Step Approach to Using the SAS System for Factor Analysis and Structural Equation Modeling. Cary, NC: SAS Institute, Inc; 1994

[40] Arrindell WA, van der Ende J. An empirical test of the utility of the observations-to-variables ratio in factor and component analysis. Applied Psychological Measurement. 1985;**9**:165-178. DOI: 10.1177/014662168500900205

[41] Kline P. An Easy Guide to Factor Analysis. Abingdon-on-Thames, UK: Routledge; 2014

[42] Castello AB, Osborne JW. Best practices in exploratory factor analysis: Four recommendations for getting the most out of your analysis. Practical Assessment, Research, and Evaluation. 2005;**10**:1-9. DOI: 10.7275/jyj1-4868

Chapter 5

The Contribution of Isoflavones in Menopausal Symptomatic as Alternative Treatment Option

Panagiotis Tsikouras, Anna Chalkidou, Georgios Iatrakis, Efthimios Oikonomou, Anastasia Bothou, Dimitrios Kyriakou, Aise Chatzi Ismail Mouchterem, Alexios Alexiou, Konstantinos Nikolettos, Nektaria Kritsotaki, Theopi Nalbanti, Sonia Kotanidou, Stefanos Zervoudis and Nikolaos Nikolettos

Abstract

Menopause should be treated as a state of alteration of estrogen metabolism. It is characterized by a decrease in progesterone and an increase in estrogen followed by a drop in estrogen. The purpose of this study is to investigate the activity of hyaluronic acid 120 mg and isoflavones MF11RCE 80 mg, in the recovery of the symptoms of menopause and the treatment of its secondary complications such as osteoporosis, urogenital atrophy and accompanying urinary incontinence and vasomotor syndrome MF11RCE isoflavones are widely used to treat various disorders related mainly to women's health and mainly osteoporosis and menopausal discomforts, based on epidemiological studies that brought the above diseases to a lower percentage, in populations with a high consumption of these plant estrogens. Isoflavones are derived from plants and structurally or functionally resemble endogenous-natural estrogens and their active metabolites. Therefore, they have significant estrogenic (agonistic/antagonistic) activity.

Keywords: isoflavones, hyaluronic acid, hormone replacement theory, alternative treatment options for climacteric symptoms, climacteric symptoms

1. Introduction

Menopause is the permanent cessation of a woman's period due to the exhaustion of the follicles, and loss of ovarian function and marks the end of a woman's reproductive age occurring during the climacteric [1]. For a woman to be considered menopausal, menstruation should have stopped for a period of 12 months from the last menstrual period without any obvious physiological or pathological cause being responsible. The climacteric period may begin approximately four years before the last menstruation, on average 50.8 years. Duration of the symptoms may continue for several years after the last menstruation. The timing of menopause does not depend on the timing of menstruation and depends on family and racial factors [1]. The true causes of the process of ovarian failure leading to menopause have not been fully elucidated. An association of genes and menopause related to the biological mechanisms of DNA self-repair was certified. Two genes in particular, Chek1 and Chek2, according to experimental research in rodents, significantly affect fertility and menopause [2, 3]. The above genes are involved in cell apoptosis. Women who have a particular variant of Chek2, which renders the gene non-functional, are at menopause 3.5 years later compared to those in whom the specific gene is fully functional. According to researchers, the genetic modification of female mice, with the Chek2 gene deactivated, the survival time of the eggs of the experimental animals was longer. It is believed that if there was a drug that blocked Chek2, it would help women have more eggs at an older age [3–6].

Hormone replacement therapy began, initially, as an attempt to alleviate specific symptoms (vasomotor) caused by changes in estrogen production during menopause.

However, when the long-term complications of menopause on women's health became known, hormone replacement, in addition to being symptomatic, also acquired a preventive character. Classical hormone replacement therapy involves the administration of estrogens in combination with progesterone.

2. Phytoestrogens

They are a large group of plant substances whose chemical molecular structure contains a phenolic ring like estrogen. The main representatives are isoflavones and lignans. Isoflavones such as genistein are found in a number of plants such as green tea and possess both estrogenic and antiestrogenic properties like tamoxifen. Other plant substances are herbs and fruits such as valerian, hops, and black beans.

Dihydroepiandrosterone is an endogenous steroid secreted from the surface of the adrenal gland and is a precursor of testosterone and estrogen. The term phytoestrogens is descriptive and is used for non-steroidal compounds, which either exhibit estrogenic activity or are metabolized to substances with estrogenic activity. Phytoestrogens are a large family of plant-derived, non-steroidal substances that structurally or functionally resemble endogenous natural estrogens and their active metabolites. Therefore, they have significant estrogenic (agonistic/antagonistic) activity. The main groups of phytoestrogens are four: isoflavones, linoleins, coumestanes and stilbenes. They are found in more than 300 plants, especially vegetables. Phytoestrogens are structurally similar to 17β-estradiol (phenol ring) and bind to the estrogen receptors Era and Erβ. There are more than 1000 types of isoflavones. The most studied are genistein and daidzein, which have the strongest estrogenic effect. They are found in vegetables such as soybeans, chickpeas, clover, lentils and beans. Secondary soy products (milk and flour) contain lower amounts of phytoestrogens than primary products. Isoflavones are found in plants as conjugated glycosides, called glucones. This carbohydrate derivative must be broken down in the intestine, by the action of the intestinal flora, in order to produce active substances, the aglycones. The bioavailability of isoflavones depends on individual differences in intestinal flora and intestinal absorption. A difference has been found in the metabolism of phytoestrogens between men and women, with the latter metabolizing them more efficiently. Isoflavones are found in their active unconjugated form in fermented soy foods. These foods are most commonly found in Asia, where the consumption of soy products is widespread. Linoids, mainly enterolactone and enterodiol, are the most common phytoestrogens in the Western diet and are found in large amounts in flaxseed, lentils, and various fruits and vegetables. Coumestans are strong activators of estrogen receptors, but they are not included in the daily diet. They are mainly found in plant stems. Of the stilbenes, the best known is resveratrol. Its protective effect against breast cancer is the subject of research [6–9].

3. Effect of phytoestrogens

Phytoestrogens can bind to estrogen receptors α and β (ERa and ER-β respectively), in the same way that selective estrogen receptor modulators (SERMs) do. Their chemical affinity for the Era and Erβ receptors may be dose-dependent but is less than that of estrogens However, some phytoestrogens show a higher affinity for Erb receptors than estrogens, which may mean that they exert their effects through different pathways.

Each phytoestrogen exhibits different estrogenic potency. For example, in the flavonoid group, genistein is stronger than biochanin A, which is stronger than daidzein. Kuiper and colleagues showed that the intensity of stimulation of transcriptional activity by the receptor varies and depends on the estrogenic potency of the phytoestrogen, which is bound. Also, phytoestrogens, as well as synthetic estrogens, show a different degree of affinity for each of the two isoforms of the estrogen receptor. In general, it appears that phytoestrogens preferentially bind to Er-β rather than Era. Phytoestrogens have limited estrogen receptor modifying ability. Studies have shown that isoflavones have agonistic and antagonistic activity but are strong ERβ and mild ERα agonists. The structural formula of the isoflavones, with the phenolic ring, is similar to that of 17β-estradiol. The similarity allows isoflavones to bind to the estrogen receptor, essentially replacing 17β-estradiol) [9–14]. Their effect can explain the way in which phytoestrogens act protectively against breast cancer, since ERβ inhibits the growth of breast cells, while ERα promotes it. However, it is not known whether isoflavones bind to the estrogen receptor competitively at the primary estrogen binding site, or whether they have a different binding site. Furthermore, genistein has been found to bind to the active estrogen binding site in ERβ. Phytoestrogens can also promote differentiation and Studies on phytoestrogens have shown that the recruitment of co-regulatory molecules may have an important role in determining their function. In particular, isoflavones appear to selectively activate transcriptional pathways, initiated by ERβ, and in particular, transcriptional repression. The affinity shown by isoflavones for ERβ results in a change in the structure of the receptor, which thus exhibits a greater affinity for specific co-regulators than Erα, which causes inhibition of angiogenesis, cell proliferation, tyrosine kinase and topoisomera Phytoestrogens also have a dual effect on signaling pathways starting with estrogen receptors. For example, protein kinase B (Akt), whose phosphorylation normally follows ERα activation, is up-regulated by genistein and daidzein in estrogen receptor-positive breast cancer cell lines, while resveratrol has inhibited the phosphorylation of act activity. In this way, they prevent the growth of tumors. Conversely, in cell lines negative for estrogen receptor expression, resveratrol and daidzein activate act, while genistein inhibits its phosphorylation. Research into the effect of phytoestrogens on cell cycle regulators and transcription factors is contributing to the creation of synthetic substances that inhibit pathways and factors that are up-regulated by estrogen receptors. Their role is not completely known even for plants (protection from UV radiation and fungi, antioxidant activity, and many others) [9–14].

Associated with the ERs (ERa, EΠβ), they have a selective modifying capacity in the final gene expression, acting on transcription factors, so that their estrogenic/antiestrogenic effect is tissue-specific and cell-specific. They are referred to as natural SERMs. They are weak estrogens, but the affinity and activation of ERβ is 100 times stronger than that of ERα. They are therefore considered to have a beneficial effect on tissues with a strong presence of Erβ (ovary, prostate, lung, CNS, bladder, gastrointestinal). In cancerous tumors, the existence of ERP is favorable for the course of the disease. They also inhibit enzymes important for the metabolism of steroids, such as 17β-H5θ5, (12 isozymes, 1,5,7 are of interest for the breast), 3β-H5D1, aromatase, sulfatase, and sulfotransferases, which convert patient estrogens and androgens, to strong estrogens with mitogenic action) [9–14].

The above results both from in vitro cell systems, and from in vivo models of hypophysectomized, ovariectomized, (depending on the ultimate goal) experimental animals.

Like estrogens, they bind to membrane receptors, but they also exert estrogen-independent action by other mechanisms. Genistein may alter the expression of progesterone, androgen, and oxytocin receptors with unknown clinical significance. It has been reported that they induce the release of hormones from SHBG, inhibit MAPkinase, topoisomerae II etc.

They exert unwanted effects on the reproductive system, female and male. The first observations were made in sheep that developed infertility by eating subterranean clover. Also, chronic exposure of spermatozoa to high doses of genistein caused infertility, by inhibiting the acrosomal reaction and affecting their motility. The ingested plant foods are digested and the phytoestrogens they contain are converted by the intestinal bacteria into biologically active components. The amount of biologically active components absorbed varies widely, while the relative potency or affinity of phytoestrogens for estrogen receptors is 0.1–0.2% of that of estradiol.

In premenopausal women with physiologically high circulating estrogen levels, phytoestrogens compete with endogenous estrogens for binding to their respective receptors. Therefore, the net effect of phytoestrogens in premenopausal women may be antiestrogenic. Correspondingly, in postmenopausal women who have naturally high levels of natural estrogens or are receiving estrogen therapy, the net effect of phytoestrogens may also be antiestrogenic. Conversely, in postmenopausal women with low levels of circulating estrogen, the binding of phytoestrogens to estrogen receptors may result in estrogenic action of these substances. The latter, i.e. postmenopausal women with low levels of circulating estrogen and without replacement therapy for their ovarian function, have the greatest risk of vasomotor symptoms, atrophy of the vaginal epithelium and osteoporosis. This group of women is expected to benefit more from taking phytoestrogens. Recently, experimental and epidemiological studies provide convincing data on the various benefits that can come from the consumption of soy and its derivatives. For example, the isoflavones it contains seem to protect against the onset of various forms of cancer or diseases of the circulatory system, as well as against the loss of bone density. Numerous research investigations have demonstrated the impact of soy isoflavones on distinct target molecules and signaling pathways, encompassing vital cellular processes such as cell growth and differentiation, regulation of cell cycle, apoptosis, angiogenesis, cell adhesion and migration, as well as metastatic ability, along with the activity of diverse enzymes. Soy isoflavones exhibit binding affinity towards estrogen receptors α and β, thereby exerting a modulatory effect. Concurrently, these same substances appear to exert an effect independent of estrogen receptor activation [14–16].

4. Phytoestrogens and their effect on estrogen biosynthesis and excretion

Human studies of the effect of phytoestrogens on estrogen synthesis and excretion usually assess urinary levels of estrogens or steroid derivatives, as well as their metabolites. In addition, many of these studies also estimate the levels of phytoestrogens and investigate the factors influencing the values. Clinical studies have conflicting results. Lu et al. fed ten premenopausal women a high-soy diet starting from the second day of the cycle to the second day of the next cycle. Blood and urine samples were taken before and during feeding. The results showed that 17β-estradiol levels decreased by 25%, however, cycle length did not change. The Kumar et al. dietary intervention study reached similar conclusions results regarding the overall effect of phytoestrogens. The women were randomized to receive 40 mg of isoflavones or placebo per day for twelve weeks. It was found, therefore, that the values of free estradiol and estrone were reduced. Sex hormone-binding globulin (SHBG) and mean cycle length increased. In contrast, in the long-term dietary intervention study by Maskarinec and colleagues in premenopausal women, no difference in cycle length or hormone concentrations was detected. All of the above studies lead to the hypothesis that dietary intake of phytoestrogens, although important, may not be a decisive factor in breast cancer prevention by itself [14–16].

The urine phytoestrogens are metabolized by the intestinal flora into more active compounds, with the result that substances that affect the flora, potentially also affect the activity of the phytoestrogens. Administration of antibiotics has been observed to cause a sustained decrease in enterolactone levels in the gut. It appears that premenopausal women who receive long-term antibiotic therapy for urinary tract infections are at greater risk of developing breast cancer, possibly because the intestinal metabolism of phytoestrogens is disturbed. The intake of phytoestrogens, in combination with several other factors, affects the levels of estrogen derivatives in the body and their excretion. In clinical studies it is difficult to determine serum levels of phytoestrogens due to their short half-life. As most phytoestrogens are excreted in the urine, measurement of their urinary metabolites can be indicative of the phytoestrogens that dominate the diet and the main sources of intake. Some metabolites of phytoestrogens, such as enterolactone and equol, are found in urine. Urinary equol excretion was suggested as an indicator of the protective effect of phytoestrogens. Duncan et al. studied the hormonal profile of women who did or did not excrete equol in the urine and found that the first group of women had lower levels of estrone, estrone sulfate, testosterone, dihydrotestosterone, as well as higher SHBG values, regardless of dietary intake phytoestrogens. This steroid profile was found to have a protective role in breast cancer. It is noteworthy that the urinary excretion of phytoestrogens is not constant, but shows a geographical distribution. Women, living in areas with a low incidence of breast cancer, have a higher value of isoflavonoids in urine. Women who do not eat meat also have a higher concentration of isoflavonoids in their urine. However, it is unknown whether urinary enterolactone has a protective role against breast cancer or is simply indicative of a healthy hormonal profile. Certainly, the amount of phytoestrogens ingested with food is not the only factor that determines their protective effect. The levels of reproductive hormones are possibly such a factor. Phytoestrogens have been observed to stimulate the production of sex steroid hormones by liver cells. In addition, they have been found to inhibit the function of enzymes involved in the synthesis of estrogen. This, in turn, leads to low free estrogen values and reduced peripheral conversion of androgens to estrogens, which are important in estrogen development [14–16].

5. Metabolism

Individual differences in the bioavailability of the isoflavones genistein, and daidzein (most common phytoestrogens), depend on the intestinal flora. They are absorbed with soy as inactive glycosides, and are converted in the intestine into biologically active aglyconic forms, by the action of bacterial β-glucosidases. After absorption they are reconstituted in the liver mainly to glucuronic acid and less to sulfuric acid. Daidzein can be further metabolized to equol (in 30–50% of people), or to o-demethylangolensin (O-DMA) in 80–90% of the population.

A metabolite of genistein is p-ethyl phenol. The main phytoestrogens detected in the blood and urine of mammals are daidzein, genistein, equol, O-DMA. Their metabolism, mainly intestinal, and hepatic differs between children, adolescents and adults, resulting in difficulty in the interpretation of the various measurements. Phytoestrogens are polyphenolic non-steroidal plant compounds with a biological activity analogous (agonistic or antagonistic) to that of estrogens [16–20].

Based on their chemical composition, phytoestrogens can be divided into four main groups: isoflavonoids, flavonoids, stilbenes and lignans. Of these, soy mainly contains isoflavones, which are the best-studied substances in this category. Since phytoestrogens are structurally very similar to 17β-estradiol, they may exhibit selective estrogen receptor modifying activity. Many structurally diverse compounds, from both industry and natural sources, have been reported to have estrogenic activity. Such substances are DDT, polychlorinated biphenyls (PCBs) and diethylstilbestrol, as well as pharmaceutical estrogens, opium and ethinylestradiol. If we exclude ovarian steroids, most substances with estrogenic action are produced by plants. In addition to the substances mentioned above, there are also some that have not been sufficiently studied, such as β-resorcyclic acid lactans produced by fungi that attack nuts and classified as mycoestrogens or terpenoids and some saponins that appear to exhibit some estrogenic activity. Isoflavonoids are, as mentioned, the most studied group of phytoestrogens. The discovery of these substances was accidental and is of historical interest. In 1932, Marrian and Haslewood isolated a substance that was thought to have "contaminated" the hormone hydroxyestrine, which was found in high levels in the urine of pregnant mares (X). As the substance was found in the urine of non-pregnant mares as well as male horses, it was considered unrelated to pregnancy. Because it came from horses, it was called equoli Characteristically, the substance was isolated in the urine during the summer months, less during the autumn and not at all during the winter. Although it was not recognized at first, we later learned that this is due to the seasonal presence of isoflavones in plants [16–20].

Soybeans are an abundant source of isoflavones, containing approximately 2 g of isoflavonoids per kilogram of fresh weight.

However, it is important to note that the content of isoflavones in soy products can vary depending on the specific soybean variety and the processing methods employed. Consequently, different sources of soy proteins may not possess equal quantities of isoflavones, and this variability should be considered in epidemiological studies. Thus, soy proteins used in the production of meat analogs tend to have low levels of isoflavones when extracted with water, and no isoflavones if extracted with ethanol. Similarly, soybean oil does not contain any isoflavones, while soy sauce generally has minimal to negligible amounts. In addition to soy, legumes such as lentils and beans also contain isoflavones, although in much smaller quantities. Numerous types of isoflavonoids have been identified, with daidzein and genistein being the primary representatives.

These isoflavonoids are derived from their β-glycoside precursors daidzein and genistin, through their enzymatic conversion by normal flora in the gastrointestinal tract. The intestinal flora then further metabolizes daidzein to an estrogenic analog, but this biotransformation varies greatly from person to person. Despite the similarities of their biphenolic structure with estradiol, their estrogenic activity is 100–1000 times less than that of estradiol. At the same time, however, their plasma concentration can be up to 100 times higher than that of estradiol [16–20].

6. Phytoestrogens clinical purposes

Clinical targets of phytoestrogens include relief of vasomotor symptoms of menopause, maintenance of bone mineral density, and inhibition of breast cancer growth in retrospective studies. Due to the concern caused by the adverse effects of hormone replacement therapy, alternative treatments for the symptoms of menopause were sought, with phytoestrogens being the most important. A recent Cochrane review highlighted that the efficacy of phytoestrogens in alleviating menopausal symptoms remains inconclusive. Furthermore, a recent double-blind, prospective study involved the randomization of 60 women into two groups: one receiving a daily dosage of 60 mg of isoflavones for the duration of three months, and the other receiving a placebo. Menopausal symptoms were assessed and documented both before and after the treatment period.

Women in the phytoestrogen group experienced reductions in hot flashes and night sweats by 57% and 43% respectively Similar results were observed in another study with a small number of women and a duration of administration of phytoestrogens for six weeks.

In Europe, phytoestrogens are used clinically to treat menopausal symptoms. Recently, locust-derived prenylated flavonoids have been developed for menopausal symptoms. One such derivative is 8-prenylnaringenin, which exhibits a strong estrogenic effect, and is already administered in Belgium. Regarding the effect of phytoestrogens on bone tissue, the results of studies are conflicting. It appears that enriching the diet with isoflavones contributes to the maintenance of spinal bone density. A randomized, double-blind, controlled study compared the effects of hormone replacement therapy with genistein on bone metabolism and mineral density after one year. When the study was completed, it was found that women receiving hormone replacement therapy and those receiving genistein had a significant increase in bone mineral density at the hip, compared to women receiving a placebo. Similar data were reported by another randomized, double-blind, controlled trial comparing bone mineral density in women receiving an isoflavone extract and in women receiving a placebo [16–20].

Akinson et al. found that women in the isoflavone group experienced reduced bone mineral loss and bone mineral density.

Although studies on the direct effect of estrogen on breast cancer are difficult to conduct, given the long time period necessary to draw conclusions, there are studies on mammary cell proliferation and mammographic density. Short-term intake of phytoestrogen supplementation stimulates the proliferation of mammary epithelial cells. The same was observed in premenopausal women who received phytoestrogens for a long time. These histological data are also supported by the observation that women who reported even low soy consumption were more likely to present high-risk ultrasound parenchymal findings. Other studies reported similar results regarding mammographic density in women with long-term intake of phytoestrogen supplements. As shown by animal studies, the age at which a woman is exposed to phytoestrogens, as well as the duration of exposure, is potentially important in determining their potential protective effect. Key et al. conducted a prospective study involving more than 30,000 women. The women filled out a questionnaire twice over a 12-year period and were then screened for breast cancer. No relationship was found between soy consumption and the development of cancer [21–24]. However, it is worth noting that the majority of women involved in the study were not adolescents. Shu et al. conducted a retrospective study focusing on women with breast cancer. Participants were asked to complete a questionnaire regarding their dietary habits during their adolescent years. The study revealed that high soy consumption during adolescence was associated with a reduced incidence of breast cancer in adulthood. This finding suggests that this factor may contribute to the observed phenomenon where women who immigrate after puberty to countries with a higher prevalence of breast cancer than their country of origin exhibit a similar breast cancer incidence rate. Nutritional supplements, particularly those containing phytoestrogens, are widely utilized for the prevention and treatment of various conditions, primarily concerning women's health. For instance, in 2000, the consumption of such supplements reached $20 billion, with 40–55% of Americans regularly using supplements, and 24% of these supplements containing plant estrogens.

In 1975–1996, 600 articles were published on the potential benefits of phytoestrogens in cardiovascular disease, cancer (prostate, breast, colon), osteoporosis, and menopausal disorders, based on epidemiological studies that brought the above diseases to a lower rate in populations with high consumption of vegetable estrogens, mainly soy. After 2002, with the restriction of the indications of hormone replacement therapy (HRT) exclusively to severe vasomotor symptoms of menopause, the role of phytoestrogens as an alternative proposal to HRT is very important [21–24].

7. Cardiovascular disease

Genistein, 54 mg daily improved glycemic and vascular indices in normoinsulinemic, and insulin sensitivity in hyperinsulinemic women. In a double-blind, randomized controlled trial of 22 women, mean age 58 years, a comparison of 60 mg raloxifene and 55 mg phytoestrogens had no effect on humeral expansion. Of the components of the metabolic syndrome, with the administration of various soy foods, only hypertension appears to be associated with mental disorders, while any protection in CHD is due, not to protein, but to other components contained in soybeans (fiber, polyunsaturated fat, vitamins) [24–26].

8. Osteoporosis

In in vitro tests they stimulate osteoblasts and suppress osteoclasts through IL-6, OPG, RANKL. In vivo models of adult ovariectomized mice have been developed to study their effect on bone metabolism. In histomorphometric studies in mice, dietary administration does not protect bone. Ipriflavone, a synthetic isoflavone, did not affect BMD and vertebral fractures in 475 postmenopausal women at a dose of 600 mg for 4 years. Other authors observed with the same formulation, an improvement in osteoporosis indicators, but there is no clinical indication for prevention of osteopenia, and reduction of the risk of fractures [25–29].

In Asia, the incidence of fractures due to osteoporosis is lower compared to that seen in Western countries. This fact can be due to many reasons such as some related to anatomical differences, but a main reason could be the high intake of phytoestrogens from foods. Asian populations consume 10–20 times more soy, a major source of isoflavones, than populations in Western societies. High dietary intake and high urinary excretion of isoflavones has been associated with high bone mineral density in Chinese, Japanese, and Korean postmenopausal women [25–29].

Small clinical studies in humans have shown the protective effect of phytoestrogens on tonic metabolism. Soy isoflavones, genistein and daidzein, prevent postmenopausal bone loss in the lumbar fate of the spine. A high dose of isoflavones, about 90 mg daily, had a favorable effect on bone density, as observed in a study of elderly postmenopausal women.

In a randomized, double-blind, one-year study, researchers evaluated the effect of genistein on ninety healthy postmenopausal women. These women were given hormone replacement therapy with estrogen and progesterone or genistein at a dose of 54 mg per day or placebo. Bone mineral density was assessed and bone metabolism products were measured in blood and urine, and their results showed that genistein and hormone replacement therapy reduced bone loss about equally.

Assessments of bone metabolism have shown that genistein enhances bone formation and simultaneously decreases bone resorption, whereas hormone replacement therapy appears to only decrease bone resorption.

The effect of phytoestrogens on bone metabolism in fifty-five postmenopausal women who had survived breast cancer was studied in a prospective controlled study. The women received 114 mg of isoflavones daily or a placebo for 3 months [25–29].

Bone resorption, as reflected in urinary pyridinoline and deoxypyridinoline excretion, was significantly reduced in the isoflavone-treated group, while bone formation indices were not affected by this treatment regimen. Indirect evidence for the potential benefits of phytoestrogens on bone metabolism also comes from studies with ipriflavone, an isoflavone derivative. At daily doses ranging from 200 to 600 mg per day, this synthetic, non-hormonal drug has been shown to be effective in increasing bone mass and preventing bone loss.

Impressive data from multiple studies in bone cell cultures as well as experimental models of postmenopausal osteoporosis in rats support the significant protective effect of the soy isoflavones genistein and daidzein on bone. Transferring these research data into clinical practice has been a challenge. Human studies have shown favorable but mixed results. Most clinical studies are of short duration and in a relatively small number of subjects, making it difficult to observe significant and detailed changes in bone. At the same time, the level of intake of soy protein and isoflavones varies in these studies, and the optimal dose of intake, so that there is a protective effect on bones, has not yet been determined. The clinical studies that have been so far can be distinguished into those that have determined biochemical evidence of reduced bone turnover by assessing markers of osteoblast and osteoclast activity and those that have examined changes in bone mineral density.

The overall results indicate that diets rich in phytoestrogens have a long-term protective effect on bone. The magnitude of their effect and their precise mechanisms of action are currently elusive or merely conjectural.

It has been known for a long time that women in certain peoples of the Far East, such as the Chinese and Japanese, are affected at much lower rates by certain diseases such as osteoporosis, atherosclerosis, but also by certain cancers such as breast and ovarian.

Also, it was shown in epidemiological studies that these women complain less about symptoms and disorders that appear during menopause, than women in the West. In the effort to detect the protective factors responsible for these differences, great importance was given to diet. After excluding some factors that seem to be associated with the increased incidence of stomach cancer in Japan, such as preserved foods and especially pastes (which contain particularly high levels of salt, nitrites and nitrates), soybeans, which are used in various ways, were evaluated in the preparation of Japanese and Chinese cuisine. In addition to proteins and lipids of high nutritional value, soy also contains some substances with structural similarities to estrogen [25–29].

Recent epidemiological and experimental studies report that diets rich in phytoestrogens may have a protective effect on estrogen-dependent conditions such as menopausal symptoms and estrogen-dependent diseases such as breast cancer, osteoporosis, and cardiovascular disease.

9. Breast cancer

The treatment of hot flashes in women with Ca mastitis is a particularly difficult clinical problem, which will increase over time, for two main reasons. (1) The increase in survival, (2) the increase in the number of very young affected women, in whom the vasomotor effects are more intense, with consequent impact on the quality of life. In in vitro, preclinical and clinical studies the results are highly contradictory. The purity of the phytoestrogen form increases the stimulatory estrogenic effect and reverses the effect of tamoxifen. In women with aromatase inhibitors, what is the action of phytoestrogens? In America they are not recommended to consume large amounts, as in Asia, but there is no concern about the usual diets [29–32].

A recent study showed a strong inhibitory effect on 17β-H5D1, which converts E1 to E2, 10 flavonoids, as well as intermediate products of their biosynthesis, while none had a proliferative effect on breast cancer cells They seem to protect only women who are exposed from an early age, from fetal possibly, in reproductive life studies come to conflicting conclusions, while for menopause there are also insufficient results for their potentially harmful effect. Of interest is a prospective study in Japan, which showed that Genistein, Daidzein, and soy have a positive dose-dependent relationship with the increase in hepatocellular carcinoma (HCC) in women, particularly those with hepatitis, while they had no effect in men. Since HCC occurs at higher rates in the male population, so endogenous estrogens may have a prophylactic role, the herbal study showed a different effect in the two sexes.

10. Mental functions

In in vitro and in vivo studies there is a neuroprotective effect through selective activation of EPβ. A study of young women given a 1-week diet rich in phytoestrogens showed no effect on various mental skills. Taking 160 mg/day of total isoflavones, in the form of powder in drinks, for 12 weeks significantly improved hot flashes, mood, physical condition, but did not affect lipids and cognitive functions at all. Some authors argue that they have an estrogen-like beneficial effect on memory if administered peri- or very early postmenopausal Another study showed that isoflavones by mechanisms independent of estrogen, had a beneficial effect in young women. Many aloe vera skin care products contain anthraquinones, while breast enlargement products 8-prenylnaringenin etc.

Their anti-inflammatory, immunosuppressive-immunostimulatory property also raises many questions. It has been reported to protect the skin (red clover) from the immunosuppression of UV radiation, through their antioxidant and anti-inflammatory action.

Genistein in vitro and in vivo has an antiviral effect on DNA and RNA viruses that infect humans and animals. It also acts on the host cell, and on the attachment, entry, replication of the virus, through inhibition of tyrosine kinases and topoisomerase II. Pharmacological and toxicological in vitro studies have shown apoptotic and toxic effects of some phytoestrogens in some cell systems. They suggest that it is important to pay attention to the consumption of concentrated amounts of phytoestrogens in the form of phytohormone supplements, although dose-dependent studies are needed to draw conclusions. In contrast there is no need for concern regarding the intake of phytoestrogens from a regular diet [29–34].

11. SERMS (selective estrogen receptor modulator)

Another class of drugs recommended for HPT are SERMS (selective estrogen receptor modifiers) that simultaneously display an agonistic and antagonistic effect of estrogen depending on the tissue. In particular, in bone tissue, the cardiovascular system, lipid metabolism, they have an estrogenic effect, which is different from that of 17β estradiol and tamoxifen SERMS exhibit endometrial estrogenic activity, inhibit breast estrogen receptor activity, and antagonize estrogen-dependent proliferation of MCF-7 cells in breast tumors.

In addition, they do not show mitotic activity in the breast, endometrium, are administered without progestogen in an existing uterus and have a satisfactory effect regarding the prevention of osteoporosis particularly noteworthy is the lack of influence on ovarian function and hypothalamic pituitary axis disadvantages include unsatisfactory treatment of climacteric symptoms and are therefore a treatment of choice for the prevention of osteoporosis in cases of breast cancer and in vaginal bleeding occurring in conventional therapy The mentioned phodioestrogens are components of students with a source of origin mainly soy. In cases of contraindications to HRT, it is suggested to enrich the diet with foods rich in phodioestrogens and lead to a remission of vasomotor symptoms, protection of the cardiovascular system, but they are less effective in osteoporosis and atrophy of the genitourinary system.

The SERMS category includes substances that act as estrogenic agonists or antagonists depending on the tissue. This category includes tamoxifen (anti-estrogenic effect on the massive mammary gland, estrogenic effect on the endometrium), Clomiphene used in cases of a afollicular infertility affects the pituitary gland with an anti-estrogenic effect in women of reproductive age, however, its action in the pituitary gland of postmenopausal women is estrogenic.

SERMS act selectively on estrogen receptors either as agonists or antagonists in a target gene and have beneficial effects of estrogen on target tissues avoiding negative off-target effects. According to recent data they act as agonists with estrogen receptors in bone tissue cardiovascular system competitively in the breast.

There are four SERMS formulations approved for clinical use.

The three formulations belong to the triphenylethylene family and are as follows:

Clomiphene
Tamoxifen
Toremifene

Raloxifene belongs to the benzothiphene family (second generation SERMS), it is the main representative of SERMS, it comes from a modification of the molecular structure of clomiphene citrate, tamoxifen and is a selective modifier of estrogen receptors.

The indication for raloxifene administration is in women at increased risk for breast cancer as an alternative treatment for HRT. The recommended dosage is 60–120 mg, the duration of treatment is 4 years and a reduction in vertebral and not vertebral fracture is observed. Indifferent from applications-modus: orally or vaginally [27–36].

The substances contained in these preparations act as antagonists in the female reproductive system (endometrium, breast) where α-estrogen receptors prevail and have an agonistic effect on the skeleton (β estrogen receptors), lipoprotein profile.

In particular, raloxifene has an indication for the prevention of osteoporosis due to the certified manifestation of estrogenic effects on bones, increasing bone density and anti-estrogenic effects on the breasts and the endometrium.

It acts competitively with the intake of calcium and vitamin D in the bones, it has a cardioprotective effect by inhibiting the oxidation of LDL, while a 1/10,000 thromboembolic event and slight side effects, seasickness myalgia, are reported. Raloxifene influences the pituitary gland and the release of gonadotropins in addition to its favorable effects in the prevention or treatment of osteoporosis. In experimental animal studies, raloxifene prevented the morning fall in LH levels induced by estradiol, while it did not affect the evening rise in the levels of the mentioned hormones.

The anti-estrogenic effect of raloxifene on the gonadotropic cells of the anterior pituitary gland was certified in these studies. Also, in other experimental studies the anti-estrogenic effect of raloxifene on the hypothalamus was certified. of the basal secretion of FSH and LH in postmenopausal women and exerts an agonistic or antagonistic effect on the estrogen receptors depending on the tissue.

The new selective estrogen receptor modulators include Bazedoxifene, Lasoxifene [27–36].

12. Vascular menopauseal symptoms

In 2007, results were published in which the clinical significance of *Trifolium pretense* (red clover) in improving hot flashes was questionable. In 2008 in a total of 1112 peri- and post-menopausal women, from various countries, also uncertain result, after taking Black cohosh (*Cimicifuga racemosa*), Cimicifuga or Botryoidus or Coriander. Their usefulness in cases of mild-moderate symptoms, at a relatively young age, is not in doubt. A 2009 meta-analysis on the side effects of phytoestrogens reported gastrointestinal discomfort (abdominal pain), myalgia and insomnia at significantly high levels, while there was no thrombosis, stroke, vaginal bleeding, myocardial infarctions, endometrial hyperplasia, or breast cancer.

In January 2009 the Cochrane Database of Systematic Reviews published results of 30 studies in peri- and postmenopausal women who received high doses of soy, soy extract, red clover extract (Promensil), and other phytoestrogens for at least

12 weeks. Of the 30 studies, few met the criteria for inclusion in a meta-analysis. In these, no significant reduction of vasomotor symptoms was found compared to placebo, which, however, in several studies, had a marked improvement in both hot flashes and night sweats. In the remaining, low-quality studies, they observed a small reduction in discomfort always compared to a placebo.

A Mayo Clinic pilot study was considered encouraging, in which 30 women received 40 g of ground flaxseed daily for 6 weeks, and recorded a significant reduction (>50%) in their hot flashes score. However, a longer study in terms of duration and number of women is needed for definitive conclusions. In the above study 50% experienced mild abdominal distention, 30% mild diarrhea, and 20% discontinued due to side effects.

The authors do not consider that there is sufficient evidence to recommend phytoestrogens in the treatment of menopausal symptoms. Hyperplasia of the endometrium, for administration up to 2 years was not observed, but intake of soy 150 mg daily, for 5 years caused hyperplasia. With what is known to date, long-term safety for the body as a whole has not been established [27–32].

It is clear that the variety and contradiction of the above is not only due to the small number of good quality studies (control group, duration, small participation, etc.), but also to inherent peculiarities, such as (1) new phytoestrogens are constantly being isolated, (2) nomenclature problems, (3) individual differences in their intestinal and hepatic metabolism, (4) different action depending on the endogenous estrogenic environment, (5) difference in action depending on dose, route of administration, duration of exposure, and age (from fetal to postmenopausal), (6) confusion between the substance and the food containing it, (7) the method of extraction from the plants probably affects their action and (8) genetic polymorphism.

The idea that "natural" is safe and beneficial is not accepted in every case. Phytoestrogens, in any form and concentration, are not indicated for the treatment of menopausal vasomotor symptoms, due to insufficient medically documented knowledge about their effectiveness. Bearing in mind, the potentially harmful effects on the body, during their long-term administration, the decision should be individualized, and in the case of insistence on the alternative route, it is necessary to explain their action, the recommendation for short-term use, and the same control as in classic HRT [27–36].

Phytoestrogens are a modern alternative, but derived from a long pharmaceutical tradition, for the treatment of osteoporosis and at the same time a holistic proposal for the treatment of the symptoms and problems of menopause. Phytoestrogens are substances present in food that have a modifying effect on estrogen receptors and may have partial estrogenic and anti-estrogenic effects [32, 37–42].

Multiple epidemiological data and experimental findings from in vivo animal studies support the protective effect of phytoestrogens on bone loss, in vitro experiments argue for their action on bone, specifically on the osteoclast and osteoblast, while some other data show that they improve the absorption of calcium in the intestine and thus may improve bone density [27–36].

Additionally, human clinical studies of phytoestrogens show that they may protect against bone loss seen during and after menopause and with age. In conclusion, as shown by the multiple research data of recent years, phytoestrogens may improve bone mass by acting diversely on bone metabolism, thus constituting a new alternative treatment for osteoporosis.

Phytoestrogens are substances present in food that may have an estrogenic effect. Phytoestrogens are divided into isoflavones, lignans and coumestans. Isoflavones are converted by intestinal bacteria into genistein and daidzein, while lignans are converted into enterolactone and enterodiol. A variety of foods contain sufficient amounts of the various phytoestrogens, such as soy and flaxseed products, which are particularly rich sources of isoflavones and lignans respectively.

Today, phytoestrogens seem to be a new alternative, but with deep roots in past centuries, a solution for dealing with osteoporosis as well as the symptoms and problems that accompany the loss of ovarian function, i.e. menopause. Epidemiological, experimental and clinical data support their protective role in osteoporosis.

13. Biological impacts of phytoestrogens

The potential of numerous isoflavonoids to interact with estrogenic receptors has been extensively examined. Research has revealed that coumestrol exhibits the strongest binding to estrogenic receptors among the isoflavonoids, comparable to that of 17β-estradiol, affecting both ERα and EIF receptors. Conversely, genistein, daidzein, and equol exhibit a higher inclination to bind with ECβ receptors rather than ERα receptors. Isoflavones are often present in higher concentrations in the body compared to endogenous estrogens. However, the methylation or glycosylation of isoflavones generally diminishes their chemical affinity for estrogen receptors.

Certain isoflavonoids can hinder key enzymes involved in the synthesis of estrogens and androgens, such as aromatase, 5α-hydroxylase, and 17-OH-dehydrogenase. This explains the observed decrease in the occurrence of hormone-secreting cancers like breast and prostate cancer. Moreover, additional effects of isoflavonoids have been documented, including the inhibition of tyrosine kinase synthesis, DNA topoisomerase I and II, and their antiangiogenic and antioxidant properties. Therefore, apart from their selective estrogen receptor modulator (SERMs) properties, isoflavonoids show potential in the prevention and treatment of various types of cancer, at least in experimental models.

Replacement therapy is administered to postmenopausal women to prevent menopausal symptoms, osteoporosis, and cardiovascular disease. Despite these benefits, after the WHI study, there are concerns about the development of various cancers in these women. Today, many studies are investigating the possibility of using phytoestrogens as an alternative replacement therapy. An important work by Potter et al., showed an inhibition of bone loss if the diet contains for six months 90 mg/day of isoflavonoids. The dose, however, was quite large and as noted in a study by Scambia et al., a daily dose should not exceed 50–60 mg, in order to avoid adverse effects. Furthermore, ipriflavone, which is an alternative replacement therapy for pre-existing low bone density or menopausal osteoporosis, also showed some results in osteoporosis. Iproflavone is a synthetic isoflavone derivative of daidzein that has been approved in several countries for the treatment of osteoporosis. It does not appear to act through a direct effect on estrogen receptors, so it could only be classified as a phytoestrogen in the broadest sense. However, a percentage of 10% after its intake by the body turns back into daidzein. However, a large multicenter study did not show its effectiveness and linked it to several side effects [32, 38–44].

There are enough data from the use of isoflavonoids in hot flashes during menopause, but without being able to unequivocally support their prescription. In a double-blind study, 177 menopausal women were randomized to receive either 50 mg/day of soy isoflavonoids or placebo. Women in the placebo group woke up an average of 1.89 times during the night due to night sweats and hot flashes, while women taking the soy isoflavonoids woke up 1.52 times, an improvement of 12.4%.

Also important was the reduction in the intensity of the vasomotor phenomenon, as assessed by the women. Various researchers have of course noted the logical observation that the reduction by 12.4% means that if a woman had ten episodes of hot flashes, with the drug the episodes would now be nine, an observation that underlines that statistical significance does not always go hand in hand with clinical effectiveness.

In a more recent work, 75 menopausal women with at least seven hot flashes/day were randomized to receive soy isoflavonoids or placebo for 16 weeks. The percentage of women reporting at least a 50% reduction in hot flashes was 65.8% in the isoflavonoid group and 34.2% in the placebo group, a difference that was statistically highly significant ($p < 0.005$). However, it must be emphasized that in this study as well as in others, no change was observed in other menopausal symptoms [32, 36–44].

On the other hand, in a very recent double-blind study of 72 women who were randomized to receive soy capsules or a placebo, no statistically significant difference was observed in the relief of menopausal symptoms or overall quality of life. Finally, in the recent position of the North American Menopause Society, it is noted that the studies published to date can neither support nor reject the administration of isoflavone supplements or the consumption of foods containing soy. Finally, however, for the relief of mild vasomotor symptoms, he recommends the administration of isoflavones in combination with lifestyle changes as an initial treatment before the administration of drugs [44–50].

14. Possible adverse effects

In general, both soy contained in foods and isoflavones contained in preparations are well tolerated. However, due to the relatively limited and often conflicting data from in vitro and experimental animal studies, a definitive safety assessment for isoflavonoid intake cannot be made. Moderate intake of isoflavonoids appears to be safe for the majority of people, whereas long-term consumption of soy products and isoflavone-containing formulations is currently recommended for women with a history of breast cancer [46–50].

15. Conclusions

The lifestyle and eating habits of Asian pigs are very different compared to the West, so even differences in the occurrence of diseases or menopausal disorders cannot be attributed to the consumption of soy and its products alone. Given how the doses of commercial preparations, phytoestrogens have not yet been clarified in large studies and the possible—long-term—side effects are generally unknown, one cannot unreservedly recommend their administration. However, the evidence from the often conflicting studies is generally encouraging and certainly indicates the need for further investigation. Regarding their use in menopausal symptoms, most researchers tend to agree that the use of substances such as soy phytoestrogens could be used as a first-line treatment for mild symptoms not associated with sleep or daytime activity disturbances, along with lifestyle changes.

Author details

Panagiotis Tsikouras[1*], Anna Chalkidou[1], Georgios Iatrakis[1], Efthimios Oikonomou[1], Anastasia Bothou[1], Dimitrios Kyriakou[1], Aise Chatzi Ismail Mouchterem[1], Alexios Alexiou[1], Konstantinos Nikolettos[1], Nektaria Kritsotaki[1], Theopi Nalbanti[1], Sonia Kotanidou[1], Stefanos Zervoudis[2] and Nikolaos Nikolettos[1]

1 Department of Obstetrics and Gynecology, Democritus University of Thrace, Greece

2 REA Maternity Hospital, Athens, Greece

*Address all correspondence to: tsikouraspanagiotis@gmail.com

References

[1] Sengos C, Iatrakis G, Andreakos C, Xygakis A, Papapetrou P. Hormonal reproductive status of women at menopausal transition compared to that observed in a group of midreproductive-aged women. Clinical and Experimental Obstetrics & Gynecology. 2000;**27**(1):54-56

[2] Ruth KS et al. Genetic insights into biological mechanisms governing human ovarian ageing. Nature. 2021;**596**(7872):393-397

[3] Burgess DJ. Dissecting the genetics of ovarian ageing. Nature Reviews. Genetics. 2021;**22**(10):623. DOI: 10.1038/s41576-021-00415-y

[4] Zondervan KT. Genomic analysis identifies variants that can predict the timing of menopause. Nature. 2021;**596**(7872):345-346. DOI: 10.1038/d41586-021-01710-8

[5] McGrath IM, Mortlock S, Montgomery GW. Genetic regulation of physiological reproductive lifespan and female fertility. International Journal of Molecular Sciences. 2021;**22**(5):2556. DOI: 10.3390/ijms22052556

[6] Laven JS. Genetics of early and Normal menopause. Seminars in Reproductive Medicine. 2015;**33**(6):377-383. DOI: 10.1055/s-0035-1567825. Epub 2015 Nov 16

[7] Chen H, Liu C, Li Y, Wang X, Pan X, Wang F, et al. Developmental dynamic transcriptome and systematic analysis reveal the major genes underlying isoflavone accumulation in soybean. Frontiers in Plant Science. 2023;**14**:1014349. DOI: 0.3389/fpls.2023.1014349. eCollection 2023

[8] Křížová L, Dadáková K, Kašparovská J, Kašparovský T. Isoflavones. Molecules. 2019;**24**(6):1076. DOI: 10.3390/molecules24061076

[9] Rietjens IMCM, Louisse J, Beekmann K. The potential health effects of dietary phytoestrogens. British Journal of Pharmacology. 2017;**174**(11):1263-1280. DOI: 10.1111/bph.13622. Epub 2016 Oct 20

[10] Rowe IJ, Baber RJ. The effects of phytoestrogens on postmenopausal health. Climacteric. 2021;**24**(1):57-63. DOI: 10.1080/13697137.2020.1863356. Epub 2021 Jan 4

[11] Kolátorová L, Lapčík O, Stárka L. Phytoestrogens and the intestinal microbiome. Physiological Research. 2018;**67**(Suppl 3):S401-S408. DOI: 10.33549/physiolres.934022

[12] Chen MN, Lin CC, Liu CF. Efficacy of phytoestrogens for menopausal symptoms: A meta-analysis and systematic review. Climacteric. 2015;**18**(2):260-269. DOI: 10.3109/13697137.2014.966241. Epub 2014 Dec 1

[13] Tempfer CB, Bentz EK, Leodolter S, Tscherne G, Reuss F, Cross HS. Phytoestrogens in clinical practice: A review of the literature. Fertility and Sterility. 2007;**87**(6):1243-1249. DOI: 0.1016/j.fertnstert.2007.01.120. Epub 2007 May 9

[14] Patra S, Gorai S, Pal S, Ghosh K, Pradhan S, Chakrabarti S. A review on phytoestrogens: Current status and future direction. Phytotherapy Research. 2023;**37**(7):3097-3120. DOI: 10.1002/ptr.7861. Epub 2023 May 29

[15] Basu P, Maier C. Phytoestrogens and breast cancer: In vitro anticancer activities of isoflavones, lignans, coumestans, stilbenes and their analogs and derivatives. Biomedicine & Pharmacotherapy. 2018;**107**:1648-1666. DOI: 10.1016/j.biopha.2018.08.100. Epub 2018 Sep 8

[16] Swathi Krishna S, Kuriakose BB, Lakshmi PK. Effects of phytoestrogens on reproductive organ health. Archives of Pharmacal Research. 2022;**45**(12):849-864. DOI: 10.1007/s12272-022-01417-y. Epub 2022 Nov 28

[17] Kuryłowicz A, Cąkała-Jakimowicz M, Puzianowska-Kuźnicka M. Targeting abdominal obesity and its complications with dietary phytoestrogens. Nutrients. 2020;**12**(2):582. DOI: 10.3390/nu12020582

[18] Suen AA, Kenan AC, Williams CJ. Developmental exposure to phytoestrogens found in soy: New findings and clinical implications. Biochemical Pharmacology. 2022;**195**:114848. DOI: 10.1016/j.bcp.2021.114848. Epub 2021 Nov 18

[19] Bennetau-Pelissero C. Risks and benefits of phytoestrogens: Where are we now? Current Opinion in Clinical Nutrition and Metabolic Care. 2016;**19**(6):477-483. DOI: 10.1097/MCO.0000000000000326

[20] Kim Y, Kim DW, Kim K, Choe JS, Lee HJ. Usual intake of dietary isoflavone and its major food sources in Koreans: Korea National Health and nutrition examination survey 2016-2018 data. Nutrition Research and Practice. 2022;**16**(Suppl 1):S134-S146. DOI: 10.4162/nrp.2022.16.S1.S134. Epub 2022 May 9

[21] Akinson et al. Methods for high-dimensional analysis of cells dissociated from cryopreserved synovial tissue. Arthritis Research & Therapy. 2018;**20**(1):139. DOI: 10.1186/s13075-018-1631-y

[22] Domínguez-López I, Yago-Aragón M, Salas-Huetos A, Tresserra-Rimbau A, Hurtado-Barroso S. Effects of dietary phytoestrogens on hormones throughout a human lifespan: A review. Nutrients. 2020;**12**(8):2456. DOI: 10.3390/nu12082456

[23] Zamora-Ros R, Knaze V, Luján-Barroso L, Kuhnle GG, Mulligan AA, Touillaud M, et al. Dietary intakes and food sources of phytoestrogens in the European prospective investigation into Cancer and nutrition (EPIC) 24-hour dietary recall cohort. European Journal of Clinical Nutrition. 2012;**66**(8):932-941. DOI: 10.1038/ejcn.2012.36. Epub 2012 Apr 18

[24] Sridevi V, Naveen P, Karnam VS, Reddy PR, Arifullah M. Beneficiary and adverse effects of phytoestrogens: A potential constituent of plant-based diet. Current Pharmaceutical Design. 2021;**27**(6):802-815. DOI: 10.2174/1381612826999200917154747

[25] Mohajer N, Du CY, Checkcinco C, Blumberg B. Obesogens: How they are identified and molecular mechanisms underlying their action. Frontiers in Endocrinology. 2021;**12**:780888. DOI: 10.3389/fendo.2021.780888. eCollection 2021

[26] Lethaby A, Marjoribanks J, Kronenberg F, Roberts H, Eden J, Brown J. Phytoestrogens for menopausal vasomotor symptoms. Cochrane Database of Systematic Reviews. 2013;**2013**(12):CD001395. DOI: 10.1002/14651858.CD001395.pub4

[27] Lethaby AE, Brown J, Marjoribanks J, Kronenberg F,

Roberts H, Eden J. Phytoestrogens for vasomotor menopausal symptoms. Cochrane Database of Systematic Reviews. 2007;(4):CD001395. DOI: 10.1002/14651858.CD001395.pub3

[28] Gencel VB, Benjamin MM, Bahou SN, Khalil RA. Vascular effects of phytoestrogens and alternative menopausal hormone therapy in cardiovascular disease. Mini Reviews in Medicinal Chemistry. 2012;**12**(2):149-174. DOI: 10.2174/138955712798995020

[29] Kang I, Rim CH, Yang HS, Choe JS, Kim JY, Lee M. Effect of isoflavone supplementation on menopausal symptoms: A systematic review and meta-analysis of randomized controlled trials. Nutrition Research and Practice. 2022;**16**(Suppl 1):S147-S159. DOI: 10.4162/nrp.2022.16.S1.S147. Epub 2022 May 4

[30] Yang SE, Lien JC, Tsai CW, Wu CR. Therapeutic potential and mechanisms of novel simple O-substituted isoflavones against cerebral ischemia reperfusion. International Journal of Molecular Sciences. 2022;**23**(18):10394. DOI: 10.3390/ijms231810394

[31] Mense SM, Hei TK, Ganju RK, Bhat HK. Phytoestrogens and breast cancer prevention: Possible mechanisms of action. Environmental Health Perspectives. 2008;**116**(4):426-433. DOI: 10.1289/ehp.10538

[32] Jayusman PA, Nasruddin NS, Baharin B, Ibrahim N, Ahmad Hairi H, Shuid AN. Overview on postmenopausal osteoporosis and periodontitis: The therapeutic potential of phytoestrogens against alveolar bone loss. Frontiers in Pharmacology. 2023;**14**:1120457. DOI: 10.3389/fphar.2023.1120457. eCollection 2023

[33] Zervoudis S, Iatrakis G, Peitsidis P, Tsikouras P, Galazios G, Liberis V, et al. Tibolone vaginal versus per os administration in the management of post-menopausal symptoms. Revista Medico-Chirurgicală a Societăţii de Medici şi Naturalişti din Iaşi. 2009;**113**(2):471-477

[34] Potter B, Schrager S, Dalby J, Torell E, Hampton A. Menopause. Primary Care. 2018;**45**(4):625-641. DOI: 10.1016/j.pop.2018.08.001. Epub 2018 Oct 5

[35] Liu Z, Chen B, Li B, Wang C, Li G, Cao W, et al. Greater consumption of total and individual lignans and dietary fibers were significantly associated with lowered risk of hip fracture-a 1:1 matched case-control study among Chinese elderly men and women. Nutrients. 2022;**14**(5):1100. DOI: 10.3390/nu14051100

[36] Lephart ED, Naftolin F. Factors influencing skin aging and the important role of estrogens and selective estrogen receptor modulators (SERMs). Clinical, Cosmetic and Investigational Dermatology. 2022;**15**:1695-1709. DOI: 10.2147/CCID.S333663. eCollection 2022

[37] Gómez-Zorita S, González-Arceo M, Fernández-Quintela A, Eseberri I, Trepiana J, Portillo MP. Scientific evidence supporting the beneficial effects of isoflavones on human health. Nutrients. 2020;**12**(12):3853. DOI: 10.3390/nu12123853

[38] Słupski W, Jawień P. Nowak B botanicals in postmenopausal osteoporosis. Nutrients. 2021;**13**(5):1609. DOI: 10.3390/nu13051609

[39] Lephart ED, Naftolin F. Menopause and the skin: Old favorites and new innovations in cosmeceuticals for estrogen-deficient skin. Dermatology and Therapy. 2021;**11**(1):53-69.

DOI: 10.1007/s13555-020-00468-7. Epub 2020 Nov 26

[40] Shi K, Liu X, Pan X, Liu J, Gong W, Pan G, et al. Unveiling the complexity of red clover (*Trifolium pratense* L.) transcriptome and transcriptional regulation of isoflavonoid biosynthesis using integrated long- and short-read RNAseq. International Journal of Molecular Sciences. 2021;**22**(23):12625. DOI: 10.3390/ijms222312625

[41] Błaszczuk A, Barańska A, Kanadys W, Malm M, Jach ME, Religioni U, et al. Role of phytoestrogen-rich bioactive substances (*Linum usitatissimum* L., *Glycine max* L., *Trifolium pratense* L.) in cardiovascular disease prevention in postmenopausal women: A systematic review and Meta-analysis. Nutrients. 2022;**14**(12):2467. DOI: 10.3390/nu14122467

[42] Wickham KA, Nørregaard LB, Oxfeldt M, Cheung SS, Gliemann L, Hansen M, et al. Short-term supplementation with fermented red clover extract reduces vascular inflammation in early post-menopausal women. Frontiers in Cardiovascular Medicine. 2022;**9**:826959. DOI: 10.3389/fcvm.2022.826959. eCollection 2022

[43] DePree B, Houghton K, DiBenedetti DB, Shiozawa A, King DD, Kim J, et al. Practice patterns and perspectives regarding treatment for symptoms of menopause: Qualitative interviews with US health care providers. Menopause. 2023;**30**(2):128-135. DOI: 10.1097/GME.0000000000002096. Epub 2022 Nov 20

[44] Ţiţ DM, Pallag A, Iovan C, Furău G, Furău C, Bungău S. Somatic-vegetative symptoms evolution in postmenopausal women treated with phytoestrogens and hormone replacement therapy. Iranian Journal of Public Health. 2017;**46**(11):1528-1534

[45] Barańska A, Kanadys W, Bogdan M, Stępień E, Barczyński B, Kłak A, et al. The role of soy isoflavones in the prevention of bone loss in postmenopausal women: A systematic review with meta-analysis of randomized controlled trials. Journal of Clinical Medicine. 2022;**11**(16):4676. DOI: 10.3390/jcm11164676

[46] Schmidt PJ, Wei S-M, Martinez PE, Ben Dor RR, Guerrieri GM, Palladino PP, et al. Randomized Controlled Trial The short-term effects of estradiol, raloxifene, and a phytoestrogen in women with perimenopausal depression. Menopause. 2021;**28**(4):369-383. DOI: 10.1097/GME.0000000000001724

[47] Aljumah R, Phillips S, Harper JC. Affiliations an online survey of postmenopausal women to determine their attitudes and knowledge of the menopause post. Reproductive Health. 2023;**29**(2):67-84. DOI: 10.1177/20533691231166543. Epub 2023 Mar 29

[48] Fait T. Menopause hormone therapy: Latest developments and clinical practice. Drugs Context. 2019;**8**:212551. DOI: 10.7573/dic.212551. eCollection 2019

[49] Glisic M, Kastrati N, Musa J, Milic J, Asllanaj E, Fernandez EP, et al. Phytoestrogen supplementation and body composition in postmenopausal women: A systematic review and meta-analysis of randomized controlled trials. Maturitas. 2018;**115**:74-83. DOI: 0.1016/j.maturitas.2018.06.012. Epub 2018 Jun 22

[50] Canivenc-Lavier M-C, Bennetau-Pelissero C. Phytoestrogens and health effects. Nutrients. 2023;**15**(2):317. DOI: 10.3390/nu15020317

Chapter 6

Role of Hormones over the Lifespan: How Hormone Balance Affects General Health and Well-Being at All Ages

Erika Schwartz and Jill Ketner Villa

Abstract

Hormones define who we are. From puberty to late post-menopause, the changes in our sex hormones affect every other hormone in our body. This article will explore the state of the science and the clinical application of hormone therapies at various ages and during various periods of female lifespan. Literature review of hormone therapies, state of the science compared to clinical practice in areas of hormone therapies, the role of class effects, the public and medical training understanding of the role of hormone therapies, and the future possibilities for education and research in the areas related to hormone therapies. Clinical correlation and relationship between scientific data published in PubMed and Google Scholar and public and practitioner understanding of hormone therapies.

Keywords: menopause, perimenopause, pre-menopause, postmenopause, puberty, lifespan, health, fertility, infertility, class effect, HRT, bHRT, bioidentical hormones, human identical hormones, pregnancy, postpartum, prevention, healthspan, women

1. Introduction

As early as 1889, the Merck manual listed "Ovariin" an oral powder derived from dried cow's ovaries, as a treatment for "climacteric, "the term used for menopause at the time. The use of hormone therapies for treatment of symptoms of menopause is not new to our generation, and research and scientific data abound in the past 30 years of PubMed, SCOPUS, or Google Scholar. However, if one went to medical school and post-graduate training in the past 50 years, one would think hormone therapies are recent developments and the research and confusion surrounding them started as recently as the year 2002 in the wake of the failure of the Women's Health Initiative.

Although we are still mired in confusion surrounding gonadal hormones the data is available to try to put some clarity into the situation. The use of nomenclature, presence or absence of class effect, various roles hormones play, use and symptoms associated with hormone changes at various ages and the safety of their usage need clarification in order to achieve our goal of accomplishing a thorough understanding leading to appropriate use of hormones in prevention and enhanced lifespan.

The confusion is primarily due to semantics and politics affecting the practice of medicine. Medical education is lacking in the area of training on female hormones. The confusion must be eliminated as much as possible so providers can have effective and safe information and training to take care of patients and focus on improving the patient's quality of life. There is dire need to provide education on the role of hormones in health and longevity, conduct more clinical and comparative studies and provide answers to questions that focus on the long term clinical application of the use of hormones and share the information we have on larger scale.

In this chapter, we will attempt to provide a scientifically sound, clinically based and research supported perspective on gonadal hormones, their roles in females at various phases and stages of their life based on the most up-to-date scientific data from Google Scholar, PubMed and Cochrane review.

2. Types of hormones and interactions

Modern science's transformative impact in the area of gonadal hormones was heralded in 1922 with Allen and Doisy's identification of the ovarian cycle and the discovery of estrogen. By 1936, pharmaceutical companies like Schering and Richter were already developing oral contraceptives (BC pills) and synthetic hormone replacement therapies (sHRT). Over the following 15 years pharmaceutical advances led to wider patient accessibility and increasing use of hormone-related interventions, such as BC pills for ovulation suppression, pregnancy prevention and conjugated equine estrogen (CEE) to alleviate menopausal symptoms (Premarin™). As synthetic (non-human identical) hormones were developed bio-identical hormones (molecularly identical to human hormones) were also manufactured. The process of manufacturing hormones is all synthetic regardless of what raw materials are used (plant based or laboratory developed). The molecular formulas vary. From the outset, as more HRT and contraceptive drugs were developed and came to the market, the distinction between their actions at the molecular level was lost. They were all regarded as one class of drugs. Although their actions may have varied, they became viewed as one, that is, estrogens and progestogens. This situation lead to the erroneous assumption that all estrogens and progestogens have the same effect.

The introduction of the BC pill (must be synthetic in order to suppress ovulation) and sHRT (sourced inexpensively for reasons of cost and availability) initially held promise. To this day BC pills work well to prevent ovulation and pregnancy and Premarin helps reduce vasomotor symptoms (VMS) of menopause. However, in time and as a consequence of numerous small studies undesirable side-effects appeared leading to a constant search for better pharmaceutical options and more research and development.

It's important to note that the impact and interactions of hormones vary in women at all ages and phases of their life. The complex interplay of gonadal hormones and their intricate and crucial roles shape human development, metabolic processes, fertility and overall health.

3. Hormones in puberty and adolescence

The onset of puberty, marked by the increase production and release of gonadal hormones, triggers sexual expression leading to maturation and gender differentiation. This hormonal upsurge typically occurring between ages 9–16 in girls, manifests physically with the development of secondary sexual characteristics. Hormonal stimulation at puberty alters specific glandular activity leading to adult body odor, pubic and axillary hair. The onset of menstruation occurs as the maturation of the reproductive system and the cyclic release of estrogen and progesterone are established. Fluctuating hormone levels also affect psychological development. Hormone changes may lead to anxiety, identity issues, mood swings, insomnia, weight gain, brain fog, even depression during puberty. Increased sebum production induced by hormonal changes, coupled with skin cell buildup may lead to acne. The hormonal shifts during puberty represent the transition from childhood to adolescence to adulthood manifested in many physical and mental changes also including hair growth and distribution, mood swings and phenotypical changes [1].

The gonadal hormones; estrogen (E1, E2, and E3), progesterone, and testosterone, play a critical role in their interaction with other hormones like insulin, thyroid, and adrenal hormones. This indelible connection between all hormones becomes clearly noticeable and continues for the rest of the woman's life although it's often overlooked during clinical patient evaluation.

With the emergence of a rhythmic hormonal journey estradiol, progesterone, and testosterone lead to regular or irregular cycles, amenorrhea, or pregnancy. The master regulator of the actions and interactions between gonadal hormones and other hormones and metabolic processes is the HPA (hypothalamo-pituitary-adrenal axis). The final product is an adult woman with gonadal hormones taking their position in the cascade of all bodily functions through bi-directional messaging up and down the HPA.

The fluctuations of gonadal hormones determine fertility, libido, moods among other metabolic processes. As a female's menstruation may become more regular in her twenties, a monthly cycle of preparing for pregnancy occurs, guided by the rise and fall of estradiol, progesterone, and testosterone.

4. Hormones in pregnancy

A complex interplay of hormones during pregnancy orchestrates massive physiologic changes to support fetal development. They include to our present knowledge human chorionic gonadotropin (b-hCG), estrogen (estradiol and estriol), progesterone, and prolactin. The placenta produces Beta-hCG and maintains the corpus luteum, which in turn continues producing progesterone to sustain and enhance the uterine lining. Estriol, the estrogen of pregnancy is produced by the placenta rising gradually, contributing to increasing uterine size, blood flow, and mammary gland development while prolactin prepares the breasts for lactation. The fine interplay between all these hormones lead to the growth of the fetus during the 40 weeks of gestation and the changes in the maternal body to accommodate the fetus and its growth.

In Vitro Fertilization (IVF), via hormonal manipulation, egg maturation and reproductive cycle control is induced with a combination of pharmaceutical and human identical hormones (bHRT). Follicle-stimulating hormone (FSH) and luteinizing hormone (LH) (both pharmaceutically manufactured yet human identical (bioidentical) in their molecular structures are administered to induce ovulation, while progesterone maintains the uterine lining ready for implantation. IVF therapy offers significant benefits (the promise of pregnancy and delivery of a viable fetus to women who are having difficulty conceiving naturally), but also presents risks. Risks include multiple pregnancies, which may lead to preterm birth and low fetal weight, ovarian hyperstimulation syndrome, potentially causing serious health issues and/or early menopause. Ethical concerns about surplus embryos and the emotional toll of failed cycles significantly impact individuals and affect relationships of couples undergoing IVF. Lastly, some research raises possibilities of increased risk of hormone sensitive cancers such as ovarian and breast and premature ovarian failure in women who undergo multiple IVF cycles [2].

5. Post partum period

Postpartum, hormone levels undergo rapid changes. Estrogen and progesterone levels drop precipitously as the placenta is expelled, triggering prolactin release and milk production. Oxytocin stimulates uterine contractions to shrink the uterus to pre pregnancy size, create the emotional bond between the mother and baby and commence the milk letdown reflex. Additionally, cortisol and thyroid hormones collaborate with gonadal hormones impacting energy levels, sleep, mood and metabolism. It takes time for hormones to return to pre-pregnancy levels, and this transition varies among individual women. The hormonal shift may contribute to mood changes and may lead to from elation and total attachment to newborn to postpartum blues and depression. An infinite number of factors influence the postpartum experience for women—vaginal simple, complicated versus Caesarian delivery, complications during gestation or birth, social and psychological support systems and often unaddressed yet highly important environmental factors.

Problems that can arise during the postpartum period include postpartum hemorrhage, infection, perineal pain or tears, breastfeeding difficulties, vaginal dryness and loss of libido. There is a glaring absence of research and provider training during this critical period or a woman's life. Once the baby is delivered and is healthy, the woman has very few medical resources to provide educational and emotional support during this life altering transition. It is crucial to address and create individualized postpartum care plans to appropriately provide help for the diverse needs of the individual woman. There is little data or research at this point in this area but the need is dire and it's no longer acceptable to discharge a woman by ob-gyn with 6 week follow up and be told she can have sex.

6. Hormones in thirties and forties; pre and perimenopause

During the late thirties and forties, hormone levels may start to change leading to irregular menses, ineffective and infrequent ovulation. While menstrual cycles continue, the hormone levels are not the same as in the 20s and 30s and the impact on the female body starts to reflect these changes. Waiting until menopause to address hormone balance misses an entire decade of life. Being mindful of these changes and addressing them correctly makes a big difference in long term outcome.

The pre and perimenopausal periods can start as early as 30s and 40s. Although fertility may still continue to varying degrees, changes in frequency of menstrual cycles, brain fog, anxiety, vaginal dryness, weight gain, insomnia, thinning hair and decreased libido are signs of the change in hormones long before the onset of menopause. As a woman gets into her later 40s and early 50s menses become more irregular and symptoms like, hot flashes, night sweats, insomnia arise and directly affect the woman's physical and emotional wellbeing. These may occur long before reaching the formal definition of menopause which is 1 year without a menstrual cycle yet symptomatically may be decades of discomfort and downward spiral in general health. Estradiol, progesterone, testosterone, thyroid and adrenal supplementation administered correctly in the right preparations treating the women's symptoms with the support of biomarkers like bloods, body composition and physical examination may increase quality of life and even help women feel well enough to lead their lives unaffected by the symptoms of hormone imbalance which herald the onset of diseases of aging.

7. Hormones in menopause

The conventional medical definition is the cessation of menstruation for 12 months or more. Most commonly this occurs in the late 40s, early 50s. However, since as described above it is the hormone imbalance and the symptoms that occur that truly define the moment in time when women need help in terms of HRT the providers need a clearer understanding of what happens physiologically to the female body in this time period and be alert to these changes and treat accordingly.

7.1 Menopause symptoms

As hormones change during the decade prior to menopause a variety of physiologic and clinically significant changes start to unfold. Fluctuating mood likely due to the complex interactions between hormones, the HPA axis, insulin, cortisol and neurotransmitters may affect these shifts. Night sweats and hot flashes, triggered by thermoregulatory changes within the central nervous system, underscore the hypothalamic involvement in temperature control and symptomatic outcomes leading to poor sleep and metabolic instability.

Rapid spikes and troughs in hormone levels manifest as insomnia, disrupted sleep-awake cycles, possibly mediated by neuroendocrine mechanisms leading to poor quality of sleep and the side-effects thereof. Weight gain may also occur due to rapid shifts in estrogen and progesterone and HPA axis interactions leading to metabolic alterations, insulin resistance, metabolic syndrome and changes in appetite and dysregulated ghrelin and leptin release. Increased frequency of urination may also be directly connected to hormone changes.

Cessation of menses, the "hallmark definition of menopause," reflects decreasing hormone production along with age and environmental factors. Painful intercourse, loss of libido often associated with vaginal dryness and atrophy also result from untreated hormonal depletion. Decrease in bone density follows decrease in estrogen levels emphasizing the importance of hormonal influence on skeletal health.

Within 10 years after menopause the risk of CV disease increases dramatically and rapidly becomes higher than in men [3, 4]. Women who are not treated with hormone therapies represent the higher end of risk for CV disease with age. At the same time, diabetes, metabolic syndrome, arthritis, hypertension and other diseases of aging start to appear.

In essence, menopause depicts myriad physiologic responses and symptomatic expressions, each intimately tied to hormonal fluctuations their eventual disappearance and its effect on all body systems. Age is the primary cause of increase risk and onset of disease but it is the lack of hormones that indelibly and invariably connects age to disease.

7.2 Menopause treatments

Sadly, menopause represents the worst season of a woman's life but does not have to be. Physically and mentally most women who do not have access to proper HRT suffer ever increasing problems leading to chronic disease of aging [5].

The abrupt halt and the medical and media frenzy that followed the Women's Health Initiative (WHI) study in 2002 essentially eliminated the HRT option for menopausal women and left in its wake millions of women suffering. The only conventional options offered at the time were antidepressants and wearing layered clothing and staying in dark cool rooms. Faced with such limited possibilities, many women turned to bioidentical-human-identical hormone therapies (bHRT) considered novel and alternative due to their intense marketing. The truth is they were pharmaceutically manufactured to mimic the exact molecular structure of estradiol and progesterone and were not novel nor alternative.

Starting in the mid 1950s to the early 2000 the most common form of hormone therapy for menopause was conjugated equine estrogen (CEE) and BC pills (initially more popular in Europe).

In 2022 *Fact or Fiction: The Role of Regulated Body-Identical Hormone Therapy for Menopausal Women*, more than 40 clinical studies that demonstrated a 30–50% reduction in cardiovascular disease (CV) and all-cause mortality among women using HRT [6]. These findings and others led to a resurgence in use of HRT even though no new large scale studies have been undertaken since the early 2000s and there have been very few studies comparing actions of various types of gonadal hormones.

]The WHI was started in the early 1990s and although a large (double blind placebo controlled) DBPC governmentally sponsored study, did not compare sHRT to bHRT and looked at a population of women more than 10 years after menopause with other pre-existing conditions [7].

The WHI study was stopped abruptly after 5.8 years in 2002 due to unacceptable side effects. Although the data proved erroneous upon deeper review, doctors, medical societies and women stopped using HRT abruptly and suffered terrible consequences. These consequences were return of symptoms: hot flashes, night sweats, insomnia, weight gain, irritability, loss of libido, as well as depression, decreased cognitive function and loss of ability to perform at work and at home at premenopausal levels.

Given that the data of the WHI study was limited to sHRT an ever increasing number of women turned to bHRT for a safer alternative to manage their symptoms. bHRT is usually manufactured from plant extracts such as soy and yams oils and have the same molecular structure as human sex hormones. They are pharmaceutically produced and thus synthetic. Only their molecular formula is identical to the molecular formula of human hormones.

Both regulated (US FDA-approved) and compounded (not FDA approved, but using the same raw materials) bHRT therapies are widely available in the United States.

Aversion to compounded bHRT is partly due to concerns that these products lack standards and evidence of purity, have not been rigorously tested, and may not be safe for women. However, to date there is no scientific evidence to support the claims of lack of safety. The most recent article on lack of reliability of bHRT comes from 2004 [8].

In contrast, FDA approved bHRT products such as 17-beta-estradiol and micronized progesterone are standardized and the active hormones are the same as the compounded ones. Since the WHI study, researchers and principle investigators have re-evaluated the results of the study reaching the conclusion it was flawed and did not truly reflect the situation in most women. In 2013, the final data was published in the BMJ by the principle investigators of the WHI study finding that all cause mortality in women on sHRT used in the study was lower than that of women on placebo [9].

Since the early 1990s many studies, some large scale have been conducted on the benefits and risks of HRT. In many of the studies, although never clearly stated there were arms that used bHRT which consistently seemed to produce better effects. These studies included the Danish Study, PEPI, and KEEPS trials. The arms of these studies that used bHRT with 17-beta-estradiol and micronized progesterone safely and effectively managed menopausal symptoms while minimizing endometrial hypertrophy, lowering risk of VTE and CV disease (improved HDL, decreased LDL) and improving insulin sensitivity [6]. Very few conventional studies on compounded hormones exist to date and most of them are limited and with low traction.

8. Class effect

The controversy between various formulations of HRT boils down to a lack of understanding of the concept of "class effect". By class effect we refer to similar outcomes, both therapeutic and adverse from various medications categorized together as "one class" for whatever reasons chosen by pharmacologists or other scientific group [10].

In the 1930s when pharma developed hormones in the form of BC pills and CEE they were all assigned to the umbrella class of estrogen and progestogen. The assumption was made that all these variety of molecules they acted the same in the woman's body. As more drugs came to market and studies were conducted, the concept of class effect swallowed up all gonadal hormones. In time, less differentiation between the effects of various hormones was made. Results of the studies that found risks like increased blood clotting, increased incidence of cancer, risk of dementia, etc. did not make any distinction between the hormone molecules involved in the studies.

When the WHI found increased risk of CV events all HRT were blamed. Apart from the fact that the study was poorly designed and the results proved incorrect, the issue of "class effect" was never addressed adding to the confusion. It was determined that all estrogens and progestogens used in menopausal women carried unacceptable risk and hence their usage was discontinued although they were not removed from the market. Their labels on the FDA approved products had to carry a black box warning albeit the WHI only studied CEE and medroxy-progesterone acetate. The human identical molecular formula estrogen- 17- beta estradiol and progesterone were lumped into this class effect melee and carried the stigma of the failed study albeit no study proven they had any negative effects. Sadly, this served to hurt millions of women since data on all studies that included the human identical formulations of estradiol and progesterone consistently demonstrated significantly lower risk profile for these drugs [7].

In 2011 at the International Menopause Society annual meeting in Rome, Italy, the issue of "class effect" came up for the first time in a global forum and scientists and researchers from around the globe agreed that neither estrogen nor progesterone were subject to class effect. The studies and clinical data proved that beyond a reasonable doubt there was no class effect in the area of HRT [11].

However, this significant information was not accepted or addressed in the US and still is not in medical training. The result has been more confusion, less education and initially, after the WHI study fiasco, the marketing of the compounded form of bHRT touted to be something new and different. That is not correct. bHRT has been around since the 1890s and the FDA approval of bHRT preparations that followed the WHI study only serves to confirm the low risk associated with bHRT.

The black box warning on FDA approved estrogens and progestogens serve to further confuse and separate from compounded bHRT.

As we continue to untangle the issue of bHRT vs. sHRT, once we understand and are no longer burdened by the class effect dilemma it becomes easier to address the use of hormone preparations at all ages and in various situations for various conditions. It is also easier to separate compounded vs. FDA approved HRT and focus on what works best for the individual patient.

9. Formulation, dosing routes, administration and safety of hormone usage

The FDA has approved all HRT for four specific uses:

1. Alleviating moderate to severe VMS

2. Safeguarding against postmenopausal osteoporosis

3. Addressing hypoestrogenism due to hypogonadism, bilateral oophorectomy, or premature ovarian insufficiency

4. Managing moderate to severe vulvovaginal symptoms.

In instances where FDA indications for systemic estrogen therapy are absent, FDA guidance recommends employing low-dose topical vaginal estrogen therapy as a solution for treating genitourinary symptoms linked to menopause.

Various synthetic estrogen formulations are available: CEE, conjugated estrogens, ethinyl estradiol. Conjugated equine estrogens, notably used in the WHI, are derived from pregnant horse urine including more than 300 estrogen like estrone sulfate, equilin sulfate, and estradiol sulfate. In postmenopaual women, estrone sulfate acts as an estrogen precursor converted into estrone (E3) and estradiol (E3) 17β-estradiol is molecularly identical to human estradiol.

Birth control pills contain many variations of sHRT because the goal is to suppress ovulation and with bHRT that cannot happen. Ethinyl estradiol, a synthetic estrogen, is primarily partnered with a progestin in hormone contraceptives.

When exogenous estrogen is used in women with a uterus, progestogens (including synthetic progestins as well as micronized progesterone) are given together continuously or in cyclical fashion. Progestogens include MPA, norethindrone acetate (NETA), norethisterone and micronized progesterone. While medroxyprogesterone acetate, levonorgestrel, and NETA are synthetic progestins, micronized progesterone is molecularly identical to progesterone produced by the corpus luteum. The rationale for progestogen usage originates from a 1975 article connecting use of unopposed synthetic estrogen to increased incidence of endometrial hyperplasia and potential risk of endometrial cancer [12].

Different progestogen types and dosages, administration routes, and regimen protocols (sequential or continuous-combined) may have distinct implications for health outcomes. Patient preference, a vital factor, must be taken into account, given that some women prefer regimens that avoid periodic menstrual bleeding.

A primary adverse outcome linked to synthetic progestins is the risk of breast cancer. Synthetic variants have the potential to stimulate and escalate the division of estrogen-related breast cells, essentially promoting the proliferation and spread of tumor cells. This unregulated cell division is considered as the genesis of cancer. Moreover, sHRT has been observed to metabolize estrogens in the body into more aggressive forms (such as 16-hydroxyestrone). These may be potentially harmful iterations of estrogen triggering the formation of cancer.

In contrast, bioidentical progesterone has demonstrated an opposing effect compared to its synthetic counterparts. Hormones that are bioidentical, like progesterone, obstruct the division of breast cells and have been associated with inhibiting breast cancer development (by interacting with kinase inhibitors). Naturally sourced progesterone has been described as having a safeguarding function within the female body by impeding the formation of breast cancer, whereas synthetic progestogens may actually encourage the onset of breast cancer. Bioidentical hormones may offer a safer, long-term alternative to the contentious synthetic alternatives [13].

10. FDA approved synthetic estrogen replacement therapy

ORAL
CEE
Conjugated Estrogen
Esterified Estrogens (Amnestrogen, Estratab, Evex, Femogen, Menest)
Estradiol Acetate (Femtrace)
Conjugated Estrogens (Cenestin, Enjuvia)
PATCHES
Alora, Climara, Esclim, Estraderm, Fempatch, Menostar
Emulsions
Estradiol hemihydrate (Estrasorb)
GELS
CEE (Premarin) –
Estradiol Acetate (Femring)
INTRAMUSCULAR INJECTION
CEE
Estradiol Cypionate (Depo-Estradiol, Estradiol Cypionate)
Estradiol Valerate (Delestrogen, Estradiol Valerate)

11. FDA approved estrogen human identical (bioidentical)

Estradiol - Minivelle, Vivelle, Vivelle-Dot)
GELS
Estradiol (Divigel, Elestrin, Estrogel)

SPRAYS
Estradiol (Evamist)
Estradiol (Vagifem)
CREAMS
Estradiol (Estrace)
Estradiol (Imvexxy)
RINGS
Estradiol (Estring)
Polyestradiol Phosphate (Estradurin) previously available in the U.S. but was discontinued

12. FDA approved synthetic estrogen and progestogen combinations

Conjugated Estrogens and Medroxyprogesterone Acetate (Premphase (Premarin, Cycrin 14/14)
Premphase 14/14, Prempro, Prempro (Premarin, Cycrin), Prempro/Premphase)
Estradiol and Drospirenone (Angeliq)
Estradiol and Norethisterone Acetate (Activella, Amabelz)
Ethinylestradiol and Norethisterone Acetate (FemHRT)
Estradiol and Levonorgestrel patch (Climara Pro)
Estradiol and Norethisterone Acetate (Combipatch)
Medroxyprogesterone acetate (Provera)
Norethindrone
Hydroxyprogesterone
Levonorgestrel (Mirena, Skyla, Kyleena)
Drospirenone (Slynd)

13. FDA approved progesterone human identical (bioidentical)

Micronized progesterone capsules or creams
Prometrium (oral micronized progesterone)
Utrogestan

14. Diseases of aging and the role of hormones

Hormones serve as signaling molecules that orchestrate physiologic responses, and their decline and eventual disappearance during the aging process brings closer the onset and progression of age-related diseases.

The aging process is characterized by alterations in endocrine function, resulting in permanent hormone decrease and disappearance. Such changes impact metabolic pathways, immune responses, inflammatory changes and tissue integrity, leading to lowered defenses against diseases, the hallmark of age. Reduction in estrogen, progesterone and testosterone contribute to bone loss and increased vulnerability to osteopenia and osteoporosis.

Age-related changes in hormone signaling pathways appear as chronic conditions such as cardiovascular disease, diabetes, cognitive dissonance and neurodegenerative disorders. Insulin resistance, a hallmark of type 2 diabetes, is linked to impaired insulin signaling and function, which may arise in conjunction with alterations in hormone receptor interactions and downstream signaling cascades [14, 15]. Dysregulated hormone levels, such as cortisol in response to chronic stress, play a role in immune system dysfunction and inflammatory responses, fostering an environment conducive to age-related diseases.

The intricate interplay between hormones and aging involves biochemical interactions that impact many physiologic processes. Understanding these relationships is crucial for elucidating and even preventing the mechanisms of age-related diseases and developing targeted interventions to mitigate their impact on age while using hormones in prevention.

15. NAMS and future research

The 2022 North American Menopause Society (NAMS) -Hormone Therapy Position Statement summarizes the most recent recommendations for hormone therapy. It emphasizes the balance of risks and benefits, along with guidance for managing menopause symptoms. NAMS position states that hormone therapy is most effective for addressing VMS, genitourinary syndrome, bone loss, and fractures. The statement underscores the importance of individualized care and shared decision-making in treatment. Patients should be regularly assessed for risk-to-benefit ratios, with appropriate doses, duration, and administration routes tailored to manage symptoms and treatment goals. No definitive time limits or type of hormone therapies are recommended.

The most recent Position Statement offers specific recommendations for clinicians, including the impact of hormone therapy on type 2 diabetes, considerations for longer-duration therapy, and the safe use of low-dose vaginal estrogen therapy for select cancer survivors. It also addresses non-estrogen alternatives for dyspareunia, the influence of age and time since menopause on risk stratification, and the nuanced breast cancer risk associated with different hormone therapies.

Evaluating benefits and risks is crucial, with NAMS highlighting that for most healthy symptomatic women under 60 within 10 years of onset of menopause, "the benefits of hormone therapy outweigh the risks and should be the first line of treatment". The Position Statement extends to female patients with ovarian insufficiency and early menopause, suggesting hormone therapy until the mean age of menopause if appropriate.

In essence, the 2022 NAMS Hormone Therapy Position Statement serves as a dynamic tool guiding both clinicians and patients through informed decision-making and individualized care. While based on current evidence, treatment approaches must consider individualized risk-to-benefit ratios to ensure the best possible care [16].

16. Summary

At all life stage, hormones orchestrate intricate processes, influencing reproduction, metabolic functions, and overall health. Always remembering the omnipresence and ubiquitous role of hormones is crucial for maintaining well-being during every phase of life. While diet, exercise, sleep, stress management, supplements and conventional medical care have integral roles in maintaining health, the lack of hormones balance make prevention and delay of diseases of aging impossible to achieve. Hormone replacement therapy is the torchbearer, managing symptoms and signaling the dawn of a new phase, where hormones and time build a story of evolution--of the female spirit's indomitable journey. For a healthier and more optimal life, it is crucial to have access to honest, research driven and informative education about hormones.

Author details

Erika Schwartz* and Jill Ketner Villa
Evolved Science, LLC, NY, USA

*Address all correspondence to: drerika@eshealth.com

References

[1] Chen M et al. Characteristics of referrals for gender dysphoria over a 13-year period. Journal of Adolescent Health. 2016;**58**(3):369-371. DOI: 10.1016/j.jadohealth.2015.11.010

[2] Li J, Shen J, Zhang X, Peng Y, Zhang Q, Hu L, et al. Risk factors associated with preterm birth after IVF/ICSI. Scientific Reports. 2022;**12**(1):7944. DOI: 10.1038/s41598-022-12149-w

[3] Prabakaran S, Schwartz A, Lundberg G. Cardiovascular risk in menopausal women and our evolving understanding of menopausal hormone therapy: Risks, benefits, and current guidelines for use. Therapeutic Advances in Endocrinology and Metabolism. 2021;**12**:3-6. DOI: 10.1177/20420188211013917

[4] Rodgers JL, Jones J, Bolleddu SI, Vanthenapalli S, Rodgers LE, Shah K, et al. Cardiovascular risks associated with gender and aging. Journal of Cardiovascular Development and Disease. 2019;**6**(2):19. DOI: 10.3390/jcdd6020019

[5] Boardman HMP et al. Hormone therapy for preventing cardiovascular disease in post-menopausal women. Cochrane Database of Systematic Reviews. 2015;**2015**:CD002229

[6] Miller VM, Naftolin F, Asthana S, Black DM, Brinton EA, Budoff MJ, et al. The Kronos early estrogen prevention study (KEEPS): What have we learned? Menopause. 2019;**26**(9):1071-1084. DOI: 10.1097/GME.0000000000001326

[7] Donnelly L, Balneaves LG. Fact or fiction? The role of regulated body-identical hormone therapy for menopausal women. Nursing for Women's Health. 2022;**26**(2):143-151

[8] Boothby LA, Doering PL, Kipersztok S. Bioidentical hormone therapy: A review. Menopause. 2004;**11**(3):356-367. DOI: 10.1097/01.gme.0000094356.92081.ef

[9] Wild Robert A, Chunyuan W, Curb JD, Lisa M, Lawrence P, Marcia S, et al. Coronary heart disease events in the women's health initiative hormone trials: Effect modification by metabolic syndrome. Menopause: The Journal of The North American Menopause Society. 2013;**20**(3):254-260

[10] Woolner D, Holford N. Class Effects and the Rational Comparison of Drugs. Department of Pharmacology & Clinical Pharmacology, University of Auckland. 27 June 2013. Available from: https://clinpharmacol.fmhs.auckland.ac.nz/docs/class-effectsarticle.pdf

[11] Singh M, Shah D. Thirteenth world congress on menopause, Rome, 8-11 June, 2011. Journal of Mid-life Health. 2011;**2**(1):45-46. DOI: 10.4103/0976-7800.83276

[12] Ziel H, Finkle W. Increased risk of endometrial carcinoma among users of conjugated estrogens. The New England Journal of Medicine. 1975;**293**:1167-1170

[13] Stute P, Wildt L, Neulen J. The impact of micronized progesterone on breast cancer risk: A systematic review. Climacteric. 2018;**21**(2):111-122. DOI: 10.1080/13697137.2017.1421925

[14] Nick P, Medical Advisory Council of the British Menopause Society. BMS–consensus statement: Bioidentical HRT. Post Reproductive Health. 2019;**25**:61-63

[15] Casanova G et al. Effects of low-dose versus placebo or conventional-dose postmenopausal hormone therapy on variables related to cardiovascular risk: A systematic review and meta-analyses of randomized clinical trials. The Journal of Clinical Endocrinology & Metabolism. 2015;**100**(3):1028-1037

[16] "The 2022 Hormone Therapy Position Statement of The North American Menopause Society" Advisory Panel. The 2022 hormone therapy position statement of the North American Menopause Society. Menopause. 2022;**29**(7):767-794. DOI: 10.1097/GME.0000000000002028

Chapter 7

Satisfaction with Antenatal Care Services and Its Associated Factors among Pregnant Women at Public Health Centers of Lemi Kura Sub-City, Addis Ababa, Ethiopia, 2022

Ayehu Kassaw Asres and Yirgalem Amogne

Abstract

Pregnant women satisfied with the provided health care services will keep using the services at a particular health institution. This study aims to assess the level of satisfaction with antenatal services and its associated factors among pregnant women. A facility-based cross-sectional study design was conducted from November 1 to December 15, 2021. Systematic random sampling technique was used to select study participants. A total of 405 pregnant women were enrolled in the study. Structured questionnaire was used to collect the data. Data were entered into Epi-Data 4.1 and exported to SPSS for analysis. Bivariable and multivariable binary logistic regression with 95% confidence interval and P value of 0.05 were deployed. Pregnant women who had 5 and more family members were 6 times more likely to be satisfied than those who had a single family member (AOR: 6.3; 95% CI = (1.78–22.39)). Pregnant women who did not have chronic diseases were 2 times more satisfied with the antenatal care services (AOR: 2.18; 95% CI = 1–4.77). Having occupation such as housewife, distance of home from health facility, and mode of transportation were factors associated with satisfaction at $P < 0.05$.

Keywords: antenatal care, health centers, satisfaction, pregnant women, health care service

1. Introduction

Antenatal care (ANC) is a branch of obstetrics that is dealing with presymptomatic diagnosis of general medical disorders, nutrition, immunological problems, health education, and social medicine, with the major focus on prevention and early detection of pregnancy disorders and other illness [1].

World Health Organization (WHO) in 2016 recommended at least eight ANC visits, and the first visit should take place before the first trimester of pregnancy [2].

IntechOpen

However, Ethiopia has launched at least four visits as standard. The first visit takes place before or at 16 weeks; the second is planned between 24 and 28 weeks; the third at 32 weeks; and the fourth at 36–38 weeks. The initial visit takes 30–40 min, and the other visits take around 20 min each [3, 4].

Antenatal care (ANC) coverage is a success story in Africa, since over two-thirds of pregnant women have at least one ANC contact. However, to achieve the full life-saving potential that ANC promises for women and babies, four visits providing essential evidence-based interventions with a package often called focused antenatal care are required [5].

Essential interventions in ANC include identification and management of obstetric complications such as preeclampsia, tetanus toxoid immunization, and intermittent preventive treatment for malaria during pregnancy, and identification and management of infections including HIV, syphilis, and other sexually transmitted infections (STIs) [2].

ANC is also an opportunity to promote the use of skilled attendance at birth and healthy behaviors such as breastfeeding, early postnatal care, and planning for optimal pregnancy spacing [5]. ANC attendance during pregnancy also has a positive impact on the use of postnatal healthcare services [6].

Satisfaction is the extent of the client's experience to the ideal care compared with expectations or the given care [7]. Patient satisfaction is accepted as one of the indicators of a health-care service, and it favors or limits the utilization of a health-care service in a certain health institution. The patients' level of satisfaction highlights the breach between health-care service providers and the anticipation of the patients. Therefore, the client who is satisfied with the provided health-care service will keep using the service at a particular health institution, and this might eventually help pregnant women to complete their ANC services' follow-up schedule correctly [8].

Assessing satisfaction is used to assess the quality of provided services with respect to health-care provider, institution, and provider–client interaction. It also indicates the effectiveness of the implemented policy. Studies have reported that satisfied service users are more likely to utilize health services, comply with services and follow-ups, and continue with the health care [6, 7, 9]. Thus, this shows that pregnant women who are satisfied with antenatal care services will have a capability to complete the recommended four visits and comply with interventions.

2. Literature review

2.1 Overview of antenatal care services

Antenatal care (ANC) continues to be one of the safest maternal care interventions aimed at significantly reducing maternal and perinatal morbidities. ANC utilization ensures effective management of prenatal morbidities, facility delivery, and postpartum care and to manage complications in order to improve the health outcomes of the mother and fetus. ANC offers pregnant women the chance to take and make appropriate lifestyle decisions and choices, respectively. Pregnant women are provided with the opportunity to have interactive engagements with nurses, midwives, doctors, and other caregivers among the broader health-care system during ANC visits. However, at which component of antenatal care pregnant mothers are satisfied or dissatisfied is not addressed well.

World Health Organization estimated that 25 percent of maternal deaths occur during pregnancy, with variability between countries depending on the prevalence of unsafe abortion, violence, and disease in the area. Between a third and a half of maternal deaths are due to causes such as hypertension (preeclampsia and eclampsia) and antepartum hemorrhage, which are directly related to inadequate care during pregnancy [5, 10].

In a study conducted in six West African countries, a third of all pregnant women experienced illness during pregnancy, of which three percent required hospitalization. Certain preexisting conditions become more severe during pregnancy. Malaria, HIV/AIDS, anemia, and malnutrition are associated with increased maternal and newborn complications as well as death where the prevalence of these conditions is high. New evidence suggests that women who have been subject to female genital mutilation are significantly more likely to have complications during childbirth, so these women need to be identified during ANC [2, 5, 10]. Maternal mortality is 412 deaths per 100,000 live births in Ethiopia, which is far higher than the global target of reducing maternal mortality to less than 70 per 100,000 live births by 2030 [10].

Antenatal care utilization is the only means that prevents morbidity and mortality related to pregnancy [11]. Utilization of antenatal care is determined by clients' satisfaction. Unsatisfied pregnant women cannot comply and continue their antenatal care services. Poor satisfaction with antenatal care services has negative outcomes on the health status of both the mother and the baby [12].

Poor satisfaction with ANC services might predispose pregnant women to home delivery rather than the delivery in health-care facilities [13] and incomplete visits. In Ethiopia, only one third of pregnant women complete the recommended visits [14]. The Ethiopian Demographic Health Survey (EDHS) 2019 mini report showed that 74% of pregnant women attended at least one ANC visit, but among these, only 48% of clients gave birth at a health facility [4].

Furthermore, dissatisfaction of women with antenatal care (ANC) services has different consequences, such as poor adherence to treatment, poor participation in their own health care, breaking the continuum of care, and increasing maternal morbidity and mortality [15]. Breaking the continuity of care lowers the recommended number of visits [16].

Visiting health facility for antenatal care services decreases not only maternal mortality but also neonatal death [17]. Antenatal care visit decreases the likelihood of under-five mortality in Ethiopia by 45.2%, while the timing of the first antenatal care within the first trimester decreases the likelihood of under-five mortality by 10% [18].

Satisfaction with antenatal care services is affected by different dimensions such as structure (physical environment and availability of adequate human resources, medicines, and supplies), process (interpersonal behavior, privacy, promptness, cognitive care, perceived provider competency, and emotional support), and outcome (health status of the mother and fetus) [19]. It is also associated with sex of the health-care provider; the religion, educational status, residence, ethnicity, and age of the mother; history of antenatal care; waiting time; transportation; distance of health facility from home; type of pregnancy; and history of abortion [19–24].

Satisfaction with antenatal care services among pregnant women at different parts of Ethiopia ranges from 33.4% to 83.9% [23]. This shows that the quality of antenatal care services is inconsistent and varied. There is no study that has assessed the satisfaction with antenatal care services at Lemi Kura Sub-City. Thus, this study is initiated to assess the satisfaction of pregnant mothers with antenatal care services at public health centers of Lemi Kura Sub-City, Addis Ababa, Ethiopia.

2.2 Satisfaction with antenatal care services

Different studies were conducted across the world on the satisfaction of pregnant mothers with antenatal acre services. A study that was conducted in Sweden reported that 82% of the total study participants were satisfied with antenatal care services [12]. Another study that was conducted at Pakistan's primary health-care facilities among pregnant women revealed that of the total study participants, 46% of them were satisfied with antenatal care services [25]. A study that was conducted in the Musandam region of Oman showed that 59% of pregnant women reported that the rendered antenatal care makes them satisfied [26]. Moreover, a study conducted in India showed that more than 90% of pregnant women who visited nurses were satisfied with antenatal care services. But in this study, only 31.8% of the mothers were satisfied with the health education on family planning [27].

A study conducted in Malaysia has reported that 75.4% of mothers reported satisfaction with the antenatal care services provided [28]. Another study conducted in Iraq reported that 85.7% of the study participants were satisfied with the care provided [29]. In Myanmar, 48% of the pregnant women were highly satisfied with ANC services [30].

A study that was conducted in Ibadan, Nigeria, on perception and satisfaction of pregnant women with antenatal care services reported that 81.1% of the respondents were satisfied [31]. Another study that was conducted at other parts of Nigeria revealed that the percentage of satisfaction with antenatal care services among pregnant women was 67% [32].

A recent cross-sectional study conducted in Ghana has revealed that 92.7% of pregnant women were satisfied with the provided antenatal care services [33]. Another study conducted on the quality of antenatal care among pregnant women in Uganda showed that 74.3% of them were satisfied [34].

A cross-sectional study that was conducted on the satisfaction of pregnant women with focused antenatal care services in Jimma Town showed that 60.4% of the study participants were satisfied with the provided antenatal services [35]. A study conducted at public health facilities in Guji Zone, South West Ethiopia, reported that 67% of pregnant women were satisfied with antenatal care services [22].

Another study that was conducted in Harari, Eastern Ethiopia, in 2017 at public health facilities reported that pregnant women's satisfaction with antenatal care services was 70.3% [36]. A comparable finding is reported by a study conducted at public health centers in Hawassa in 2017. In this study, 79.2% the total study participants were satisfied with the ANC service. As per specific components, 74.2% of the respondents were satisfied with the information provided [8]. Moreover, a study conducted in Sidama Zone and Arba-Mich Zuria districts, South Ethiopia, reported that 33% and 68% of pregnant women were satisfied with antenatal care services, respectively [21, 24].

A cross-sectional study that was conducted in the Tigray region in 2019 reported that 83.9% of pregnant women were satisfied with antenatal care services [37]. Furthermore, a study conducted in Hossana, Ethiopia, in 2020 showed that 74% of mothers were satisfied with antenatal care services rendered in the public health institutions of Hossana town [38].

A recent study published in 2021 in Hawassa, South Ethiopia, has revealed that 79.2% of the total respondents were satisfied with antenatal care services provided by health-care professionals [8]. Another recent cross-sectional study that was conducted at public health facilities of Debre Tabor showed that 53.8% of pregnant women were satisfied with antenatal care services [39]. A study that was conducted in the northwest part of Ethiopia showed that 68.3% of pregnant women were satisfied with antenatal care services [40].

2.3 Factors associated with satisfaction with antenatal care services

Satisfaction with antenatal care service is associated with different factors that are categorized as client related, health-care provider related, and health facility related. Studies show that age has a significant association with the satisfaction with antenatal care services. For example, a study conducted in Debre Tabor indicated that study participants whose ages were 25–29 years were 6 times more likely to be satisfied compared with those whose ages were 35 years and above [39]. In another study that was conducted in Hosanna, younger mothers were more likely to be satisfied than their counterparts [38].

A study conducted in Guji Zone, Ethiopia, reported that pregnant women who were students were 6 times more likely to be satisfied compared with those who were government employees [22]. Besides this, pregnant women who lived in urban areas were 2 times more likely to be satisfied compared with women who lived in rural areas [22]. Furthermore, studies conducted in Ghana revealed that the satisfaction of pregnant women with antenatal care services is increased when the charges of services are increased [33]. This is also reported by a study conducted in Nigeria [41].

Different studies showed that educational status is also associated with the satisfaction with antenatal services [28, 32, 40]. Women who had no formal education and attended primary education had 2.53 and 2.17 higher odds of satisfaction with ANC services compared with those who had secondary education and above, respectively [36]. Similarly, in a study conducted in Hosanna, study participants who are illiterate were four times more likely to be satisfied than those who were in primary school and above [38].

Family monthly income is also associated with the level of satisfaction [32]. A study conducted in Jimma town revealed that pregnant women whose family monthly income is below Ethiopian Birr (ETB) 500 were 8 times more likely to be satisfied compared with pregnant women whose monthly income is above ETB 1000 [35].

The level of satisfaction is increased while pregnant women visit health facilities repeatedly [22, 40]. This is supported by a study conducted in Debre Tabor. In this study, pregnant women who had 4 and above visits were 3.3 times more likely to be satisfied [39]. Moreover, pregnant women who had more than one ANC visit had 4.62 times the odds of being satisfied with ANC services than those who had the first visit [36]. Furthermore, the odds of pregnant women's satisfaction were 1.74 times higher among women who initiated their ANC in the first trimester of pregnancy compared with those who had initiated the same after the first trimester of their pregnancy [36].

Another factor that has an association with satisfaction is the type of pregnancy. Women became more satisfied with antenatal care services when their pregnancy was planned and wanted [39]. This finding is supported by a study conducted in Jimma Town. In this study, pregnant women whose pregnancy was planned were 5 times more likely to be satisfied compared with their counterparts [35]. Pregnant women who had no history of stillbirth had 2.52 times the odds of being satisfied with ANC services compared with their counterparts [36].

In a study conducted in Hawassa, South Ethiopia, pregnant women waiting for their health-care providers for 30 minutes and less than 30 minutes were 2.6 times more likely to be satisfied than their counterparts [8]. Besides, pregnant women who waited for less than 30 minutes in the health facility to get the services had 2.31 times higher odds of satisfaction with ANC than those who waited for more than 30 minutes [36].

The commitment and interaction of the health-care provider is the other factor [40]. Timely and complete adherence by the provider to the protocol during the first ANC visit has been shown to increase the women's level of satisfaction, enhance their motivation to attend subsequent follow-up visits, increase the likelihood of institutional delivery, and improve perinatal outcomes [40, 42]. Despite this, in a study conducted in Guji Zone, Ethiopia, major attributes for the overall satisfaction with focused antenatal care services were in relation to the service providers [22]. Pregnant women who got services from female health-care providers were more likely to be satisfied compared with those who got the same from male health-care providers [22]. Satisfaction increases when pregnant women access health facility easily [33].

In study conducted in West Guji Zone, Ethiopia, most attributes of the overall dissatisfaction of mothers during antenatal care services were received from health facilities and transportation, that is, toilet-related structural dimensions, electric power availability, laboratory services, water availability, transportation, waiting area, service room cleanness, and others [22]. Distance of the health facility from home is significantly associated with satisfaction [40]. Pregnant women who travel less than 30 minutes to reach facilities were two times more likely to be satisfied than those who travel more than 30 minutes [38].

In study conducted in Hareri, pregnant women who had no history of stillbirth had 2.52 times the odds of being satisfied with ANC services compared with their counterparts. In another study that was conducted in Jimma Town, pregnant women who had no history of stillbirth were 5.47 times more likely to be satisfied compared with those who had it [35]. Presence of chronic disease is explored as a factor for satisfaction with antenatal care services [29].

3. Obejectives

3.1 General objective

To assess the level of satisfaction with antenatal care services and its associated factors among pregnant mothers at public health centers of Lemi Kura Sub-City, Addis Ababa, Ethiopia, 2021.

3.2 Specific objectives

- To determine the level of satisfaction with antenatal care services at public health centers of Lemi Kura Sub-City, Addis Ababa, Ethiopia, 2021

- To identify the factors associated with the satisfaction with antenatal care services at public health centers of Lemi Kura Sub-City, Addis Ababa, Ethiopia, 2021

4. Methods and materials

4.1 Study area and study period

The study was conducted at public health centers of Lemi Kura Sub-City, Addis Ababa, Ethiopia. Lemi Kura Sub-City is one of the 10 sub-cities of Addis Ababa. The sub-city covers 118.08km^2 with total population of 451,631. Among the total population, one-third of them are women under the reproductive age. There are one public hospital, nine public health centers, and three private hospitals. Public health centers in the sub-city are Summit Health Center, Amoraw Health Center, Merry Health Center, Goro Health Center, Arabsa Health Center, Raey Health Center, Hidasa Health Center, Abado Health Center, and Woreda 13 Health Center. The total number of health-care providers who are working in these public health centers is near to 750 [43]. The study was conducted from November 1 to December 152,021.

4.2 Study design

Institution-based cross-sectional study design was employed.

4.3 Source population

All women who were utilizing antenatal care services in public health centers of Lemi Kura Sub-City were the source population.

4.4 Study population

All women who were utilizing antenatal care services in selected public health centers of Lemi Kura Sub-City during the data collection period were the study population.

4.5 Eligibility criteria

4.5.1 Inclusion criteria

All women whose ages were 18 years and above and who were utilizing antenatal care services at public health centers of Lemi Kura Sub-City were included.

4.5.2 Exclusion criteria

- Women who were unable to communicate,
- Women who were seriously ill, and
- Women referred to other public health centers and hospitals were excluded from the study.

4.6 Sample size calculation

Sample size for the first objective is calculated by using single population proportion formula with 95% confidence level, 5% margin of error, and proportion of pregnant mothers' satisfaction toward antenatal care services at a similar setting. Proportion, which was 60.4%, is taken from a study conducted on the satisfaction of pregnant women with focused antenatal care services at public health centers of Jimma town [35].

$$N = \frac{\left(Z_{\frac{\propto}{2}}\right)^2 (P)(1-P)}{d^2} \tag{1}$$

N: Sample size.

$Z_{a/2}$ = 1.96 (standardized normal distribution curve value for the 95% confidence Interval).

P = 0.604 (proportion of satisfaction with antenatal care services).

D = 0.05 (degree of margin of error)

$$= \frac{(1.96)^2 (0.604)(0.396)}{0.05^2}$$

= 368 by adding 10% nonresponse rate, the final sample was 405.

4.7 Sampling procedure

First, from the nine public health centers, 5 of them were selected by lottery method. Selected health centers were Summit Health Center, Goro Health Center, Merry Health Center, Amoraw Health Center, and Arabsa Health Center. Then, the total sample was allocated to each public health center proportionally based on the previous 2 months' report. The previous 2 months' antenatal care visit reports for Summit Health Center, Goro Health Center, Amoraw Health Center, Merry Health Center, and Arabsa Health Center were 152, 202, 171, 186, and 160, respectively. Study participants were selected by using systematic random sampling in every K value. K value was calculated by dividing the reported number of pregnant mothers to sample size, which is 2. The first client was selected by lottery method from the first visitors.

4.8 Study variables

4.8.1 Dependent variables

Satisfaction with antenatal care.

4.8.2 Independent variables

- **Socio demographic and economic characteristics**: age, marital status, educational status, occupation, ethnicity, religion, address, monthly family income, family size, presence of chronic disease

- **Obstetric history**: gravid, parity, type of pregnancy, history of ANC follow-ups, number of visit, gestational age at first visit, history of abortion, history of still birth

- **Health-care provider-related factors**: sex of health-care provider

- **Others**: cost of service, waiting time, distance of health facility from home, mode of transportation, payment for transportation, reason for visit

4.9 Data collection tool

Data were collected using a structured questionnaire, and a face to face interview was used for data collection. The tool had three parts. The first part was focused on the sociodemographic status. The second part assessed the services related to healthcare providers and health institutions. The third part assessed pregnant women's satisfaction toward antenatal care services. Satisfaction tool was adapted from previous researches [22, 36, 38] and was presented using a 5-point Likert scale (1 – very dissatisfied, 2 – dissatisfied, 3 – neutral, 4 – satisfied, and 5 – very satisfied). It has a total of 29 items that assessed the process, structure, and outcome. In this study, the internal reliability of the tool was 0.924. For the purpose of description, the 5-point Likert scale was categorized into two: strongly dissatisfied, dissatisfied, and neutral were categorized as dissatisfied, while satisfied and strongly satisfied were categorized into satisfied. After calculating the total score, the cut point for satisfaction and dissatisfaction was calculated by using demarcation formula: [(highest score – lowest score) divided by 2 + lowest score] [8]. All parts of the questionnaire were prepared in English version initially and translated into Amharic and then back to English to check their consistency.

4.10 Data collection procedure

After preparing the questionnaire, 5 BSc nurses for data collection and 1 BSc nurse for supervision were recruited. Two days' training was given to each of them on the meaning of every item in the questionnaire and the techniques of data collection such as ways of greeting, ways of taking consent, ways of data-quality monitoring, and ways of addressing ambiguous items. After this, data were collected by face-to-face exit interview. To prevent repeated interview, the data collectors verified with the clients whether they were interviewed before or not. Supervisor and principal investigator monitored closely the data collection process.

4.11 Operational definition

Satisfied: pregnant women who responded to the items at or above the cut point (demarcation point) were categorized as satisfied.

Dissatisfied: pregnant women who responded to the items below the cut point (demarcation point) were categorized as dissatisfied.

4.12 Data quality control

The quality of data was assured by training data collectors and supervisors, designing questionnaire carefully, monitoring the data collection process, and checking completeness of data during the data collection time. In addition to these, before reaching the respondents, all questionnaires were pretested on 5% of sample size at Hidasa Health Center to address confusing items and to increase the quality of data. Necessary amendment was made on the questionnaire based on the result of the pretest. Supervisors closely supervised the completeness and consistency of gathered information, and timely corrections were made.

4.13 Data processing and analysis

After data collection, data was entered into EpiData version 4.1 and exported to Statistical Package and Service Product (SPSS) version 26 for analysis. The results of the study were presented by using text, tables, and figures, and binary logistic regression model was enrolled by considering 95% confidence level and

P value of 0.05. Multivariable binary logistic regression was done by taking variables that had P value of ≤0.2 from bivariable logistic regression by using backward stepwise likelihood ratio method to identify the factors associated with the satisfaction with antenatal care services. Hosmer and Lemeshow test was utilized to check whether the data fit with model or not before data analysis, and its result was 0.924.

4.14 Ethical consideration

Prior to data collection, ethical clearance was obtained from Unity University, Addis Ababa Campus and proceeded to Addis Ababa Health Bureau and Public Health Research directorate. Then, a supportive letter was obtained from Lemi-Kura Sub-City Health Department and attached to the managers of each health centers. The purpose and importance of the study were explained to each of study participants. Informed consent was obtained from each participant. Confidentiality was maintained at all levels of the study. To keep confidentiality, names of respondents were not registered. Participation in the study was on voluntary basis. If participants were unwilling, they can quite their participation at any stage of the data collection.

5. Result

5.1 Sociodemographic characteristics

From a total of 405 study participants, 399 participated in this study with a 98.5% response rate. The mean of age of study participants was 29.15 (SD ±5.22). Among the total study participants, 265 (66.4%) were in the age group of 25–34 years. Educational status of 192 (48.1%), or nearly half, of the total study participants was above grade 12. But 82 (20.6%), or one-fifth, of them were single in their marital status. One hundred and twenty-five (31.3) of the study participants had a family size of five and above. Thirty-eight (9.5%) of the study participants had a history of chronic diseases, and among these, 22 (5.5%) had a history of hypertension (**Table 1**).

Variables	Category	Frequency (n)	Percentage (%)
Age	18–24	63	15.8
	25–34	265	66.4
	> = 35	71	17.8
Educational level	Unable to read and write	35	8.8
	Informal school	33	8.3
	Primary school (Grade 1–8)	61	15.3
	Secondary school (Grade 9–12)	78	19.5
	Above grade 12	192	48.1
Marital status	Single	82	20.6
	Married	271	67.9
	Widowed	20	5
	Divorced	26	6.5

Variables	Category	Frequency (n)	Percentage (%)
Residence	Urban	316	79.2
	Rural	83	20.8
Occupation	Farmer	63	15.8
	Merchant	93	23.3
	Student	44	11
	Employee	174	43.6
	Others (housewife, no permanent job)	25	6.3
Monthly income (ETB)	≤2500	103	25.8
	2501–5200	98	24.6
	5201–8000	99	24.8
	>8001	99	24.8
Family size	1	18	4.5
	2	63	15.8
	3–4	193	48.4
	≥ 5	125	31.3
Presence of chronic disease	Yes	38	9.5
	No	361	90.5
Type of chronic disease	DM	12	3
	Hypertension	22	5.5
	Others	4	1

Note: Monthly income was categorized based on quartile range; separated couples are added to divorced.

Table 1.
Sociodemographic and economic status of study participants in public health centers of Lemi Kura Sub-City, Addis Ababa, Ethiopia, 2022 (N = 399).

5.2 Obstetrics history

Among the total study participants (399), 79 (19.8%), or nearly one fifth, were null Para. One hundred and seventy-nine (44.9%) of the total study participants had no history of antenatal care (ANC) follow-up. Three hundred and fifty-four (88.5%) of them had started their visit at first trimester, and 329 (82.5%) of them had a history of more than one visit. However, 45.4% of the total study participants had started their ANC visit because of reasons such as getting sick and pressure from others. The current pregnancy was unplanned for 110 (27.6%) of the total respondents (**Table 2**).

5.3 Health service-related factors

From the total study participant, 139 (34.8%), or slightly higher than one third, participants had contact with a male health-care provider. Two hundred and nine (52.4%) of the study participants had spent more than 30 minutes at the health center to be seen by the health-care provider. Two hundred and sixty-four (66.2%) respondents took more than 30 minutes to arrive at the health center. One-tenth of the total study participants (10.8%) had paid a charge for the services (**Table 3**).

Variables	Category	Frequency(N)	Percentage
Parity	Zero	79	19.8
	One	78	19.5
	Two	133	33.3
	Three or more	109	27.3
Gravida	One	82	20.6
	Two	82	20.6
	Three or more	235	58.9
Having history of ANC follow-up	Yes	220	55.1
	No	179	44.9
Number of visit for current pregnancy	First visit	63	15.8
	Repeated visit	329	82.5
Gestational age during first visit	<16 weeks	354	88.7
	16-24 weeks	32	8
	25–32	7	1.8
	> 32 weeks	6	1.5
Type of pregnancy	Wanted	289	72.4
	Unwanted	110	27.6
History of abortion	Yes	55	13.8
	No	344	86.2
History of stillbirth	Yes	24	6
	No	375	94

Table 2.
Obstetric history of study participants in public health centers of Lemi Kura Sub-City, Addis Ababa, Ethiopia, 2022 (N = 399).

Variables	Category	Frequency (n)	Percentage (%)
Sex of health-care provider	Male	139	34.8
	Female	260	65.2
Waiting time before being seen by health-care provider	≤30 minutes	190	47.6
	>30 minutes	209	52.4
Distance of home from health institutions	Takes up to 30 minutes	135	33.8
	Takes more than 30 minutes	264	66.2
Way of transportation	Ambulance	6	1.5
	Public transport	177	44.4
	Private	116	29.1
	On foot	100	25.1
Payment for transportation (ETB)	Free	138	34.6
	Paid	261	65.4
Charge for service (drug, laboratory request...)	Free	43	10.8
	Paid	356	89.2

Variables	Category	Frequency (n)	Percentage (%)
Reason for ANC visit	Pressure from family and friends	54	13.5
	Heard from media	24	6
	Got sick and needed health care	100	25.1
	I feel it is necessary	218	54.6
	Other reasons	3	0.8

Table 3.
Health service-related factors in public health centers of Lemi Kura Sub-City, Addis Ababa, Ethiopia, 2022 (N-399).

5.4 Satisfaction of pregnant women with antenatal care services

High proportions of pregnant women were satisfied in some areas of antenatal care services. From the total study participants, 311 (77.9%), 288 (72.2%), 276 (69.2%), 272 (68.2), and 272 (68.2) were satisfied with the welcoming environment of the health center starting from the gate, performance of procedures with clean and safe manner, effort of health-care providers to involve them in decision-making and asking concerns and interests, respectively. On the contrary, only 157 (39.3%), 160 (40.1%), 164 (41.1%), and 183 (45.9%) were satisfied with the availability of functional toilet, availability of hand-washing facility, the way of the health-care provider to introduce himself/herself, and waiting time to be seen by health-care provider, respectively (**Table 4**).

Variables	Women satisfaction	
	Satisfied N (%)	Dissatisfied N (%)
Welcoming environment of health center starting from the gate	311(77.9)	88(22.1)
Politeness of health-care providers	211(52.9)	188(47.1)
The way a health-care provider introduces himself/herself	164(41.1)	235(58.9)
Adequate explanation of procedures	186(46.6)	213(53.4)
Keeping privacy during examinations	255(63.9)	144(36.1)
Cleanness of examination room	288(72.2)	111(27.8)
Light and space of examination room	247(61.9)	152(38.1)
Effort of health-care provider to give comfort	228(57.1)	171(42.9)
Easiness of understanding their explanation	236(59.1)	163(40.9)
Talking in clear and straightforward manner.	231(57.9)	168(42.1)
Ease of accessibility of antenatal care room	252(63.2)	147(36.8)
Effort to involve you in decision-making	272(68.2)	127(31.8)
Asking interests and concerns	272(68.2)	127(31.8)
Cleanness of waiting room	264(66.2)	135(33.8)
Light and space of waiting room	214(53.6)	185(46.4)
Waiting time to be seen by health-care provider	183(45.9)	216(54.1)
Cooperativeness of health-care providers	228(57.1)	171(42.9)
Listening carefully during conversation	256(64.2)	143(35.8)
Antenatal care advices given	269(67.4)	130(32.6)

Variables	Women satisfaction	
	Satisfied N (%)	Dissatisfied N (%)
Duration of advice	261(65.4)	138(34.6)
Laboratory and other diagnostic services	254(63.7)	145(36.3)
Explain adequately about the result or finding of examination	256(64.2)	143(35.8)
Availability of drug and medical supplies	202(50.6)	197(49.4)
Explain about the drug adequately.	244(61.2)	155(38.8)
Availability of functional toilet	157(39.3)	242(60.7)
Availability of hand-washing facility	160(40.1)	239(59.9)
Performing procedures with clean and safe manner	276(69.2)	123(30.8)
The overall cleanness of health facility	268(67.2)	131(32.8)
Administrative process of the institution	235(58.9)	164(41.1)

Table 4.
Level of women's satisfaction with antenatal care services in public health centers of Lemi Kura Sub-City Addis Ababa, Ethiopia, 2022 (N = 399).

5.5 Overall level of satisfaction of women with antenatal care services

The overall satisfaction of pregnant women is calculated by using demarcation formula. According to the finding, from the total study participants, 230 (57.6%) were categorized as satisfied toward antenatal care services (**Figure 1**).

5.6 Factors associated with women satisfaction with antenatal care services

Variables that have an association with satisfaction with antenatal care services at P value ≤0.2 in bivariable logistic regression were age, educational status, marital status, residence, occupation, family monthly income, having chronic disease, family size, history of abortion, history of stillbirth, distance of home from health facility, mode of transportation, type of pregnancy, and charge for services. All these variables were entered in multivariable logistic regression to identify the factors associated with satisfaction. However, in multivariable logistic regression, only occupation, family size, having chronic disease, mode of transportation, and distance of home from health facility were associated with the satisfaction with antenatal care services at P value of 0.05. According to the finding of the study, pregnant women whose occupation is other than farmer, merchant, student, and employee were 5 times likely to be satisfied with the given antenatal care services compared with pregnant women who are merchants (AOR: 5.08; 95% CI = (1.63–15.87). On the other hand, pregnant women who had 5 and more family members were 6 times more likely to be satisfied compared with those who had a single family member (AOR: 6.3; 95% CI = (1.78–22.39)). Pregnant women who were coming to the health center by public transport were 2 times more likely to be satisfied with the given antenatal care services compared with those who used private transport (AOR: 2.33; 95% CI = (1.38–3.91)). Pregnant women whose house is far from the health center were 2 times more likely to be satisfied with the given antenatal care services compared with those whose house is near to the health center (AOR: 1.72; 95% CI = 1.08–2.74)). In addition, pregnant women who did not have chronic diseases such as hypertension, diabetes, and others were 2 times more likely to be satisfied with the antenatal care services compared with their counterparts (AOR: 2.18; 95% CI = 1–4.77) (**Table 5**).

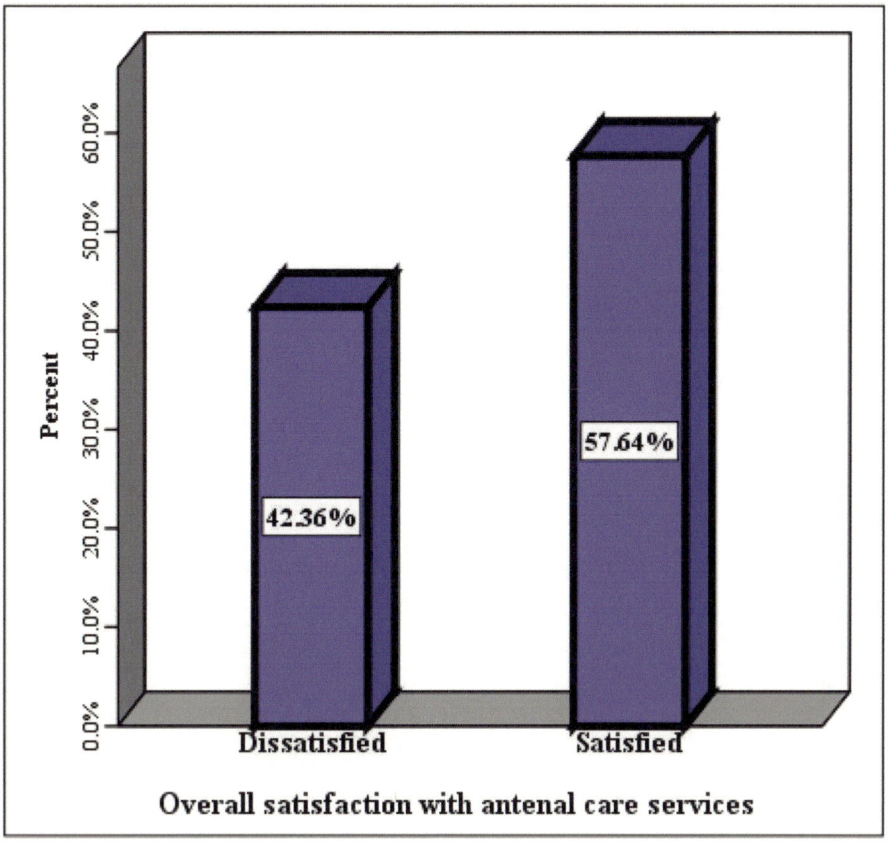

Figure 1.
Level of overall satisfaction with antenatal care services in public health centers of Lemi Kura Sub-City, Addis Ababa, Ethiopia, 2022.

Variables	Category	Satisfaction		COR at 95% CI	AOR at 95% CI
		Satisfied	Dissatisfied		
Age	18–24	28	35	0.40(0.20–0.82)	
	25–34	110	155	0.72(0.41–1.24)	
	> = 35	47	24	1	
Monthly income (ETB)	<2500	60	43	1.81(1.04–3.17)	
	2501–5200	63	35	2.34(1.31–4.15)	
	5201–8000	64	35	2.38(1.34–4.22)	
	>8001	43	56	1	
Type of pregnancy	Wanted	180	109	1.98(1.27–3.09)	
	Unwanted	50	60	1	
Educational status	Unable to read and write	13	22	0.31(0.15–0.67)	
	Informal school	19	14	0.72(0.34–1.54)	
	Grade 1–8	27	34	0.42(0.23–0.76)	
	Grade 9–12	46	32	0.77(0.45–1.32)	

Variables	Category	Satisfaction		COR at 95% CI	AOR at 95% CI
		Satisfied	Dissatisfied		
	Above grade 12	125	67	1	
Occupation	farmer	27	36	0.87(0.45–1.66)	0.87(0.43–1.76)
	Merchant	43	50	1	1
	Student	23	21	1.27(0.62–2.61)	1.7(0.75–3.86)
	Employee	117	57	2.38(1.42–3.99)	2.3(1.31–4.03)
	Others(house wife, no job)	20	5	4.65(1.60–13.44)	5.08(1.63–15.87)
Marital status	Single	38	44	0.38(0.15–0.98)	
	Married	167	104	0.71(0.30–1.7)	
	Widowed	7	13	0.23(0.06–0.82)	
	Divorced	18	8	1	
Family size	1	4	14	1	1
	2	38	25	5.32(1.57–18.02)	4.58(1.23–17.17)
	3–4	108	85	4.44(1.41–14.00)	3.49(0.99–12.27)
	≥5	80	45	6.22(1.93–20.04)	6.3(1.78–22.39)
Residence	Urban	190	136	1.61(0.99–2.63)	
	Rural	40	43	1	
Mode of Transport	Ambulance	1	5	0.23(0.02–2.09)	0.49(0.51–4.79)
	Public transport	120	57	2.50(1.54–4.05)	2.33(1.38–3.91)
	Private	53	63	1	1
	On Foot	56	44	1.51(0.88–2.59)	1.55(0.85–2.83)
Abortion	Yes	22	33	0.43(0.24–0.78)	
	No	208	136	1	
Stillbirth	Yes	8	16	0.34(0.14–0.82)	
	No	222	153	1	
Distance of home	Takes less than 30'	66	69	1	1
	Takes more than 30'	164	100	1.71(1.17–2.60)	1.72(1.08–2.74)
Charge for services	Yes	20	23	1	1
	No	210	146	1.65(0.87–3.12)	
Chronic disease	Yes	14	24	1	1
	No	216	145	2.55(1.27–5.10)	2.18(0.99–4.77)

Table 5.
Bivariable and multivariable logistic regression output on the association between satisfaction with antenatal care services and factors, 2022 (N = 399).

6. Discussion

This study was aimed to assess the level of satisfaction with antenatal care services among pregnant women at Lemi Kura Sub-City public health centers. The finding of this study will be helpful to different bodies by showing areas that dissatisfy pregnant women.

Based on the study finding, the level of satisfaction with antenatal care services among pregnant women was 57.6% (95% CI: 53% -63%). This finding is in line with study conducted in Jimma, Ethiopia (60.4%) [35], Oman (59%) [26], and Debre Tabor (53.8%) [39]. However, this finding is higher than the study conducted in Sidama, South Ethiopia (33%) [24], Pakistan (46%) [25], and Myanmar (48%) [30].

In contrast, there are studies that have reported higher findings. For example, a study conducted in Arba Minch, Ethiopia (68%) [21]; Hawassa, Ethiopia (79.3%) [8], Gujji, Ethiopia (67%) [22]; Harare, Ethiopia (70.3%) [36]; Uganda (74.3%) [34]; and Nigeria (67%) [9]. The possible reason for this discrepancy might be the difference in sample size, study design, and sociodemographic status. Additionally, the difference in the study area might be another reason for the discrepancy.

In this study, satisfaction among pregnant women was assessed in only public health centers. But in other studies, satisfaction was assessed in both public hospitals and health centers.

Unlike the previous studies, this study revealed that pregnant women who were housewives or did not have permanent job were 5 times more likely to be satisfied with the given antenatal care services compared with pregnant women who were merchants (AOR: 5.08; 95% CI = (1.63–15.87)). The possible justification for this might be the decreased workload and stress. Women who do not have any permanent job will take the responsibility of childbearing. Thus, when they are coming to health facility, they become relaxed and cooperative with the care given.

Family size has shown an association with the level of satisfaction. Pregnant women who had 5 and more family members were 6 times more likely to be satisfied compared with those who had a single family member (AOR: 6.3; 95% CI = (1.78–22.39)). Women who have many children might have repeated exposure to antenatal care services and understand their meaning and use the given services. These women come to health centers for the same purpose by themselves. In spite of this, the previous studies did not show the association between family size and satisfaction.

Pregnant women who were coming to the health center by public transport were 2 times more likely to be satisfied with the given antenatal care services compared with those who used private transport (AOR: 2.33; 95% CI = (1.38–3.91)). This might be due to the fact that public transport is cost-effective, easily accessible, and quick. This finding is supported by a study conducted at West Gujji zone, Ethiopia [22].

In this study, pregnant women whose house is far from the health center were 2 times more likely to be satisfied with the given antenatal care services compared with those whose house is near the health center (AOR: 1.72; 95% CI = 1.08–2.74). Unlike to this study, a study that was conducted in Hossana, Ethiopia, reported that pregnant women who traveled less than thirty minutes were more likely to be satisfied. This discrepancy might be related with women's preparedness and plan for their antenatal care. On the other hand, women who are near the health center might plan to return home quickly [38].

In addition, pregnant women who did not have chronic diseases such as hypertension, diabetes, and others were 2 times more likely to be satisfied with the antenatal care services compared with their counterparts (AOR: 2.18; 95% CI = 1–4.77). This might be related with anxiety and fear from the adverse effects of chronic diseases. Women who do not have chronic diseases will not have any anxiety and fear for the outcome of their pregnancy when compared with those who do have chronic diseases. This finding is supported by a study conducted in Iraq [29].

In this study, the level of satisfaction with antenatal care services ranged from 39.3% to 77.9%. Availability of hand-washing facility and toilet and health-care providers introducing themselves to their clients were areas of poor satisfaction among pregnant women. This finding is in line with the study conducted in Harare, Ethiopia [36].

7. Conclusions

In this study, the level of satisfaction with antenatal care services among pregnant women was low. Occupation, family size, mode of transportation, distance of home from health center, and having chronic diseases were factors associated with the level of satisfaction. Welcoming environment of health center starting from the gate, performance of procedures in a clean and safe manner, and the effort of health-care providers to involve clients in decision-making and asking concerns and interests were areas that pregnant women were highly satisfied with.

Based on the findings, the following recommendations are given to different bodies.

Health-care workers: Pregnant women whose family size is single need extensive and detail discussion. Thus, health-care workers have to discuss with them in detail. Additionally, pregnant women who are merchants need to receive care immediately.

Health centers: Adequate advice and counseling is needed for pregnant women who have a history of chronic diseases to decrease their stress due to the concomitant diseases. To make this feasible, health centers better prepare additional antenatal care rooms and deploy health-care workers who are experts in chronic diseases.

Governmental and non-governmental organizations: The most dissatisfying area of antennal care services is the unavailability of functional toilet and hand-washing facility. Thus, organizations should give attention to these facilities in every health-care center.

Researchers: The finding of the study will be strong if researchers use a mixed research method. Factors that are found in quantitative study will be explored in qualitative research methods.

Conflict of interest

This is the original work, and there is no form of competing interests of authors. And authors have agreed to the publication of this article.

Author details

Ayehu Kassaw Asres[1]* and Yirgalem Amogne[2]

1 Wollo University, College of Health Science, Department of Nursing, Dessie, Ethiopia

2 Addis Ababa University, College of Health Science, School of Nursing, Addis Ababa, Ethiopia

*Address all correspondence to: ayehu1213@gmail.com

References

[1] Chakravarti SU, Pai M, Kushtagi P. Holland and Brews Manual of Obstetrics E-book. Elsevier Health Sciences; 15 Oct 2015

[2] World Health Organization. WHO recommendations on antenatal care for a positive pregnancy experience: Summary: Highlights and key messages from the World Health Organization's 2016 global recommendations for routine antenatal care

[3] Phillips E, Stoltzfus RJ, Michaud L, Pierre GL, Vermeylen F, Pelletier D. Do mobile clinics provide high-quality antenatal care? A comparison of care delivery, knowledge outcomes and perception of quality of care between fixed and mobile clinics in central Haiti. BMC Pregnancy and Childbirth. Dec 2017;**17**(1):1

[4] Institute, E.P.H. Mini Demographic and Health Survey 2019. Addis Ababa, Ethiopia, and Calverton, Maryland, USA. 2019. Available from: http://www.moh.gov.et/ejcc/sites/default/files/Complete_KIR_EMDHS20Final.pdf [Accessed: December 14, 2019]

[5] Lincetto O, Mothebesoane-Anoh S, Gomez P, Munjanja S. Antenatal Care. Opportunities for Africa's Newborns: Practical Data, Policy and Programmatic Support for Newborn Care in Africa. 2006. pp. 55-62

[6] Nimi T et al. Prenatal care and pregnancy outcomes: A cross-sectional study in Luanda, Angola. International Journal of Gynecology & Obstetrics. 2016;**135**:S72-S78

[7] Morris BJ, Jahangir AA, Sethi MK. Patient satisfaction: An emerging health policy issue. American Academy of Orthopaedic Surgeons. 2013;**9**:29

[8] Lire T, Megerssa B, Asefa Y, Hirigo AT. Antenatal care service satisfaction and its associated factors among pregnant women in public health centres in Hawassa city, Southern Ethiopia. Proceedings of Singapore Healthcare. 2021;**1**:8

[9] Anikwe CC, Ifemelumma CC, Ekwedigwe KC, Ikeoha CC, Onwe OE, Nnadozie UU. Correlates of patients' satisfaction with antenatal care services in a tertiary hospital in Abakaliki, Ebonyi State, Nigeria. The Pan African Medical Journal. 2020;**37**:342

[10] World Health Organization. World health statistics 2016: Monitoring health for the SDGs sustainable development goals. WHO's annual compilation of health statistics for its 194 Member States. 8 Jun 2016

[11] Abou Zahr C, Wardlaw T. Antenatal Care in Developing Countries: Promises, Achievements and Missed Opportunities-An Analysis of Trends, Levels and Differentials, 1990-2001. 2003. p. 32

[12] Hildingsson I, Rådestad I. Swedish women's satisfaction with medical and emotional aspects of antenatal care. Journal of Advanced Nursing. 2005;**52**(3):239-249

[13] Rani M, Bonu S, Harvey S. Differentials in the quality of antenatal care in India. International Journal for Quality in Health Care. 2008;**20**(1):62-71

[14] Muchie KF. Quality of antenatal care services and completion of four or more antenatal care visits in Ethiopia: A finding based on a demographic and health survey. BMC Pregnancy and Childbirth. 2017;**17**(1):1-7

[15] Ejigu T, Woldie M, Kifle Y. Quality of antenatal care services at public health facilities of Bahir-Dar special zone, Northwest Ethiopia. BMC Health Services Research. 2013;**13**(1):1-8

[16] Mohammed AY, Wanamo TE, Wodera AL. Prevalence of antenatal care services satisfaction among mothers attending antenatal Care in Goba Hospital, bale zone, Oromia region, Southeast Ethiopia. Health Science Journal. 2021;**15**(7):1-8

[17] Alkema L et al. Global, regional, and national levels and trends in maternal mortality between 1990 and 2015, with scenario-based projections to 2030: A systematic analysis by the UN maternal mortality estimation inter-agency group. The Lancet. 2016;**387**(10017):462-474

[18] Oduse S, Zewotir T, North D. The impact of antenatal care on under-five mortality in Ethiopia: A difference-in-differences analysis. BMC Pregnancy and Childbirth. 2021;**21**(1):1-9

[19] Srivastava A et al. Determinants of women's satisfaction with maternal health care: A review of literature from developing countries. BMC Pregnancy and Childbirth. 2015;**15**(1):1-12

[20] Gudu W. Factors influencing antenatal care utilization in Ethiopia: A systematic review. Ethiopian Journal of Reproductive Health. 2018;**10**(3):29-33

[21] Lakew S, Ankala A, Jemal F. Determinants of client satisfaction to skilled antenatal care services at southwest of Ethiopia: A cross-sectional facility based survey. BMC Pregnancy and Childbirth. 2018;**18**(1):1-13

[22] Selgado MB, Dukele YH, Amamo DD. Determinants of focused antenatal care service satisfaction in public health facilities in Ethiopia 2018: A mixed study design. Journal of Public Health and Epidemiology. 2019;**11**(8):158-169

[23] Seyoum K. Determinants of antenatal care service satisfaction among women in ethiopia: A systematic review and meta-analysis. Obstetrics and Gynecology International. 13 Apr 2021;**2022**

[24] Tesfaye T, Mekonnen H, Negesa L. Maternal antenatal care service satisfaction and factors associated with rural health centers, Bursa District, Sidama zone, southern Ethiopia: A cross-sectional study. Journal of Women's Health Care. 2017;**6**(363):4-20

[25] Majrooh MA et al. Coverage and quality of antenatal care provided at primary health care facilities in the 'Punjab'province of 'Pakistan'. PLoS One. 2014;**9**(11):e113390

[26] Ghobashi M, Khandekar R. Satisfaction among expectant mothers with antenatal care services in the Musandam region of Oman. Sultan Qaboos University Medical Journal. 2008;**8**(3):325

[27] Pricilla RA et al. Satisfaction of antenatal mothers with the care provided by nurse-midwives in an urban secondary care unit. Journal of Family Medicine and Primary Care. 2016;**5**(2):420

[28] Rahman MM, Ngadan DP, Arif MT. Factors affecting satisfaction on antenatal care services in Sarawak, Malaysia: Evidence from a cross sectional study. Springerplus. 2016;**5**(1):1-6

[29] Al-Abedi GA. Identification of pregnant Women's satisfaction among antenatal health Care Services in Primary Health Care Centers at Al-Amara City/Iraq. Bahrain Medical Bulletin. 2021;**43**(2):492-493

[30] Hsai NM et al. Satisfaction of pregnant women with antenatal Care

Services at Women and Children Hospital in south Okkalapa, Myanmar: A facility-based cross-sectional study triangulated with qualitative study. Patient Preference and Adherence. 2020;**14**:2489

[31] Nwaeze I et al. Perception and satisfaction with quality of antenatal care services among pregnant women at the university college hospital, Ibadan, Nigeria. Annals of Ibadan Postgraduate Medicine. 2013;**11**(1):22-28

[32] Sufiyan M, Lawal S, Suleiman N. Client satisfaction with quality of antenatal care services among attendees of university health services medical center, Ahmadu Bello University Zaria, Kaduna state Nigeria. Journal of Medical and Basic Scientific Research. 2021;**2**(1):125-138

[33] Asafo AJ, Adoma DB. Determinants of women's perceived satisfaction on antenatal care in urban Ghana: A cross-sectional study. Clinical Journal of Obstetrics and Gynecology. 2019;**2**:38-52

[34] Tetui M, Ekirapa EK, Bua J, Mutebi A, Tweheyo R, Waiswa P. Quality of Antenatal care services in eastern Uganda: Implications for interventions. The Pan African Medical Journal. 2012;**13**:27

[35] Chemir F, Alemseged F, Workneh D. Satisfaction with focused antenatal care service and associated factors among pregnant women attending focused antenatal care at health centers in Jimma town, Jimma zone, south West Ethiopia; a facility based cross-sectional study triangulated with qualitative study. BMC Research Notes. 2014;**7**(1):1-8

[36] Birhanu S et al. Pregnant women's satisfaction with antenatal care services and its associated factors at public health facilities in the Harari region, Eastern Ethiopia. SAGE Open Medicine. 2020;**8**:2050312120973480

[37] Fseha B. Assessment of mothers level of satisfaction with antenatal care services provided at Alganesh health center Shire, North West Tigray, Ethiopia. Biomedical Journal of Scientific & Technical Research. 2019;**16**(1):11798-11802

[38] Kebede DB et al. Maternal satisfaction with antenatal care and associated factors among pregnant women in Hossana town. International Journal of Reproductive Medicine. 2020;**2020**:4-6

[39] Ayalew MM et al. Women's satisfaction and its associated factors with antenatal Care Services at Public Health Facilities: A cross-sectional study. International Journal of Women's Health. 2021;**13**:279

[40] Ejigu Tafere T, Afework MF, Yalew AW. Antenatal care service quality increases the odds of utilizing institutional delivery in Bahir Dar city administration, North Western Ethiopia: A prospective follow up study. PLoS One. 2018;**13**(2):e0192428

[41] Sufiyan M, Umar A, Shugaba A. Client satisfaction with antenatal Care Services in Primary Health Care Centres in Sabon Gari local government area, Kaduna state Nigeria. Journal of Community Medicine and Primary Health Care. 2013;**25**(1):12-22

[42] Seyoum T, Alemayehu M, Christensson K, Lindgren H. Client factors affect provider adherence to guidelines during first antenatal care in public health facilities, Ethiopia: A multi-center cross-sectional study. Ethiopian Journal of Health Sciences. 2020;**30**(6):903

[43] Debela EB. An overview of squatter settlements in addis ababa, Ethiopia. Journal of Governance and Development. 31 Jul 2021;**17**(2):77-101

Chapter 8

Pioneers against Stigma: Access to Family Planning in the Caribbean

Tonia Frame, Patricia Sheerattan-Bisnauth, Yvette Delph and Fred Nunes

Abstract

In the English-speaking Caribbean, internationally-funded local NGOs pioneered the introduction of family planning, a game-changer in women's empowerment, ensuring access to women who cannot afford private physicians. These NGOs faced social controversy and cleared the space for governments to introduce the service in primary care clinics. As governments have cautiously stepped into this space, Family Planning Associations have lost clientele and not benefitted from significant government contributions. After 50 years, they remain fragile and dependent on foreign funds. They have been buffeted by the winds of the US Gag Rule, the COVID-19 pandemic, and the drive from IPPF to provide more comprehensive services, including abortion. Small size and stigma are obstacles to attracting high quality board members, and grant reductions make staff salaries unattractive to skilled professionals. The purpose of the paper is to explore the history, growth, gender bias, and the struggles for sustainability among family planning associations across the Caribbean region.

Keywords: NGOs, pioneers, stigma, family planning, sustainability, Caribbean

1. Introduction

The story of family planning in the Caribbean is a fascinating one of several faces and phases. What started as independent, indigenous activism is more than 50 years later a charity industry still mired in dependency on international funding. In our colonial period, members of the middle- and upper-classes pioneered the drive for social service and social change by attacking stigma. Today the charity industry has matured. In the era of national independence, the new leaders no longer challenge the status quo. They are the status quo. They have become so conservative that they sometimes resist advances of inclusion, equity, and service. In some instances, they have become the captive of religious forces hostile to their core mission, while others ride on Boards to extract social status. Across the region, the exceptions to this pitiful tale can be counted on one hand.

2. Women step forward

In Jamaica—as early as 1937—two Jamaican women, May Farquharson, a social worker and Amy Bailey, a social worker, educator and women's rights activist, started working to improve women's and children's lives. They created the Save the Children Fund, Mother's Welfare Clinic, and in 1939 established the Jamaica Birth Control League (JBCL). The goal of the JBCL was to advance women's social and economic welfare through birth control and to win government's support for their programme. Farquharson, who had studied in the UK and the US developed strong links with activists on both sides of the Atlantic: Vera Houghton in the United Kingdom (UK) and Margaret Sanger in the United States (US), both of whom were associated with the eugenics movement. It was no surprise then, that the JBCL ran into strong opposition from the Catholic Church, Marcus Garvey's Universal Negro Improvement Association and, expediently, the Jamaica Labour Party. Bailey pushed back forcefully against the notion that birth control was a plan to kill or limit Black people and argued instead that birth control would advance their social and economic wellbeing [1].

Two other Jamaicans, Lenworth Jacobs, a physician and his wife, Beth Jacobs, also saw the rapid birth rate and the need for women to have the means to control their childbearing, reach broader audiences, and more community integration. This led to the opening of the Beth Jacobs Clinic from 1939 to 1967 in St. Ann's [1]. So once again, the focus on population control was at least equal to the concern for women's control. By 1957, the JBCL and the Beth Jacobs' clinic merged, forming the Jamaica Family Planning Association, becoming the eighth member of IPPF. Believing that family planning should not be the sole province of a charitable organization, they promoted family planning as integral to the government's services. This led to a series of efforts at integration with and separation from primary care over various political regimes [1].

In Grenada, Helen Saftel, an expatriate from the United States of America and a member of a birth control organization in Boston recognized that birth control was a problem in Grenada. In an interview with a former Executive Director of the Grenada Planned Parenthood Association (GPPA), it was reported that "Saftel influenced a diverse group of professionals and privileged lay people to develop an NGO to support birth control for women." Helen Saftel convinced retired Chief Justice of the Windward and Leeward Islands to help organize a committee and chair the Association. Together, in 1964, they formed the Grenada Planned Parenthood Association (GPPA). They sought help to prepare committee members for their first meeting from those connected to family planning in Barbados, such as Lady Grace Thorne Adams, Sir Aubrey Gordon Leacock, known as 'Jack', and Mr. Clyde Gollop [2]. In April of that same year, on their way to the Western Hemisphere Conference on Planned Parenthood, Helen and her husband met Sir Colville Deverell, former Governor of World Planned Parenthood who provided US $2000.00 to the GPPA. In February 1964 Grenada became a member affiliate of IPPF [2]. At that time, family planning services were not being offered by the Government of Grenada, but most of the community health nurses referred women to the GPPA for family planning services. In an interview with first author, TF, a senior nurse at the time recalled (Best S 2023, personal communication, Jan 22), there was no real objection from the Ministry of Health, but some doctors and nurses objected or at least objected to the use of methods such as the intrauterine contraceptive device (IUCD) and Depo-Provera [3]. The main opposition came from the religious sector, specifically the Catholic Church on grounds of morality. She described the government's support for family planning as being driven by the need to promote child health. The focus was pediatric - on the child rather than the mother. There was less concern with poor women and more interest in providing for the nutritional and educational needs of their children in an effort to address high infant mortality [3].

In 1966, all on her own, Theresa Louisy, a registered nurse in St. Lucia saw the high birth rate and malnutrition in her rural community, Bexon. She contacted the Chief Medical Officer, John Gibling and together, they started family planning in St. Lucia. In 1967, they commenced information and education programs, and individual counseling in rural areas. With her husband Raymond Louisy, they engaged in public education called *Market Steps* to reach new communities. In 1968, St. Lucia Planned Parenthood Association (SLPPA) sought Associate Membership in IPPF. Although Mrs. Louisy led the SLPPA, it was Raymond Louisy, her husband, who became the Executive Director at that time. Almost 30 years later, in 1996, the first woman, Mrs. Audrey George became Executive Director of SLPPA [4]. SLPPA remains the only non-governmental organization offering SRH services on the island.

The story was similar in Guyana. Olga Byrne, a Trinidadian by birth who migrated to Guyana, was a teacher who organized her colleagues, expanding access to education, adult suffrage, and family planning. Byrne was a pioneer in breaking the glass ceiling by becoming the first female President of the Guyana Teachers Union in 1961; she also led the Women's League of Social Services and the International Alliance of Women (IAW). While her focus was on women, she appreciated the need to develop boys, hence the youth centre in her name for training in joinery, masonry, and welding. She contended that there was little point in women having the right to vote if they could not control their own bodies. Again, a woman of privilege using her status to help the poor. Her work leading the Women's League of Social Services gave birth to the Guyana Responsible Parenthood Association (GRPA) in 1973. The GRPA was rooted in concern with, "fostering better family life and not with contraception" [5]. The Association received funding from IPPF in 1974 and through membership in the Caribbean Family Planning Affiliation (CFPA) became a member affiliate of IPPF [6].

Essentially, across the Caribbean, the initial thrust for family planning and women's reproductive health advocacy and services was home-grown. It was largely the work of privileged middle and upper-class women who leveraged their social status and social connections to advocate for services primarily for the poorer members of their societies. In doing so, they were venturing into an arena of controversy scarred by religious dogma (St. Lucia, Guyana, Jamaica, Barbados, Grenada), disfigured by racial tension (Jamaica, Guyana), and torn by partisan opportunism (Jamaica, Antigua). It was an area spurned by private business primarily because of the controversy. Any profitability was certainly not worth the noise. With few exceptions, Caribbean businesses were still largely family owned. So, they were more sensitive to community pressure. Family planning associations (FPAs) were in a field that was at best unpopular and unprofitable. While private businesses avoided the area, governments were even more circumspect. They either stayed away or offered arms-length support. They outsourced a fundamental health service to NGOs. It is into this void that courageous women stepped and stood ever so boldly. We agree with Bourbonnais' that despite their pivotal role in the international birth control movement in the 1950s, FPAs in the Caribbean, such as Barbados, Trinidad, and Jamaica, are yet to receive due recognition [7].

3. From passion to professionalism

Passion and professionalism are not incompatible. In the best circumstances they make wonderful companions and yield great benefits. But this is not always the case. As FPAs bodies joined the IPPF, there was a gradual shift from the passionate volunteerism through which clinical services were made available in the early days to more settled operations based on paid employees. Inevitably and entirely understandably, with funding from IPPF, there came an ever-increasing need for accountability—reports and performance standards. How well these standards were adjusted to small island developing states (SIDS) is an important issue, but not one within the scope of this chapter. One example will suffice. The cost of an external audit is considerable and in some cases in small countries could amount to a third of the budget. That is onerous. Another major challenge is that volunteerism remains the mechanism through which governance of FPAs occurs, even today. In small societies with very small professional classes, the pool from which one can attract volunteers is quite limited. From our observation, this has had a tremendous negative impact on the growth and operation of associations in small poor countries, like those in the Caribbean.

Even greater than the remarkable contribution to the dramatic decline in birth rates, we contend that the real and lasting success of the associations in the Caribbean is that they persisted. They did not bend to the noise of the church, politicians, or quite commonly, the sensationalism of the media. For example, in 1977 the news that there was a plan to train a few doctors in Antigua in vasectomies resulted in quite a brouhaha [8]. In Trinidad and Tobago, many Roman Catholic officials mounted opposition to Dr. Eric Williams' People's National Movement (PNM) at the 1956 general election, on the grounds that the party supported birth control. This forced the PNM's denial of the party's official position in lieu of the statement that "birth control was a private matter for private decision rather than government policy" ([9] p. 5). According to Bourbonnais [7], Sir Grantley Adams, at the time, the Premier of Barbados and an ardent advocate for family planning and Barbados' global leadership in family planning was under attack by the politicians at home and across the region, led by the Roman Catholic Church, as illustrated below:

> *'our embryo Prime Minister would begin his Federal term without the blessing of the Christian church. What a sickening thought?' (Secretary of Bustamatne's JLP [Jamaica Labor Party] p. 272]*
>
> *'Birth control is for the white man, not for the black man.' (Premier of Antigua Vere Bird) [p. 272]*

The fact is that there was a great demand from women wanting to control their fertility, even before the rise of the family planning movement in some countries. Bourbonnais quotes a 38 year old domestic worker in 1956 Trinidad who stated, "We, the several young women of the community, have been practicing birth control in Trinidad long before Little Eric came on the scene." ([7], p. 272). Historically, the English-speaking Caribbean countries did not experience very high fertility levels as measured by crude birth rates, however, between 1950 and 1960 crude birth rates increased, somewhat representing a baby boom. Nonetheless, between 1960 and 1965 the rates remained fairly stable with a downward trend [10]. Except for a brief period at the outset, when the passion was still there, most FPAs assumed a quite passive posture. They waited for clients to arrive at their doors. Charismatic advocates like Raymond Louisy in St. Lucia, Beth and Lenworth Jacobs in Jamaica, and Clyde Gollop in Barbados, who walked the streets and played dominoes in police stations, soon vanished and were replaced by largely office-bound technicians. Those larger-than-life entrepreneurs were usually replaced by timid administrators.[1]

Still the associations stayed the course, local advocates applied constant pressure on officials and in doing so, normalized reproductive health services amidst the changing social and political dynamic of the region [7]. They made contraception such a routine component of women's health that the very governments that were hands-off in the 1950s would later begin to provide family planning services in their primary care clinics. Herbert Eldemire, a physician, was Jamaica's first Minister of Health after independence in 1962. After years of pressure from JFPA, he threatened to demit office unless his Ministry was allowed to announce its support of family planning. His coercion worked and he created birth control clinics at hospitals and primary health care facilities. The Ministry also created a Family Planning Unit within the Ministry in 1966, and the National Family Planning Board (NFPB) in 1968 [1]. This is undoubtedly the major accomplishment of the pioneers: they vanquished the stigma of contraception sufficient to win strong partnerships in government.

Of course, this very success would haunt the associations. Potential clients could obtain services for free at public health clinics. While this was good news for the society, it inevitably signaled a measure of competition for the associations whose market was depleted. The ultimate goal of associations was ensuring women's access to family planning services, and so they found ways to adapt to this changing context. In Jamaica, for example, JFPA continued to work alongside and with the government in promoting birth control, and Dr. Lenworth Jacobs of the Beth Jacobs Clinic and the JFPA became the first Director of the NFPB [1]. With very few exceptions, Caribbean governments did not readily see the value of contributing to the livelihood of the associations. In Barbados, due to vehement political opposition internal and external to his party (Barbados Labour Party), Sir Grantley Adams, in 1955 refused initiating a government-run wide-scale birth control program, but instead provided a government grant of 5000 Barbados dollars to the BFPA and allowed operations out of maternity hospitals and government health centers, increasing it to $12,000 in 1956 and to $20,000 by 1959. Governments of Jamaica (1966) and Trinidad (1967) later provided financial support [7].

The idea of integrated reproductive health services is attractive. Although there are different approaches to integration [11], it was generally viewed as providing a more convenient one-stop service for clients. But this form of integration often proved difficult at the clinic level. Working together in a single clinic there were significant differences in salaries of nurses with the same qualifications, one working with the association the other with the government. Typically the public employees were better paid, with more security and benefits. Pharmacists would struggle to fill prescriptions depending on whether drugs were available from one channel or another. Some felt that integration was the best way to serve the client, others contended that integration depleted family planning. Jamaica went back and forth—swinging between, integrating, separating and back again [1]. In some countries the commitment to integration was frustrated by funding. Governments were unable

---

[1] A stark example of this passivity is evident in an unpublished analysis by Fred Nunes, Yvette Delph, Dane Abbott, and Sheila Roseau of new acceptors in one FPA from Jan- Dec 2006. As many as 80% of the new acceptors joined after their first pregnancy. They were joining to delay their next pregnancy and for many to end childbearing rather than to plan it. Even more indicative of the Associations passivity is the fact that no client joined because of outreach from the association. Some 75% were influenced by their social network; only 15% reported being influenced by a health worker and less than 5% by a doctor.

to provide the budget for contraceptives. So, the service gradually reverted to the associations by default; one example of this is Dominica.

But there was more to be done. The hostility to unwed pregnancy persisted. Unwed mothers lost their jobs. High adolescent birth rates (ABR) persisted, declining at a much slower rate than other age groups [10], and pregnant teenagers were expelled from school. All the while the men involved in these pregnancies remained untouched and invisible. Lacking data, associations persist in a focus on teenagers to reduce teenage pregnancy. That is a focus on the vulnerable. Some 77% of teenage pregnancies result from relationships with men 20 years and older and 56% with men 20–24 [12]. The focus should be on young men. But FPAs have been generally timid about outreach to men. They have lived within the mistaken notion that Caribbean men have a cultural resistance to vasectomy when their own evidence shows no basis for that view [13].

In the broader society, the Caribbean has experienced a major shift in religious affiliation. In the 1960s the 'established' churches typically formed the Council of Churches, Anglican, Methodist, and Roman Catholic, who were routinely consulted by governments. By the 1980s, Associations of Evangelical Churches had emerged with at least equal voice—Baptist, Pentecostal, Seventh Day Adventist, Independent—and far more energy. In an interview with the fourth author, FN, in December 2020, one observer stated, "In the early 70s as a student at UWI [Jamaica], the Intervarsity Christian Fellowship (IVCF) was little more than a handful; by 2000 it was the dominant group." Some of these evangelical groups have benefited from substantial funding from their counterparts in the US. The growth of this religious right would represent a major challenge to associations in the face of IPPF policies.

Within the associations two challenges emerged as they matured. First, the passion of volunteerism was gradually replaced by employed professional staff. Second, once contraceptive service had become a widely accepted norm, associations became status conferring organizations rather than pioneers fighting stigma. The first transition for staff meant that a more contractual relationship replaced volunteerism. Services were delivered from paid staff. The alignment with the mission was no longer the primary driving force. For some of the staff it was economic; employment was mere livelihood. There was the problem of staff retention as the salary packages and recruitment policies were often inadequate to attract and retain suitable staff. In more than a few cases, staff members successfully sued the associations for considerable sums. The fact that the associations were successfully sued also exposed real deficiencies in governance. This takes us to the second transition, voluntarism at the Board level. In far too many cases, board members were no longer attracted to serve a mission that involved taking risks and lending their status and influence in a battle for social justice. Quite the opposite: Some members were climbing on to an established, recognized, reputable charity to extract status and enrich their résumés. Sadly some board members were focused on status and extraction—what's in it for me (WIIFM). It is not surprising that the boards were suboptimal if not downright dysfunctional in their governance and oversight mandate, and their ability to collaborate with management for the sustainability of the associations. Over the years, this has resulted in an absence of accountability, poor performance and closure of some FPAs, as resulted in Grenada between 2019 and 2021 [14].

4. International push and pull

Being a small island developing state is one thing. Being a small region in the shadow of a dominant world power is another, which makes the old adage fitting—"when the US sneezes, the Caribbean gets pneumonia." Of course, US foreign policy on family planning, known as the Mexico City Policy (MCP) and referred to as the Global Gag Rule (GGR) is like a windscreen wiper. It flips from one extreme to another with each change of political regime resulting in consequences for the Caribbean and globally [15, 16].

In the 2020s, it will be interesting to see how the wave of White, male supremacy in the US manifests itself in our predominantly Black region. Only a few days after the leak of Justice Alito's draft US Supreme Court decision that would vanquish 50 years of women's right-to-choice, the Rev. Dr. Hensworth Jonas, Presiding Elder of the Eastern Caribbean Baptist Mission, was gloating in the media. In a television interview, he made the most bizarre statement in saying why abortion should not be allowed in any circumstance whatsoever, not even for rape: "If women want to be pro-choice, they should choose well about their sexuality. Don't choose abortion to cover up your sin. Basically, a woman's choice should be not to conceive children" [17]. This was his bizarre, uncompromising statement in a region where a substantial proportion of women's first sexual experiences are coerced—not of their choosing. For example, studies on the prevalence of partner and not-intimate partner violence among women in the Caribbean show that among respondents 25% of women in Grenada, 30% of women in Guyana, and 32.3% of women in Jamaica reported being coerced, going along or forced to have sex at sexual debut. Sexual debut in the Caribbean is reported to start early, with 10.9% in Grenada and 13.7% in Jamaica of respondents reporting sexual debut before age 15. In Jamaica 7.7% and 10% of women, and in Grenada 9.5% and 10% of women had in their lifetime, experienced sexual violence by their male partner and a non-partner, respectively [18–20].

The tiny Caribbean basin is home to every shade of abortion law in the world—all six stages from total prohibition to fulsome choice. Half of the 10 countries in the world that have total abortion bans are in the Caribbean basin [21]. What is even more ironic is the colonial contradiction of The Netherlands Antilles which holds fast to a total ban as against The Netherlands which provides with complete access. Frankly pathetic.

The Kissinger Report (1974) is a clear example of the relationship between US political power and population policy [22]. The report, which was confidential until the 1990s, aimed to protect US, military and business interests by controlling population growth in poor countries. Known as National Security Study Memorandum (NSSM) 200, the policy proposed to constrain political power in poor countries so US business could more easily extract resources. The report reasoned that by restricting population growth, the risk of restless, anti-establishment youth, hostile to America and prone to communism would be minimized. The Study Memorandum became a Decision Memorandum under President Richard Nixon. The policy rested on four ugly pillars: [22].

1. Population growth in poor countries threatens US political power

2. The US needs poor countries to remain poor so it can extract resources

3. High birth rates yield younger populations more likely to be anti-establishment

4. American business will be threatened by governments that need to provide for growing populations

In practice, the policy was driven through the United States Agency for International Aid (USAID), by funding United Nations (UN) programmes, and by influence on national leaders. It is little wonder that even in the 1970s, persons seeing the strong USAID support for family planning across the Caribbean—although it was not listed in the 13 target countries mentioned in the Kissinger Report—were ambivalent about this new-found US interest.

Of course, Vatican II, had concluded only a few years earlier in 1966, and 2 years later in July. Pope Paul VI issued his encyclical, Humanae Vitae, declaring the church's opposition to artificial birth control and its absolute condemnation of abortion and sterilization, for the promotion of natural family planning (NFP) [23]. The stage was set for a conflict between the US National Bishops Conference and the US population policy.

Stephen Mumford has documented how rapidly the Catholic Bishops responded to the US Supreme Court's decision in 1973 (Roe v Wade) making abortion legal and NSSM 200 [22]. By 1975 the bishops had issued a Pastoral Plan for Pro-life Activities. It was a remarkably strategic document that in great detail set out how the church would finance, organize, lobby and infiltrate every level of political activity. And they did. They were persistent and relentless and, finally, in 2022, they had gained such control over the US Supreme court, that they won.

Perhaps no US policy has more directly and immediately affected the conduct of reproductive health services in the world than the Mexico City Policy, also known as the "Global Gag Rule" [24]. At first, this policy merely applied to US funds and required any NGOs receiving funds from the US to declare that they were not actively promoting or providing abortion services using US Government funding. In nearly 40 years since President Ronald Reagan introduced it in 1984, it has been enforced for 21 years [24]. But the most aggressive use was under Republican President Donald Trump from 2017 to 2021. His administration expanded it to apply to NGOs receiving funds from any source, including non-US funds and their own funds—not just US funds. Even worse, Trump extended this to programmes with no link to family planning, such as malaria and nutrition [15, 24]. Basically saying to the international community: You want my money? Then you swallow my values. Not the values of the American people, but the values of the Republican Party. An ironic anecdote exposes the unique features of the Caribbean. The late Dr. Ivor Heath of Antigua, recounted how, under the hammer of the Gag Rule, a colleague in the USVI called him, "We know you can't do them over there, just send them to us". Predictably, as history has shown, Democratic President Joe Biden reversed the Gag Rule as one of his first acts [24].

The 1990s was a period of intense international meetings of population and reproductive health and rights. In addition to several rounds of preparatory UN meetings there was the International Conference on Population and Development and Programme of Action in Cairo in 1994, the 1995 Beijing Declaration and Platform for Action, and of course Cairo+5 and Beijing+5 [25]. These meetings provided platforms for government and non-government representatives and organizations to explore the leading edge of provisions to ensure women's equality. They equally offered space for conservative groups to block those negotiations. A distinct minority of conservative states and their NGOs sought to thwart the negotiations at every turn. They were invariably assisted by the US which recorded reservations on several matters [25]. When it became clear that a small group might impede progressive positions from reaching the Group of 77 (G-77), a group of Some Latin American Countries (SLAC) emerged. They faced intense pressure from the Vatican. Soon, 14 Caribbean CARICOM countries joined this group which then became SLACC. The group worked with India, and countries in East and West Africa to advance a progressive women's rights agenda.

The Montevideo Consensus on Population and Development in the Caribbean and the preparatory meetings that preceded it, were yet another round of government and non-governmental meetings [26]. They were designed to assess the region's accomplishments since Cairo, set new targets and confirm commitment to the wide scope of social goals. Governments adopted more than 100 "priority areas" on a very broad range of topics – sexual and reproductive health, comprehensive, rights-based sexuality education for young people, provision of SRH services including contraceptive methods for adolescents, gender equality, population planning, aging, indigenous peoples, and so on [26]. The Caribbean is known for ratifying conventions and then walking away from those obligations. There are good reasons why this happens so easily.

These platforms were spaces in which Caribbean advocates displayed their passion, intellect, negotiating skill, discipline, and commitment to the mission of women's human rights. In these international meetings, they were calm, forthright and unambivalent. Yet, once back at home in their small countries, most of these very same vociferous advocates were seldom visible. The international platforms were a safe space, free of the risks and costs of speaking up. For example, in 2000, the fourth author, FN, attempted to recruit an advocate in Trinidad to join Advocates for Safe Parenthood: Improving Reproductive Equity (ASPIRE), one advocate explained, "My child goes to an excellent Catholic school. This is no time for me to jeopardize my child's education" [27].

Democracy is a good deal more than ceremonial signing of documents. Those documents have little or no meaning without a culture of accountability, which requires constant vigilance by civil society [28]. Based on our observations, in the Caribbean, there is precious little sustained noise from non-governmental organizations to hold the government accountable. Governments are not under any real public scrutiny. NGO's typically lack the resources [29] for research, so they seldom have the data essential for meaningful dialog. Therefore, in practice then, "sovereignty" becomes one party's five or so years to do as they please. Then it's either more time or another party's turn. Democracy in form, but not in substance. While small scale offers the advantage of familiarity, small scale also means easy visibility and little opportunity for the social distance that anonymity provides in larger societies. Therefore, making it hard to find allies and harder for individuals to speak up, especially so in respect of controversial and stigmatized issues.

Two major global health phenomena also left their footprint on FPAs—HIV/and AIDS, and COVID-19. The first recorded HIV/AIDS case in the Caribbean was in Haiti in 1979 [30]. Initially the disease spread among homosexual contact with bisexual males, but by the early 80s the spread was mostly by heterosexual males. This was evident throughout the region, and gradually more women became infected than men. HIV/AIDS became the leading cause of death among adults 15–44. Today the Caribbean still has the second highest prevalence of HIV/AIDS in the world; only Sub-Saharan Africa is higher [31, 32]. By the mid-1980s the disease was spread more widely among heterosexuals and, gradually in the Caribbean, more women became infected than men. HIV/AIDS became the leading cause of death among adults 15–44.

During this crisis of stigma, poverty, and sex tourism, it was the Medical Association that took the lead in Barbados. Through leadership from Professor Errol "Mikey" Walrond, Barbados became only the second country in the world to start testing blood donations for HIV. The US poured funds into the region and supported condom use. The Pan Caribbean Partnership Against HIV and AIDS (PANCAP) was established by a Declaration of CARICOM Heads of Government to support the region's response to the threat of HIV [33]. In Jamaica, there was a massive increase in condom use, largely as a result of government promotion. The same was true in Barbados. In fact, the barbados family planning association (BFPA) was not happy with the focus on condoms because it had invested heavily in more reliable methods—injections and IUDs—and saw the condom drive as undermining its hard work. Preservation of gains took precedence over the opportunity to meet a new social need.

The impact of COVID-19 was quite different. It was indirect and economic. Caribbean economies rely on tourism, with between one third and half of the gross domestic product (GDP) of The Bahamas, Barbados and Jamaica being derived from tourism [34]. When travel shrinks by 75% the impact is devastating. And when the only available approach for month after month is strict masking or staying at home or both, similar to other businesses [34], FPAs shuddered under the shrinkage of demand for services. In an interview with the Caribbean Family Planning Affiliation (CFPA) in January 2023, it was stated that "the shrinkage in service demand due to fear of COVID-19 meant a sharp drop in revenue for FPAs. Notwithstanding, supply chain challenges resulted in low contraceptive supply to meet the already low demand. Notably, in some countries family planning and SRH services were not deemed as part of the essential health services, and family planning health care providers were reassigned as part of the COVID-19 response teams." Anecdotal evidence from some FPAs indicated that during the pandemic, some women were engaging in self-harm practices to end unwanted pregnancies due to lack of access to contraceptives. Recognizing the negative impact of the COVD-19 pandemic on SRHR, CFPA together with international donor agencies, such as the United Nations Population Fund (UNFPA) [35] advocated for governments in the region to include SRH care and family planning as essential health services.

Stresses are seldom isolated. Along with the COVID-19 pandemic came the tumultuous internal conflict in IPPF [36, 37]. Allegations of fraud in London resulted in friction between London and WHR New York. That friction resulted in Caribbean countries being faced with a choice—London or New York. Typical of the region, we could not find a common position and so some chose to stay with WHR and others went with IPPF (London). IPPF then created the Americas and Caribbean Regional Office (ACRO) to work in the region and a separate office of ACRO in Trinidad to focus on the Caribbean.

Finally, the Russian invasion of Ukraine and European support for Ukraine seemed to signal a sudden and major shift of resources away from family planning and away from the Caribbean. The alarm clanged when IPPF shared the likelihood of this prospect. This time it was not simply the colossus to our north whose sneeze would cause our pneumonia. This time it threatened to be global. The Caribbean was utterly unprepared. There were anxious moments of concern for finding other sources of funds, especially at the level of national and regional governments. But as the threat subsided and the normal flow of funds resumed, the feverish interest in the initiative to be more self-reliant faded away.

5. Impact

Notwithstanding the wretched problems of governance that have plagued many FPAs in the region, their pioneering action created the space for making contraception and more broadly sexual and reproductive health acceptable. Nonetheless, the journey for sexual rights remains. The net result is that while some associations suffered debilitating problems of governance, several governments, private medical practitioners and private pharmacies provided contraceptive services. The real impact of the FPAs cannot be measured merely in the number of services or the number of advocacy events they conducted. Their far greater value was creating the social space for other actors, including non-governmental organizations (NGOs), government and private sector. They established family planning as a central and acceptable component of health care. Using fertility data from The World Bank Databank [38], **Figure 1** shows the fertility rates at 10 year intervals from 1950 to 2020 in select countries in the Caribbean region. The decline in fertility rates, starting in the 1960s, are inseparable from the path-breaking work of the FPAs. Indeed, such is the normalization of family planning that it is not easy to recall the measure of hostility and opposition the pioneers faced.

This success was so dramatic that in some cases it turned against the service. In Jamaica, a former Senior Medical Officer at Victoria Jubilee Hospital (VJH), recounted that when he started there in 1972, "We were doing 16,000 plus deliveries per year. By 2000, we were barely doing 7000. So, by the time I took over, we were no longer focused on family planning. Instead, I concentrated on modernizing obstetric and gynecological services. In fact we closed the family planning service at VJH and converted that room into a dental clinic."

Although the name had changed from birth control to family planning, the appreciation of reproductive health had not yet taken root. Even in sophisticated medical circles, family planning was still linked to population control. The HIV pandemic was a catalyst in the shift from family planning to sexual and reproductive health, and the International Conference on Population and Development (ICPD, 1994) in Cairo reiterated the expansion of family planning beyond mere contraceptive services to sexual and reproductive health—education, prevention and treatment of HIV, other

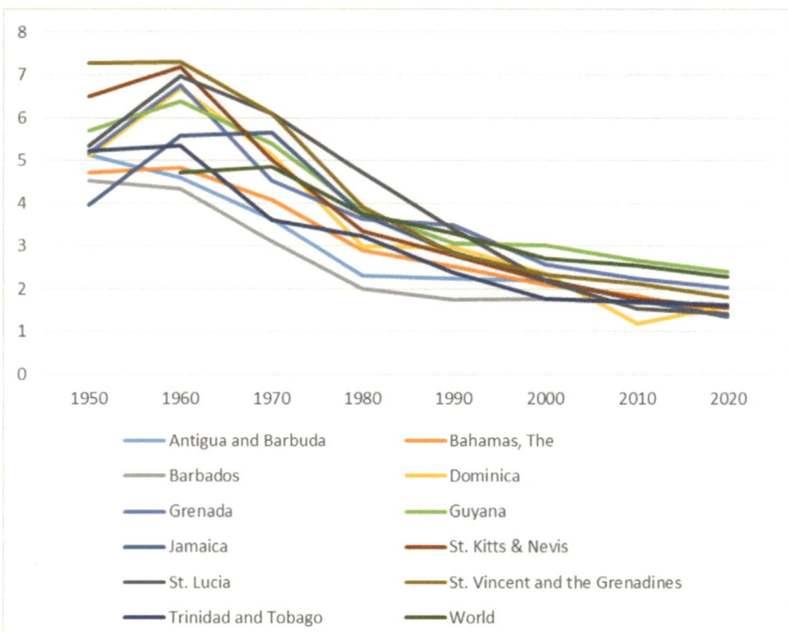

Figure 1.
Fertility rates in select Caribbean countries for 1950–2020.

STIs, and reproductive cancers, gender equity, intimate partner violence, safe pregnancy, and safe abortion in a right-based environment free of coercion, discrimination and violence [39].

5.1 Abortion law reform and services

In 1980, Belize modified its Offenses Against the Person Act to provide for a wide range of exceptions, including the expansion of legal access to abortion [40]. The changes not only codified Bourne [41], making provisions for protection of the woman's physical and mental health, but they also allowed abortion where the child was likely to be born with severe mental and physical abnormalities. Further, in assessing the impact on the woman's health, it allowed consideration of her actual and foreseeable social and economic circumstances [40]. We had expected that this remarkable advance, 3 years before the Medical Termination of Pregnancy Act in Barbados (1983), was the result of women's activism and pressure from the Belize Family Life Association (BFLA). Not so. In fact, there was no public discussion whatsoever.

On the verge of independence, 1981, with the threat of invasion from Guatemala, British Harrier jets flying overhead and an intense political campaign for general elections in December, the Criminal Code was revised without a whisper. The Attorney General, Said Musa, contracted Professor Nicholas Liverpool in the Faculty of Law at the University of the West Indies in Cave Hill, to review the Criminal Code. He did. It is his revisions that appear in the law. The Code was passed without discussion along with 10 other bills presented to the House in November 1980 [42]. This significant advance in women's health occurred without so much as a murmur. In 1980, Belize was 62% Roman Catholic. Given that process, it is little wonder that in 2023 there is almost no public knowledge of this level of legal access to abortion in Belize.

We should pause to describe the landmark Bourne UK case [40] since it also bears witness to courage and a focus on women's health, but not on women's rights. Aleck Bourne was a distinguished Harley Street surgeon. Parents asked him to perform an abortion on their 14-year-old girl who had been raped by five officers of the Royal Horse Guards. He examined her and satisfied himself that she was sufficiently well developed to bear the child. He nevertheless, performed the abortion. He then called the Chief Constable, reported his action and was promptly arrested. At the Old Bailey, his defense was that he could not distinguish between a woman's life and her health and that if the child had been forced to carry the pregnancy, it would have made her a "mental wreck." Justice Macnaghten advised the jury that life includes physical and mental health. Bourne was acquited [41]. This decision has been upheld in every Commonwealth jurisdiction in which it has been tested—Canada, Australia, and so on. While it has not been tested in any Caribbean country, Attorneys General in several Caribbean countries felt it would be upheld [43]. Bourne was not what we would call pro-choice. In fact, he opposed the 1967 Abortion Act in the UK which he considered too liberal. He favored doctors making decisions on therapeutic grounds, not women exercising their choice.

The process of law reform in Barbados was almost an exercise in stealth. Billie Miller, Minister of Health and the first woman to serve in the Cabinet of Barbados, quietly met with religious leaders and shared the facts of the harm of unsafe abortions with them. Meeting with them one-on-one, she explained the social reality and the damage poor women faced because of a law that did not in any way restrict others from obtaining safe abortions, whether from local doctors or by travel abroad. She defused the religious opposition [44]. Once again, it is not clear that the Barbados Family

Planning Association was at the forefront of this major advance in reproductive health, even though Miller had been a member of the Board and President of WHR.

In 2013, under new leadership, GRPA showed itself as an exception to this trend of withdrawal. Although Guyana's 1995 abortion law made provision for mid-level providers to perform early non-surgical abortions, no action had been taken to put this in practice. GRPA organized a workshop for midlevel providers and invited Women on Waves and Family Planning Association of Guyana (FPAG) to conduct the training. The Chief Medical Officer and the Attorney General claimed that the workshop was illegal. FPAG went to court to seek its interpretation of the clause and GRPA was an equal partner in that action. In 2016, the court ruled unequivocally in favor of the associations [45]. Allowing mid-level health professionals to provide medication abortion is important generally. It eliminates the sole reliance on doctors, removes the focus on hospitals, and radically shifts the gender of providers to women. In a large country like Guyana, with 20 percent of the population sparsely spread over a vast hinterland with very few doctors, provision of abortion services by mid-level health professions makes a world of difference for access.

Twenty years earlier, in the early 1970s, there was also a moment of real excitement in Jamaica. Kenneth McNeil, as Minister of Health was a former medical officer at VJH. He had seen at first hand the horrible conditions in which poor women arrived on the "abortion ward" or "slip and fall ward". These women could not afford doctors, but had nevertheless sought help to end their unplanned and unwanted pregnancies. The Minister for Health attempted to persuade the Cabinet to change the law [46]. When that failed, he worked with other doctors in his Ministry, notably Dr. Wynante Patterson, and Dr. Deanna Ashley to establish the Glen Vincent Clinic (GVC), a clinic that would provide abortion services. The guidelines for the GCV were carefully sculpted by Gloria Cumper—a barrister and social reformer, and Dr. Ashley. They were carefully constructed and included rape, statutory rape, referrals from the Family Court, and failed contraception (supported by her clinic record). There were provisions for Tubal Ligations (TL) following counseling [47]. Of course, once the clinic opened, the guidelines were employed with sensible elasticity. They are still used today almost 50 years later by private physicians referring patients to providers "in order to give them some legal cover." The GVC operated from 1976 to 96. It is unclear why it stopped providing abortions. Certainly, one difficulty was recruiting a doctor to replace the one who had functioned there for two decades, performing services and teaching colleagues.

The GVC's impact is only known through anecdotes. In an interview with the fourth author, FN, in 1993, the late Professor Hugh Wynter wryly remarked that the establishment of the clinic "created problems for me. Before '76 I had all the septic cases I could want. Once the clinic was established, I had problems. How could I teach my students to manage septic cases when there were none?" [48] Professor Wynter, who had recommended the physician who served there for almost its entire existence, was pleased at the service of the GVC. Wynter's experience at the University Hospital of the West Indies was fully corroborated by Dr. Douglas McDonald, former Senior Medical Officer at VJH in an interview with FN in 2022. According to McDonald, "almost immediately after GVC opened, the incidence of septic cases at VJH fell. In the early 70's women would arrive almost at the point of death, in truly horrible conditions. There is no question that GVC definitely had a huge impact in reducing the number of cases we encountered" [49].

Unfortunately, in spite of our best efforts, we have been unable to recover records for those years—not from GVC, or UHWI or VJH. Paper records take up a great deal of space. It appears that in all of the locations, dockets have been culled. Based on the anecdotal evidence provided by Wynter and MacDonald, the authors hypothesize that if records were recovered from 1965 to 2020 (x-axis) they would yield a stark picture of the number of abortion (y-axis) demonstrating the public value of creating safe access to abortion (**Figure 2**).

Our purpose for the note on the GVC is to show first how rapidly the associations had normalized family planning so that the government could easily enter that space. But also, to show that the spirit of entrepreneurship had slipped away from the 'established' associations. The government was exercising more leadership and taking bigger risks.

5.2 Lack of accountability

So much for the positive aspects. What about those associations who have performed so poorly that they have been suspended or defunded? In almost every instance this has been the consequence of poor governance, other words, Boards that did not function and Executive Directors who went off on a course of their own. One obvious metric of Board operations is attendance at meetings. Several associations struggle to get members to attend meetings, and are seldom engaged between meetings. Meaningful volunteerism has become a rare phenomenon. Nor, in several instances, is it clear that Board members truly understand their role.

The composition of Boards is critical. Let us be clear, in small, poor societies it is not easy to attract people with the competencies required. Constructing a strong Board of individuals with skills in law, finance, research, strategy, fundraising is never an easy task. Few Boards have managed to attract persons with business experience, specifically in areas of finance and strategy. This is difficult even in resource rich environments. It must be exponentially more challenging in small, poor societies. Some Boards have been rich with conservative religious leaders comprehensively misaligned with the FPA's mission. And by default, in more than a few cases, the Executive Directors essentially fill the Board with persons from their own social network. This is a recipe for non-accountability. When IPPF sets criteria for gender, age and the inclusion of

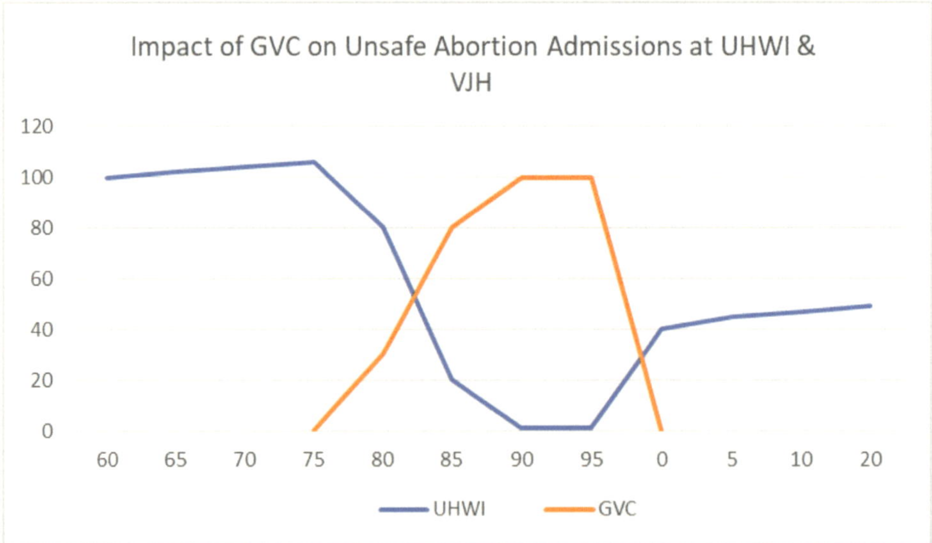

Figure 2.
Anecdotal impact of safe abortion services at GVC on unsafe abortion admissions at UHWI & VJH.

marginalized groups, the task becomes nearly impossible. It is not surprising that governance remains one of the major challenges, perhaps the major challenge of FPAs.

6. Caribbean family planning association (CFPA): colonial legacy or regional strength

The Caribbean Family Planning Association (CFPA) was created in 1971 with a clear mission: To advocate for sexual and reproductive health and rights (SRHR) through information and services including family planning, gender equality and freedom for physical and psychological, and institutional abuse. But this is exactly the mandate of the national organizations, so what was the added value of CFPA? Two decades before, Barbados, Jamaica and Trinidad had already become members of IPPF. During the 1960s the family planning movement had found roots in organizations in several other Caribbean countries—St Kitts, Grenada, St. Vincent, St. Lucia, Suriname, among others. Each of these national bodies wanted membership and so a seat on IPPF-WHR's Regional Council. Such an arrangement would have been consistent with UN-style democratic relationships.

However, the decision makers felt that the Caribbean would then have voting rights out of proportion to its population. In order to contain the voting power of the Caribbean, the CFPA was created as an umbrella for the nine affiliates. The decision did not affect the three 'larger' countries—Barbados, Jamaica and Trinidad—that had enjoyed membership since the 1950s. Subsequently, in the 1990s, Belize, Guyana and Suriname became a part of the group that had gained IPPF membership.

This arrangement through CFPA would prove problematic. First, it served to reinforce the divisive big island-small island politics of the Caribbean which had led to the downfall of the West Indies Federation in 1962—a political union of 10 Caribbean territories. Second, the decision was not aligned with established practice among international organizations. The arrangement had all the trappings of a colonial incubus.

The question then remained, what was the value proposition of the CFPA? What could it do that would make it attractive and an asset to the countries—small and large alike? The CFPA would have to deliver where the national associations could not perform. For example (i) raise funds, (ii) provide technical assistance to staff and Board alike, (iii) conduct research to nurture evidence-based approaches to reproductive health (iv) engineer deals with suppliers for the region as a whole that would yield economies no one member could command (v) foster a sharing of best practices—including any in the larger countries (vi) raise the profile of SRHR across the Caribbean, and (vii) be a voice for members in regional and international meetings.

The strength of the CFPA and its capacity to deliver added value cannot reside in the CFPA alone. Any secretariat, any collective body, is only as strong as the vibrancy of its members. That collective commitment must be a dominant characteristic. The real strength of any federal body lies in the willingness of members to work together in pursuit of a shared mission. Given the weaknesses at Board level, this is no easy task. Those weaknesses are also real in the so-called larger countries. Small countries do not have a monopoly on absenteeism, indiscipline, and unaccountability.

When the CFPA has been properly resourced, it has delivered on its value proposition—conducting research, raising the profile of sexual and reproductive health, and successfully raising millions of dollars for its members. When staff resources shrink from 16 to 2, it is absurd for anyone to expect the same level of output. Further, we do not believe that even the most insightful observer could have anticipated the spread of governance issues that have emerged in recent years. Improving governance is not a technical fix. It is an adaptive challenge that needs behavioral change. It takes and drains time.

The CFPA has not recently enjoyed the cohesion among its members that it needs to flourish. As too often happens in the Caribbean, we have broken into little pockets of comfort and division. We seem to lack the maturity for forthright dialog. We do not seem to have the appetite for high quality discussion and resolution of disagreement, without which we cannot forge the level of commitment to tackle our mission.

With IPPF's new willingness to give a vote to each country that meets certain criteria, several countries are exercising that option. That is entirely progressive. In this regard, several countries have already graduated from CFPA. They now have direct membership in IPPF. That is wonderful. Like physical fitness, graduation is not a permanent condition. Anyone who thinks otherwise is living an illusion. Several Caribbean countries are reliant on tourism, a very fickle industry. Beaches and hotels can be destroyed in a hurricane. Some countries are disrupted by volcanoes. In many ways our economies are fragile. Membership in a larger group is one way to manage the risks each country faces.

The invitation of separateness, of graduation to IPPF membership and individual votes is entirely parallel to the process that set the gears for the dissolution of the West Indian Federation. When the islands thought that their only path to separation from the UK was a federation, they hung together. As soon as they learned that the UK was only too happy to cut them loose one at a time, the fissure started to appear. We could be walking that same path again. Our short-sighted parochialism could be blinding us to the bigger picture of collectivism. Graduation does not mean abandoning a broader engagement. After all, the independent nation states in Europe saw the wisdom of forming a union in the face of global economic strength and political self-interest. Sovereignty does not imply isolation. Graduation can lead to a stronger CFPA.

The question for us is simple: Do we have the courage and the skill to convert a damnosa hereditas into a magnificent asset? Or do we prefer to see the CFPA wither away?

7. Culture of mendicancy

The first steps at birth control were driven largely by Caribbean nationals of status, privilege and means, based entirely on the realities in their immediate communities—frequent pregnancies and poverty. They were locally initiated and locally nurtured. We did what we could with what we had. The drive was rooted in empiricism, passion and good faith. The pioneers soon realized that the magnitude of the problem they faced required far more than mere good faith. So, they tried to attract support first from their governments. The toil of these pioneers was not isolated. It has to be seen as part of a broader national struggle. Across the Caribbean, the labour unrests of the 1930s had forced the creation of the Moyne Commission which addressed the problems of poverty and made recommendations for social and political reforms. The emergence of family planning was part of a nationalist, anti-colonial movement. But precisely because birth control was so controversial, even with the force of the Moyne Commission [50], Caribbean governments were largely hesitant to support the fledgling bodies. The pioneers, in some cases led by middle class women who had been educated in the UK and the USA, then turned to foreign sources for funds. Although the pioneers were women, and the mission was women's health, once the funds started to flow, it was men who occupied the posts.

Relatively easy access to funds changed the game. Self-reliance was quenched. During the severely constrained colonial period, while the colonialists extracted wealth, the national population lived by the ethic of living within your means. Incurring debt was to be avoided. That message was neatly conveyed by Charles Dickens in David Copperfield:

'Annual income 20 pounds, annual expenditure 19, 19 and 6, result Happiness.

Annual income 20 pounds, annual expenditure 20 ought and six, result Misery'.

However, that sentiment of self-sufficiency was sharply inverted upon Independence. Borrowing, seeking credit, which was once shameful, became a hallmark of accomplishment. The more one could borrow, the greater the signal of one's worth. Indeed, one of the attractions to political independence was precisely that—direct access to more channels of international funding. We celebrated our independence by significantly expanding our dependence on international borrowing. In a sense, if the World Bank, United Nations Development Programme (UNDP), Inter-American Development Bank (IDB), Pan American Health Organization (PAHO), and others would lend us money, "we had arrived". This was mendicancy on a national scale. This became the norm in our associations. Writing proposals became the important skill. Whether directly or indirectly through CFPA, IPPF became the steady source of funding for Caribbean FPAs. Naturally, with that dependence came IPPF's priorities, standards, and reporting requirements. This relationship became its own reinforcing cycle. FPAs had found a comfort zone in which we needed IPPF for our financial survival and IPPF needed us for their fundraising.

One unfortunate consequence of this relationship is that our associations were required to keep certain records of service and finance. Unfortunately, for the most part, those records were used to satisfy the reporting requirements for IPPF. They were seldom used to inform strategic planning or to guide management decisions about programme outreach or service delivery. The associations learned how to use data to placate donors but lost the capacity to turn those data to serve the mission. It is hardly surprising then that after more than 50 years of ties to IPPF, for the most part, the associations remain as dependent as ever. We have become victims of a culture of mendicancy. We no longer seem to seek to become self-sufficient.

8. Conclusions: creeping toward self-sufficiency

FPAs in the Caribbean region must try to move toward a measure of self-sufficiency and sustainability. Some Caribbean associations have shown the way, notably Barbados. We should learn from each other. There is a need to attract individuals with professional skills in finance, fund raising, and strategic planning to our Boards. The widespread Caribbean diaspora is an untapped reservoir that should be mobilized to endow our work. The associations have not tapped into the working-class and corporate organizations whose members have benefitted from their services for decades. The associations have not yet made a sufficiently strong, evidence-based case to national governments. Even if the associations cannot each become entirely self-sufficient, surely, they can set themselves the target of a sliding scale of becoming less dependent, less reliant, and less vulnerable to the shocks and whims of our international partners. If the alarm generated by the threatened decapitation of funding because of the threatened redirection of European resources following the Russian invasion of Ukraine was not a sufficient wake-up call, perhaps no alarm will be loud enough.

For most associations, ground zero is governance. This challenge must be faced and tackled head-on. Without this, there is no prospect of establishing a clear shared vision of the associations' role in 10 or more years. Without vision there can be no meaningful strategic planning or rigorous discipline of accountability. Proper governance is pivotal. There is no easy fix. Probably 90% of the work in organizations is technical, routine and managed by rules and standard procedures. That is the day-to-day busyness of the business. The other 10% requires facing uncertainty and ambiguity. That is the realm of adaptive leadership. Success in this area involves fostering disagreement, challenging the status quo, risk-taking, failure and innovation. This involves reflection—the antithesis of busyness [51]. Resolving the challenge of governance requires adaptive leadership. It will be a struggle of discovery and will require painstaking search for persons with the skills the associations need and whose values are aligned with their mission. It means building Boards of members with an appetite for constructive disagreement. This will be difficult in all countries but even more so in the smaller ones. Leaders in associations need to think outside the box. The Caribbean has lost a huge chunk of its technical skill. The fact that people have emigrated from their home country is not a statement of disinterest. In an internet connected world it is entirely possible to attract some of these persons to function as Board members. In terms of sheer numbers, there may be a pool of at least equal size in Canada, the UK, and the US. We believe this resource pool should be explored for the strength it could add to our governance.

Further, they could be a source of both direct and indirect financial support. Finance is arguably the associations' second weakest leg. By linking national expertise with their overseas cousins, literal and metaphorical, it is possible to begin to address the chronic financial challenges. No one should underestimate the willingness of Caribbean people living abroad to contribute to the region from their pockets and through their skills. There are Caribbean nationals at the leading edge of digital technology, finance, law, health care, and social justice movements who can be reached for support. The diaspora is potentially a rich source for unrestricted donations—the funds most sought by charities, because they can be used at their discretion, free of specific reporting. Attracting unrestricted funds is a function of reputation. Given their 50-year-old reputation, the associations should be well placed to explore this trove in the diaspora.

Between governance and finance is the generation of a shared vision. This is not an esoteric, pie-in-the-sky exercise. Too often it is given short shrift. Get the vision wrong and the result can be catastrophic. Railroads in the US were a phenomenally wealthy and powerful group. But they defined their business by what they did, running trains, rather than the purpose they served, moving goods and people. So, in the 1950s as then President Eisenhower built highways, they campaigned against large container trucks and missed a huge opportunity. They were in transportation, not railroads. This story has been repeated so often—Parker pen and ballpoint pens; Kodak and digital photography, and so on. IBM showed both phases—success in mainframe computing, missed out entirely on laptops and has rebounded with digital technology. FPAs need to address the far wider range of factors affecting reproductive health and justice—gender-based violence, male reproductive health, the stigma of abortion, homophobia, LGBTQ inclusion, etc. The associations need to apply their reputation for high quality and confidential services they have acquired over the years to advance justice on these frontiers. Then beyond that, what next? In some countries, FPAs were among the first charities established. They should be setting about to lead reform in other areas of social justice.

Internally, we need to learn from our mistakes. We need to invest in the diagnosis of the collapse of associations and study the dynamics of their recovery. We seem to prefer to dismiss these events rather than to document them and school ourselves in the lessons we can extract. Or worse, we imagine we are immune from a similar experience. We do not construct serious after-action reviews. This is a serious weakness and bleeds into thin 'strategic' planning. Similarly, we should learn from those associations that have soared. Sharing best practices is a neat way of building relationships and sparing under-resourced organizations from having to re-invent the wheel. But to do this sincerely, we need to care about each other. And caring about each other means vaulting over our parochialism.

One of the crushing day-to-day burdens associations face is the struggle to provide reports to a range of different donors, each with its own format and priorities. This is a paradox: it's the price we pay for our success in attracting funds from a variety of donors. No one country by itself can push against this tide that both feeds and then drains us. This surely is an area in which acting together, the region can propose some standard approach or template that makes economic sense to the associations and yet satisfies the donors. We have no doubt that this has been tried, we do not know whether it has been pushed as a collective, Caribbean wide initiative. We think reducing this burden is well worth a further effort. In some countries FPA staff are paid lower salaries than government staff. This situation exacerbates opportunities for collaboration. This is yet another area in which associations could, with real advantage, act collectively.

The way forward rests in purpose-driven, united, inclusive, collective action. "Going it alone" was a non-starter for Caribbean nations nearly 70 years ago. The word is far more connected today. Any national association that believes it can manage on its own with little or no regard for its neighbors, is simply delusional. Each national body needs to see the strong added value of a regional organization, whether CFPA or another, and work together to strengthen it. The national bodies must work together to define and create the "CFPA" that the region needs—one that has a voice because all the associations in the region are solidly aligned and speak with one voice. A regional body that can help with negotiations with individual governments precisely because it can leverage information of advances in government relations in one country with others in the region. A secretariat that is empowered because of the support it enjoys from all Caribbean countries regardless of size or status, whether affiliates, recent graduates, or long-existing postgraduates.

Advocacy rests on facts and values. Without empirical research we are stuck with our blindness and our beliefs. The lack of research, whether conducted by the associations or inspired by them in liaison with tertiary institutions, is one of the significant, persistent deficiencies of the FPAs. This lack of evidence depletes advocacy, diminishes professionalism, and erodes relevance, and leaves them blind to oncoming threats and opportunities alike. This is an easy area for the associations to quickly earn short term wins.

No one imagines any of this will be easy. If that were the case, it would have almost certainly happened long ago. But the leadership of FPAs must bend their efforts to make a clear turn in the road, so the next 15 years is distinctly unlike the last 50.

Acknowledgment

The Caribbean has not yet developed a grand tradition of record keeping. Further, as with any drive for social change, actors are far more focused on forward movement than on documentation. Not surprisingly, in our search for origin stories across the region, we relied on several individuals, a few of whom we are happy to acknowledge. From Jamaica, Professor Peter Figueroa, Dr. Douglas McDonald, and Dr. Deanna Ashley provided crucial insights to the early history and to the twenty years of government-provided abortion services. Dr. St. Rachel Ustanny, enlightened us about the politics of primary care and family planning. In Antigua, Dr Dane Abbott was a crucial source not only for his perspective but also for the leads to other contributors. Mr. Anderson Langdon helped us to appreciate the unique story of the role of government in Barbados. Ms. Joan Burke, Ms. Rosalie Saldivar and Dr. Natalia Largaespada-Beer educated us about the unusual story in Belize. Mr. Winston Duncan and Retired Nurses Best, Telesford and Moore who shared with us stories from Grenada. Finally, we are grateful to Mr. Christopher Price for his discernment of international funding and fundraising for development and/or dependence.

Conflict of interest

The authors declare no conflict of interest.

Notes/thanks/other declarations

We express gratitude to everyone across the Caribbean region who shared their stories of the history of FPAs in the Caribbean with our team. We also express thanks to the management, staff and board members of FPAs who understand the mission and work tirelessly to ensure no one is left behind.

Author details

Tonia Frame[1*], Patricia Sheerattan-Bisnauth[2], Yvette Delph[3] and Fred Nunes[4]

1 St. George's University, Grenada Planned Parenthood Association, St. George's, Grenada

2 Caribbean Family Planning Affiliation, St. John's, Antigua

3 Health Research Consultant, Silver Spring, M.D., USA

4 ASPIRE: Advocates for Safe Parenthood: Improving Reproductive Equity, St. John's, Antigua

*Address all correspondence to: tframe1@sgu.edu

References

[1] Class BN. Colour and contraception: The politics of birth control in Jamaica, 1938-1967. Social and Economic Studies. 2012;**61**(3):7-37. Available from: http://www.jstor.org/stable/41803766. [Accessed: January 14, 2023]

[2] Saftel H. History of Grenada planned parenthood: How it all began. In: Annual General Meeting. St. George's (Grenada): Grenada Planned Parenthood Association, Annual General Meeting; 1964. Report No: 2 (Unpublished report)

[3] Best S. History of the Grenada Planned Parenthood Association. [Interview, 22 January]. St. George's Grenada; 2023

[4] St. Lucia Family Planning Association. History of St. Lucia Planned Parenthood Association. 2023. Available from: https://sluplannedparenthood.com/about-us/history/#:~:text=Sister%20Theresa%20Louisy%20contacted%20Dr,gain%20formal%20recognition%20by%20government. [Accessed: January 22, 2023]

[5] Harewood J. Population policies in the Caribbean. In: Report of the 2nd Meeting of Planning Officials in the Caribbean, Kingston, Jamaica, 29 May - 2 June 1980. Santiago (CL); United Nations. Santiago Chile: Economic Commission for Latin America Office for the Caribbean; 1980. pp. 1-18. Report No.: CEPAL/CARIB 80/7

[6] GRPA. Guyana Responsible Parenthood Association Strategic Plan 2016-2022. Georgetown (GY): GRPA; 2017. p. 40

[7] Bourbonnais N. Out of the Boudoir and into the Banana Walk: Birth Control and Reproductive Politics in the West Indies, 1930-1970. Pittsburgh: University of Pittsburgh; 2013. Available from: https://repository.graduateinstitute.ch/record/286965

[8] Worker's Voice. Family planning gone Berserk: Sterilization Order of the Day. Worker's Voice Antigua. 09 Apr 1977

[9] Roberts DE. Family Planning Policy and Development Discourse in Trinidad & Tobago: A Case Study in Nationalism and women's Equality. Illinois: Law and Institute for Policy Research, North Western University; 2003. p. 43. Report No.: (WP-04-06) Available from: https://www.ipr.northwestern.edu/our-work/working-papers/2004/ipr-wp-04-06.html. [Accessed: January 15,2023]

[10] Ebanks GE. Mortality, Fertility and Family Planning: Dominica and St. Lucia. Santiago (CL): Centro Latinoamericano de demographia (CELADE); 1985. pp. 1-124. Report No.: 171

[11] WHO, Dehne KL, et al. Integrating sexual and reproductive health-care services. SRH Reproductive Health and Research Policy Brief. 2006;**2**. Available from: https://apps.who.int/iris/bitstream/handle/10665/73707/RHR_policybrief2_eng.pdf?sequence=1&isAllowed=y. [Accessed: June 19, 2023]

[12] Nunes F. Male Responsibility and Teenage Motherhood: An Analysis the Records of Teenage Mothers at Georgetown Hospital in 1994. Georgetown Guyana; 1994 (Unpublished report)

[13] Nunes F. The Vasectomy Experience at Barbados Family Planning Association (BFPA) 1980-94: The Myth of Resistance,

presented at Commonwealth Caribbean Medical Research Conference (CCMRC). Kingston, Jamaica; 21-23 April 1994

[14] Family Planning Closed 06 01 20 [Television]. Grenada Broadcasting Network. Grenada: GBN; 2020. Available from: https://www.youtube.com/watch?v=mA6o7mW9IIY

[15] Ahmed Z. The unprecedented expansion of the global gag rule: Trampling rights, health and free speech. Guttmacher Policy Review. 2020;**23**:13-18. Available from: https://www.guttmacher.org/gpr/2020/04/unprecedented-expansion-global-gag-rule-trampling-rights-health-and-free-speech. [Accessed: June 19, 2023]

[16] Mavodza C, Goldman R, Cooper B. The impacts of the global gag rule on global health: A scoping review. Glob Health Res Policy. 2019;**4**:26. DOI: 10.1186/s41256-019-0113-3

[17] Big Stories[Radio]. Observer Radio. Antigua: Antigua Observer by Newco Ltd; 2022

[18] Nicholson C, Deshong H. Grenada Women's Health and Life Experiences Study 2018 Report. UN Women: Barbados; 2020. p. 168. Available from: https://caribbean.unwomen.org/en/materials/publications/2020/8/grenada-womens-health-and-life-experiences-study-2018-report

[19] Contreras-Urbina M, Bourassa A, Myers R, Ovince J, Rodney R, Bobbili S. Guyana Women's Health and Life Experiences Survey Report. Barbados: UN Women; 2019. p. 120. Available from: https://caribbean.unwomen.org/en/materials/publications/2019/11/guyana-womens-health-and-life-experiences-survey-report

[20] Watson-Williams C. Women's health survey 2016 – Jamaica. UN Women. 2016:109. Available from: https://caribbean.unwomen.org/sites/default/files/Field%20Office%20Caribbean/Attachments/Publications/2018/AF%2020180618%20Jamaica%20Health%20Report%20for%20web.pdf

[21] Center for Reproductive Rights. The World's Abortion Laws. New York: Center for Reproductive Rights; 2023 Available from: https://reproductiverights.org/maps/worlds-abortion-laws/ [Accessed: January 26, 2023]

[22] Mumford SD. The Life and Death of NSSM 200: How the Destruction of Political Will Doomed a US Population Policy. North Carolina (US): Center for Research on Population and Security; 1996. p. 580

[23] Paul VI Pope. Encyclical Letter: Humanae Vitae. 1968. Available from: https://www.vatican.va/content/paul-vi/en/encyclicals/documents/hf_p-vi_enc_25071968_humanae-vitae.html

[24] KFF. The Mexico City Policy: An explainer. 2021. Available from: https://www.kff.org/global-health-policy/fact-sheet/mexico-city-policy-explainer/

[25] Center for Reproductive Rights. Beijing +5: Assessing Reproductive Rights. New York: Center for Reproductive Rights; 2000. p. 8. Available from: https://www.reproductiverights.org/sites/default/files/documents/pub_bp_Beijing+5.pdf [Accessed: January 26, 2023]

[26] United Nations. Economic Commission for Latin America and the Caribbean. Montevideo Consensus on Population and Development. Montevideo (UY): CEPAL; 2013. p. 40. Available from: https://repositorio.cepal.org/bitstream/handle/11362/21860/15/S20131039_en.pdf

[27] Anonymous. Personal Communication. 2000

[28] Ahmad R. Governance, social accountability and the civil society. JOAAG. 2008;**3**(1):10-21. Available from: https://controlatugobierno.com/archivos/bibliografia/ahmad.pdf [Accessed: June 19, 2008]

[29] United Nations. Report of the Special Rapporteur on the Rights to Freedom of Peaceful Assembly and of Association, Clément Nyaletsossi Voule General Assembly A/HRC/50/23. 2022. Available from: https://documents-dds-ny.un.org/doc/UNDOC/GEN/G22/337/82/PDF/G2233782.pdf?OpenElement

[30] Deschamps MD. AIDS in the Caribbean. ARCH – Alcohol Research Consortium in HIV. 1988;**2**(1):51-56

[31] The HIV Pandemic. In: Eduard J, Mays BN, Whiteside AW, Zuniga JM, editors. Local and Global Implications. Oxford University Press; 2007

[32] Joint United Nations Programme on HIV/AIDS (UNAIDS). World AIDS Day Report 2020: Prevailing against Pandemics by Putting People At the Centre. Switzerland: UNAIDS; 2020. Available from: https://aidstargets2025.unaids.org/assets/images/prevailing-against-pandemics_en.pdf

[33] Pan Caribbean partnership against HIV and AIDS (PANCAP). History of PANCAP. 2023. Available from: https://pancap.org/who-we-are/about-pancap/history-of-pancap/ [Accessed: January 26, 2023]

[34] Rosenblatt D, Mooney H, Zegarra A. Caribbean economies in the time of the coronavirus Caribbean economies in the time of coronavirus. Inter-American Development Bank. Available from: https://flagships.iadb.org/en/caribbean-region-quarterly-bulletin-2020-q1/caribbean-economies

[35] UNFPA. Provision of Sexual and Reproductive Health Care and Family Planning During the COVID-19 Pandemic Health Emergency in Latin America and the Caribbean. Panama: Interim Technical Brief; 2020. Available from: https://lac.unfpa.org/sites/default/files/pub-pdf/3-Covid-SSRyPF_ENG%20%281%29.pdf

[36] Sanger A. IPPF/WHR Statement on Separation from the Global IPPF. 2020. Available from: https://alexandersanger.com/2020/08/12/ippf-whr-statement-on-separation-from-the-global-ippf-august-5-2020/ [Accessed: June 19, 2023]

[37] IPPF. IPPF statement on Western Hemisphere The Region 2020 Aug 5. Available from: https://www.ippf.org/news/ippf-statement-western-hemisphere-region [Accessed: June 19,2023]

[38] The World Bank. Fertility Rates, Total (Births per Woman). 2023. Available from: https://data.worldbank.org/indicator/SP.DYN.TFRT.IN

[39] Roseman MJ, Reichenbach L. International Conference on Population and Development at 15 years: Achieving sexual and reproductive health and rights for all? American Journal of Public Health. 2010;**100**(3):403-406. Available from: https://www.ncbi.nlm.nih.gov/pmc/articles/PMC2820060/ [Accessed: January 24, 2023]. DOI: 10.2105/AJPH.2009.177873

[40] Belize Criminal Code, Ordinance No. 33 of 18 December 1980, Sections 108-110

[41] Rex v. Bourne (1938) 3 All England Reports, 615 (CCC)

[42] Eleven Bills Presented to House. The Belize Sunday Times. 1980. p. 8

[43] Cook RJ. Abortion laws in commonwealth countries. IPPF Medical Bulletin. 1976;**10**(2):1-2

[44] Delph Y. The Process and Benfits of Abortion Law Reform in Barbados: Lessons for Guyana. [video-recorded interview]. Bridgetown Barbados; 1994

[45] FPAG v AG. 2013. no. 849/SA 2016-01-15 (High Court of Guyana)

[46] Abortion: Statement of Policy. Kingston, Jamaica: Ministry of Health M.P. No. HH 490/01. 15th January 1975

[47] Deanna A. (Senior Medical Officer, Maternal and Child Health, Victoria Jubilee Hospital, JA). Memo to: Dr. M. Reid, Senior Medical Office for the Kingston and St. Andrew Health Department, and others (Jamaica). Kingston Jamaica; 2 May 1989

[48] Winter H. Impact of Glen Vincent Clinic. [Interview]. Kingston Jamaica; 1993

[49] McDonald D. Impact of Glen Vincent Clinic [Interview, 14 Jan]. Kingston Jamaica; 2023

[50] Wikipedia. Report of West India Royal Commission (Moyne Report). 2023. Available from: https://en.wikipedia.org/wiki/Report_of_West_India_Royal_Commission_(Moyne_Report)

[51] Heifetz RA, Linsky M, Grashow A. The practice of adaptive leadership: Tools and tactics for changing your organization and the world. Harvard Business Press; 2009

Section 3

Sexual Health

Chapter 9

Modeling Female Sexual Desire: An Overview and Commentary

Abigail L. Kohut-Jackson, Johnathan M. Borland and Robert L. Meisel

Abstract

Hypoactive sexual desire disorder (HSDD) in women is a condition of low sexual desire that develops over time. Sexual desire normally diminishes over long-term relationships, but is also negatively affected by a demanding lifestyle, poor self-esteem and body image, and loss of intimacy in a relationship. HSDD elevates to a disorder when it is a concern for the woman, arising from conflict with a partner who is interested in a greater frequency of sexual interaction. Two drugs have been marketed (Addyi and Vyleesi) to treat HSDD. Neither drug was originally developed for this purpose, nor is either drug particularly effective. The lack of rational development of drugs to treat sexual disorders in women is due to the mistaken belief that components of female sexuality, such as sexual desire, cannot be effectively modeled in animals. To the contrary, sexual interest, desire, arousal, and reward are measurable aspects of sexual behavior in female rodents. Going forward, basic research using these pre-clinical models should be the starting point for drug development. At the same time, it is not clear that drug development represents the primary therapeutic approach to the problem, with behavioral therapies providing good options for first line of treatments for HSDD.

Keywords: sexual arousal, sexual interest, sexual reward, hypoactive sexual desire disorder, Addyi, Vyleesi, animal models, mesolimbic system, nucleus accumbens, dopamine, glutamate, melanocortin receptors

1. Introduction

Sexual intimacy is an important component of ongoing, stable relationships. When one of the partners loses interest in sex or loses the ability to be sexually aroused, the relationship can be strained. A reduction or absence of sexual interest is the most reported sexual dysfunction for cis-gendered heterosexual women [1]. This loss of sexual desire and interest in having sex becomes a source of distress for which women seek treatment [2]. Because a constellation of environmental, contextual, relationship, and stimulus conditions impact sexual desire, interest and arousal in women, there is no clear cut therapeutic approach, limiting the development of medical interventions for treating women who raise concerns about their low levels of sexual desire and interest.

2. Models of sexual responses in women

Masters and Johnson [3] developed the first model of human sexual responses which were applied to both men and women. For Masters and Johnson there was a linear progression from excitement to plateau, which was followed by orgasm, and ultimately resolution (the refractory period until the re-initiation of sexual activity). In their model sexual desire initiates excitement (or pleasure) which leads to

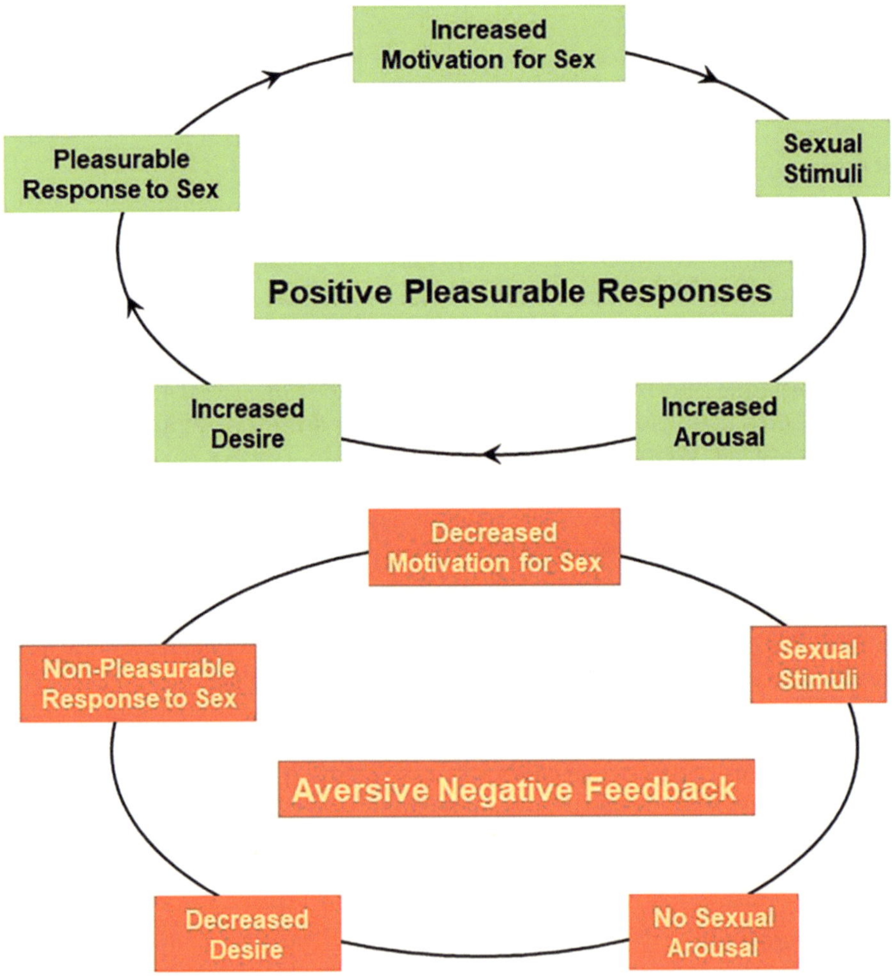

Figure 1.
Sexual Response Cycle in Women. Pictured here is a model of a woman's sexual response cycle based on Basson (2004). When a woman has a positive, pleasurable response to the components of sex, she maintains her interest and desire in sex, as well as her arousal to sexual stimuli. This becomes a positive, feed-forward process that maintains sexual activity in a relationship. The model highlights that there are a number of different components of a woman's sexual response, with all of them interacting. When one of the components is no longer a positive experience and pleasurable, it breaks the cycle, resulting in an negative-feedback reaction that diminishes future sexual activity. Notably, any of the points in the cycle can become dysfunctional, leading to different causes of female sexual dysfunction. When the primary underlying cause is a loss of sexual desire, the condition is termed 'hypoactive sexual desire disorder'.

sexual arousal. Sexual arousal is primarily associated with activation of vaginal autonomic physiological responses. In the intervening years it has become clear that sexual desire and arousal are independent of a woman's psychophysiological responses (e.g., [4–7]. The physiological responses are not coupled to a woman's subjective sexual state [6], and are still activated in response to sexual imagery that women do not find arousing [4].

Early simplified models of sexual responses in women have gradually given way to more intricate models that highlight the complexity of a woman's sexual response [8]. Basson [9, 10] proposed a comprehensive model of sexuality in women that takes into account contextual determinants of sexuality and the role of sexual and nonsexual stimuli in the initiation of sexual desire, interest, and arousal (**Figure 1**). The contextual dependence combined with a number of interacting components gives rise to large variations in the sequences and patterns of the woman's sexual response. What this means is that there are in reality a corresponding variety of potential bases for sexual dysfunctions in women, each depending on its underlying cause.

Embedded in the understanding of the underlying components of the female sexual response is a mechanism through which prior sexual experiences can either promote or interfere with future interest and desire for sex. Both Masters and Johnson's [3] and Basson's [9] models highlight pleasurable responses to sex. These pleasurable experiences become part of a feed-forward process through which desire and interest in sex are maintained (**Figure 1**). In contrast (**Figure 1**), a decrease in pleasure or even aversive responses to sex (e.g., involuntary sex) can feed-back to decrease future sexual interest and desire [1, 11]. As we will discuss, both of these processes can be modeled in animals.

3. Clinical problem

The variety of the components of the female sexual response identify a number of psychological processes that can be disrupted, leading to individual sexual dysfunctions in women (**Figure 1**). With this broad set of definitions for sexual dysfunction, there can also arise different subtypes of these disorders depending on the underlying cause [9]. Classification and diagnostic criteria for hypoactive sexual desire disorder (HSDD) have evolved over the past few decades, with this disorder being the primary target for drug therapies.

3.1 Description and incidence of HSDD

The International Society for the Study of Women's Sexual Health (ISSWSH) has provided guidelines for classifying HSDD in women [2]. Included in the description is the notation that HSDD can be lifelong or acquired. A lifelong lack of sexual desire may be more appropriately thought of being 'asexual', though the ISSWSH view may be beneficial in that it is more broadly encompassing of the range of women who meet the diagnosis of HSDD. In addition, HSDD may be generalized or situational. For the descriptive diagnosis, the criteria for HSDD must have been manifest for at least 6 months. Women classified as having HSSD have some element of low sexual desire, which includes reduced sexual thoughts or fantasies, reduced response to erotic stimuli or sexual stimulation, or a loss of desire to participate in sexual activity [2]. The diagnosis of HSDD requires that the decreased sexual desire is a source of personal distress.

A limitation in determining the causes of low sexual desire and interest is the degree of inter-individual variability among women. Still, it is striking that studies from across the globe report a rather comparable incidence of low sexual interest and desire. A large scale analysis of data from over 6000 women obtained from Britain's National Survey of Sexual Attitudes and Lifestyles reported that approximately 35% of women had drastically reduced interest in sex for at least a 3 month period in the previous year [1]. This is similar to the frequency among US women of which approximately 30% were dissatisfied with their level of sexual desire [12]. In China about 21% of women have low interest in sex [13], 46% have low interest/desire among Palestinian women [14], approximately 27% of Brazilian women report low sexual desire [15], and 30% of Australian women do so as well [16].

Although viewed as a unified disorder, it is not surprising that there are a number of causes of HSDD [17]. A common complaint among women is that they have very demanding lifestyles with their jobs, family responsibilities, financial issues and general stress [18, 19]. As a result, simple fatigue is a common cause of the loss of sexual desire as the daily demands on a woman increase [18]. Time in a relationship is another key variable, as sexual desire decreases in women the longer they are in a stable relationship [1]. In this context, Basson [9] has noted that assessments of sexual desire should take into account what are normal longitudinal progressions in a woman's sexuality across her life cycle and relationship duration.

Despite the noted variability among women, there are commonly reported underlying causes of low sexual desire and arousal. For example, many women expect intimacy, emotional closeness and their personal self-esteem to emerge from their sexual desires [6]. An exception to this is women with high levels of personal insecurity who do not necessarily seek out sex to achieve emotional closeness [19]. Feelings of intimacy and emotional closeness typically are avoided in women with a negative body image and low self-esteem, leading to decreased levels of sexual desire [12]. Women who feel less connected in their relationship [12] or express low relationship satisfaction [20], may find that their partner disregards their needs in a sexual relationship [21], with the combination of these factors producing low sexual desire.

A psychological mechanism underlying low sexual desire in women (at least in heterosexual cis-gendered women) may be based on how they view male facial attractiveness and male sexual imagery. Among women not reporting sexual problems, their inherent level of disgust predicted their responses to sexually arousing stimuli [22]. When divided by a median split for disgust as a variable, sexual arousing stimuli increased the report of disgust in women with a high disgust trait. In contrast, women with a low disgust trait reported that sexually arousing stimuli were desirable and further reduced their levels of disgust. General levels of disgust are not different between women with low sexual desire and controls [23]. However, when viewing erotic male imagery the low sexual desire group exhibited more negative facial affect (as measured by facial EMG recordings) and reported increased levels of disgust. Similarly, women classified as having hypoactive sexual desire disorder reported lower ratings of facial attractiveness for male faces than did the control females [24].

3.2 Diagnostic criteria

Hypoactive sexual desire disorder first appeared in the Diagnostic and Statistical Manual of Mental Disorders, DSM-III, and was characterized by reduced or absent sexual fantasies and/or interest in sexual activity. The diagnostic criteria were expanded on in the DSM-IV. Here, Criterion A included reduced sexual fantasies and desire for sexual activity. Criterion B noted that there had to be personal distress or relationship concerns that resulted from reduced sexual desire. Finally, the reduced sexual desire is not better accounted for by another Axis I disorder, a physiological reaction to medication, or medical condition (Criterion C). Because the frequency of sexual activity may be primarily determined by the demands of a partner, rather than intrinsic levels of sexual desire, the number of sexual encounters was not included as a criterion. Interestingly, distinctions were made as to whether the reduced sexual desire was situational or generalized, as well as whether it was lifelong or acquired. The DSM-5 perhaps took a step back in characterizing sexual disorders (e.g., [25]) by combining previously distinct components of sexuality (e.g., sexual desire and sexual interest) into single categories, thus failing to recognize the complexities of a woman's sexual response. Criteria for duration of reduced sexual desire or interest and the frequency of sexual interactions were added. Those critical of the combination of sexual arousal and interest into a single category in the DSM-5 (e.g., [25]) argued that this would not improve diagnostic accuracy and make it more difficult to diagnose these sexual dysfunctions in women, though an analysis by O'Loughlin et al. [26] did not support this contention. Embedded in these clinical criteria is the interesting notion that there are disconnects between how clinicians or women themselves view sexual desire and the problems associated with sexual desire [27].

4. Current drug therapeutics

Since 2015 there have been two FDA approved drugs for HSDD, Addyi and Vyleesi. These drugs differ in their mechanisms of action on the nervous system, the routes of administration, and the frequency of administration. The drugs share the feature that they are minimally effective, at best, for treating HSDD.

An interesting trait of women who report HSDD is that they are particularly susceptible to the placebo effects of administered drugs [28–31]. A meta-analysis was conducted that reviewed studies of women enrolled in clinical trials for various sexual dysfunctions [31]. The trials included approximately 2000 women receiving various drug treatments. Across these trials, placebo effects accounted for approximately 68% of the treatment effects in the studies. The magnitude of the placebo effect makes it more difficult to detect specific contributions of individual drugs to any clinical benefit and highlights the role of cognitive processes in HSDD.

4.1 Addyi (Flibanserin)

Deeks [32] reviewed the timeline for the development and approval of Addyi for the treatment of HSDD in premenopausal women. Flibanserin was first developed by Boehringer Ingelheim as an antidepressant. Though the drug was abandoned as an antidepressant, there were reports from some of the women in the clinical trials of a libido-boosting effect of the drug. Boehringer Ingelheim sold the rights to flibanserin to Sprout Pharmaceuticals who conducted clinical trials on premenopausal women with HSDD. Based on these trials, Sprout submitted a new drug application to the US FDA for flibanserin in 2013. The drug was not approved and Sprout appealed the decision. A second new drug application was filed in early 2015, and the drug, branded Addyi, was approved (with some restrictions) by the FDA later in 2015.

The FDA restrictions included warnings against using alcohol or cytochrome P450 enzyme inhibitors while taking Addyi, and also provided a warning for women who had impaired liver function.

4.1.1 Mechanism of action (receptor specific)

The mechanism of action of flibanserin has been comprehensively reviewed by Stahl et al. [33]. Flibanserin is primarily an agonist at serotonin $5HT_{1A}$ receptors and an antagonist at $5HT_{2A/2B}$ receptors [34]. In addition, it has mixed actions at dopamine D4 receptors. The idea behind developing a drug that acts at different receptor sites is that it can be clinically effective at lower doses, thus mitigating some of the off target side effects. Besides the specific receptor binding, flibanserin has indirect effects on synaptic communication by increasing release of other neurotransmitters, primarily dopamine and norepinephrine [35]. Because the brain operates through functional circuits, it is not surprising that flibanserin modulates activity at a number of brain regions and local circuitry. Stahl [36] has gone on to hypothesize that the microcircuits modulated by flibanserin underlie its therapeutic effectiveness, though this has not been demonstrated.

4.1.2 Therapeutic effectiveness

Thus far, flibanserin has been clinically tested in premenopausal women in stable cis-gendered heterosexual relationships who reported either generalized or acquired HSDD [37]. In the clinical trials of flibanserin, women self-reported moderate improvements to the baseline assessment of HSDD [38, 39]. One primary outcome measured was the number of "satisfying sexual events" per month. Women taking 50 mg flibanserin reported an average increase of 1.4 sexual events per month, slightly higher than the 0.8 events per month for the placebo group. Women on the higher dose of 100 mg flibanserin reported an increase of 1.6 events. Despite the statistically significant increase in the 100 mg dose compared to controls, calculations of effect size ($d = 0.18$ to 0.22) and odds ratios (1.5 to 1.67) were small, indicating minimal effects on sexually satisfying events [40]. The other primary outcome measure, monthly change in "desire score" on a scale of 0–3, did not reveal significant differences between women taking placebo and those taking flibanserin. These analyses, despite FDA approval, provide little evidence that flibanserin either improves sexual desire or the frequency of sexual interactions for women with HSDD.

4.1.3 Clinical considerations and adverse effects

Flibanserin is typically prescribed as a daily oral dose taken in the evening [41]. As typical of serotonergic drug treatments, it takes a period of weeks for the positive effects of the drug, though the side effects can occur earlier. The differential between the onset of the drug's effectiveness and the side effects causes about 12% of the women to discontinue use of the drug. The recommendation is that women continue a daily course of treatment for 8 weeks before discontinuing the medication [41]. Because of potentially harmful drug interactions, women are advised to avoid consumption of alcohol or several other prescription medications, and women who are breastfeeding or have liver complications are advised not to take flibanserin [42, 43]. Sleepiness and sedation are possible side effects of the drug. As we noted, flibanserin was rejected twice by the FDA prior to its eventual approval in 2015, due to the FDA's own assessment of the clinical effectiveness versus safety of the drug.

4.1.4 Incongruence of mechanism with a benefit for low sexual desire

As noted, the primary actions of flibanserin are as an agonist at $5HT_{1A}$ receptors and an antagonist at $5HT_{2A/2B}$ receptors. Pre-clinical studies in rodents consistently demonstrate that $5HT_{1A}$ agonists *inhibit* different components of female sexual behavior [44]. Thus, developing a drug that acts as a $5HT_{1A}$ receptor agonist to treat low sexual desire in women makes little sense neurobiologically. Further, serotonergic systems in women are also associated with inhibition of sexual interest and arousal, as low libido is a common complaint of women taking SSRIs for depression and is a basis for discontinuing use of the antidepressant medication [45]. Besides its primary actions on serotonin receptors, flibanserin has secondary effects on a number of transmitter systems [35]. Further, as flibanserin needs to be taken daily for weeks prior to seeing any benefit for HSDD, it may be that synaptic compensations, and not the initial actions of the drug on neurotransmission underlie potential therapeutic benefits for HSDD. Regardless, these are after-the-fact arguments that disregard a rational development of a drug to treat HSDD would not include $5HT_{1A}$ receptor agonism as part of its pharmacological profile.

4.2 Vyleesi (Bremelanotide)

Vyleesi is the first and only FDA-approved as-needed treatment for premenopausal women with acquired, generalized hypoactive sexual desire disorder [46]. "Acquired" means that the woman was happy with her level of sexual desire in the past, but it has over the years declined to a point of concern. "Generalized" means that the woman's level of sexual desire remains the same, no matter the sexual activity, situation, or sexual partner.

4.2.1 Mechanism of action

Bremelanotide (earlier known as PT-141), is a synthetic variant of α-MSH which was developed as a proerectile drug [47]. As a peptide, the thought was that the drug would be broken down and rendered inactive in the digestive tract. As such the drug was formulated to be given either intranasally or by self-injection. Levels of the drug peak after about 30 min when administered intranasally. The half-life of bremelanotide following injection is about 3 hours [48]. There are 5 subtypes of the melanocortin receptor, and bremelanotide has high affinities at the MC1, MC3 and MC4 receptors. The MC1 receptor is primarily in the periphery and is related to skin pigmentation. Consequently, hyperpigmentation is a side effect of bremelanotide administration [48]. The MC3 and MC4 receptors reside primarily in the central nervous system and are thought to mediate the effects of bremelanotide on sexual desire, with MC4 receptors receiving the greatest attention.

4.2.2 Therapeutic effectiveness

Phase III clinical trials were conducted on premenopausal women with generalized or acquired HSDD to test the effectiveness of bremelanotide to improve low sexual desire. In these trials women self-reported that bremelanotide increased sexual desire and reduced distress significantly more than placebo [46]. Notably, the desire score, rated on a 6-point scale, improved by either 0.5 or 0.6 points (in each respective trial) in the bremelanotide groups, while the sexual desire score improved by 0.2 points in the placebo group in each trial. Similarly, the sexual distress score, rated on a 4-point scale, was reduced by 0.7 in the bremelanotide groups and 0.4 in the placebo groups in each trial [46]. Though statistically significant, it has been questioned whether differences of 0.4 points in desire and 0.3 points in distress between the placebo and drug treatments are clinically meaningful. One limitation in assessing the true therapeutic effectiveness of the drug was that 8 of 11 efficacy outcomes that the authors of the study planned to investigate were never discussed, while several others were reported that were not planned prior to the study [49]. These changes in the planned outcome reporting between the a priori and post-hoc outcomes raise concerns regarding the objective evaluation of the drug's efficacy.

4.2.3 Clinical considerations and adverse effects

The data on side effects of repeated administration of bremelanotide come from two clinical trials. One consideration is that the drug needs to be injected subcutaneously about 45 minutes prior to engaging in sexual activity [46]. Further, the side effect profile of the drug is notable, with 40% of women experiencing nausea. Other side effects reported are flushing, injection-site reactions, changes in skin pigmentation (based on the affinity for peripheral MC1 receptors), headaches, and even vomiting.

4.2.4 Incongruence of mechanism with a benefit for low sexual desire

Bremelanotide was originally developed as a permanent skin tanning agent. One of the developers of the drug injected himself to see if it would work. He was surprised to discover that the injection produced a long-lasting erection [50]. As a consequence, the drug received further interest as an adjunct to treat male erectile dysfunction [51]. Bremelanotide works by imitating the effects of α-MSH on melanocortin receptors in the central and peripheral nervous system resulting in increased blood flow, which causes an erection. The (misguided) thought was that bremelanotide would become the female "Viagra", despite clear evidence that HSDD does not arise in women from impaired genital physiological arousal [52]. Instead of being a physiological issue, HSDD has at its roots complex psychological issues. Unsurprisingly, independent analyses of the few clinical trials which investigated the effects of bremelanotide for women with HSDD conclude that the drug is at best minimally effective [53].

5. Preclinical models of female sexual desire

Colloquially the belief is that animals have sex for the purpose of reproduction, whereas people primarily have sex for the pleasure they receive. This dichotomous view has been rejected both from neurobiological [54] and anthropological [55] perspectives. Instead, the parsimonious view is that (at least) all mammals engage in sex for the pleasurable/rewarding consequences. Neurobiologically, this view focuses on the mesolimbic system as the hub integrating external stimuli and experiences into subjective reward and pleasure [33]. Others have effectively reviewed the underlying neurobiology of female sexual behavior in rodents. In this section we will focus on how rodents have been effectively utilized to model components of female sexuality and how these models can be used to develop a rational translational strategy for developing therapeutics for women with sexual dysfunctions.

5.1 Rodent models

Female rats and hamsters have been the primary rodent models for dissecting components of the female sexual response, with each species providing a somewhat different insight. For both rats and hamsters, males approach the female from the rear and initiate a mounting attempt. This mount triggers the female's sexual posture, lordosis, which makes her vagina accessible for penile insertion (**Figure 2**). This mount only lasts up to a few seconds and may end with penile insertion (termed mount with intromission, or just intromission), or not (mount without intromission, or just mount). The intromissions are key and after a number of mounts with intromission, the male will intromit and ejaculate. The female's behavior while the male is approaching and mounting differs greatly between rats and hamsters. Female rats, after a male mounts escape the male and will actively run around with the male in pursuit. The female then stops, permitting the male to catch her and mount with or without intromission. If the male mounted without intromission the female will let the male catch up to her more quickly than if the male intromitted. This frequency of intromissions and their temporal patterning is important reproductively as there

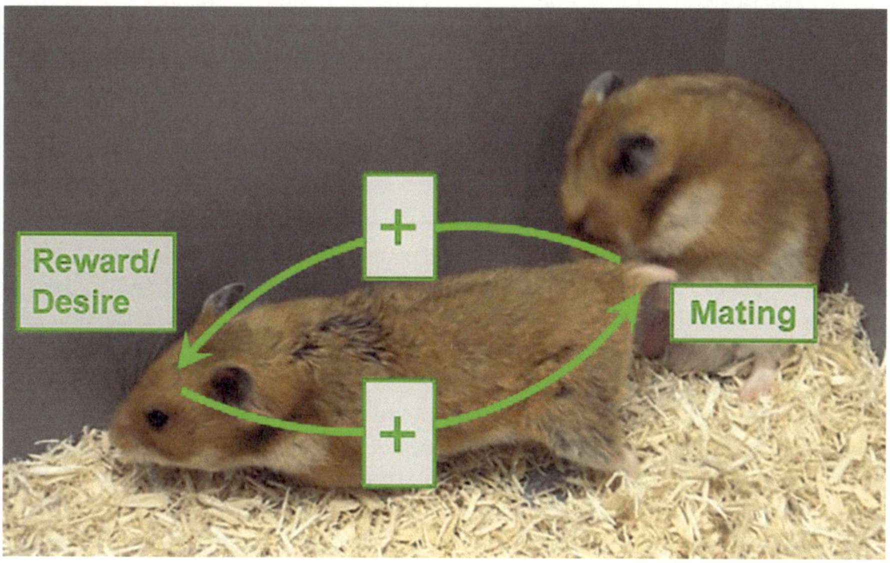

Figure 2.
Rodent Sexual Response Cycle. Sexual behavior in the female hamster involves a relatively immobile posture (termed 'lordosis') in which the female arches her back, making her vagina accessible to the mounting male. Vaginal intromission by the male is a sexually-rewarding stimulus for the female. Sexual experience produces a positive feed-forward process increasing the female's interest in and desire for sex in future encounters with males. With multiple sexual interactions with male hamsters, the female develops increased sexual interest and motivation for sex, as measured in a conditioned place preference paradigm. During sex with the male the female makes subtle perineal movements (a measure of sexual desire) that align her vagina with the point of contact of the male's penile thrusts. These movements become more efficient with repeated experience, increasing the male's ability to achieve insertion. In female hamsters, the combination of the rewarding/motivating consequences of sex (sexual interest) and the ability to regulate the likelihood of the male gaining vaginal intromission (sexual desire) are both dependent on mesolimbic dopamine neurotransmission.

is an optimal pattern that ensures fertilization upon ejaculation. In contrast, female hamsters retain a rather immobile lordosis posture between mounting attempts by the male (**Figure 2**). The male hamster may mount with or without intromission. For female hamsters there is no temporal component to receiving optimal stimulation for fertilization, rather it is the percentage of mounts that include intromission that impacts successful reproduction. As we will see, the female hamster can influence the percentage of intromissions by the male.

5.1.1 Behavioral paradigms for assessing interest

An incentive motivation testing arena consists of a large oval area with two small cages fitted to the outside wall. A wired mesh separates the small cages from the oval arena [56, 57]. The female rat is placed in the oval arena and the opposite-sex rat is placed in one of the two cages. The amount of time the female spends touching and in close-proximity to the cage with the male is used as the assessment of sexual interest [58–60]. A critical component of this test is that no sexual interactions occur, meaning that motivation is tested in the absence of actual copulation.

Similar to the incentive motivation testing arena, the three-compartment test box consists of a large Plexiglas arena divided into three equal sized compartments. The two dividers separating the middle from the outer chambers contain a small opening that allows the female subject to move freely between the three compartments. The stimulus male is confined because of the size of the opening or physically restrained in one of the two outer compartments. The amount of time the female spends in the compartment containing the stimulus male is used as the assessment of sexual motivation. Here too, physical interaction between the male and female is prevented, thus this is a measure of motivation in the absence of sexual behavior.

5.1.2 Behavioral paradigms for assessing arousal

Pacing chambers are arenas that have been optimized in such a manner that it allows the female rat control over the timing of sexual interactions with a male. One example is the bilevel arena, which consists of two elevated platforms that are separated on either side by narrow ramps [61, 62]. The male is placed on the bottom platform and the female is placed on the top platform. Because an adult female rat is smaller than adult male rats, the female can move freely either up or down between the two platforms to approach or escape the male, pacing the interaction. A variation of this testing arena utilizes a two-compartment unilevel pacing chamber [63] that has a small aperture which because of its size is accessible only by the female. Collectively, these pacing chambers result in the female controlling, limiting and terminating the number and amount of sexual interactions by the male [64, 65]. In these set-ups the active behavioral displays by the females are an accurate representation of their internal arousal state.

5.1.3 Behavioral paradigms for assessing sexual desire

Female hamsters assume the lordosis posture in the presence of a male even without physical contact. When an inexperienced male is tested with an inexperienced female, the male achieves intromission approximately 40–50% of the time [66]. The female's immobility gives an observer a misleading impression that the female is not an active participant in the sexual interaction. If the female's perineum (the area around the vagina) is treated with a topical anesthetic, the male will not achieve intromission [67]. Indeed, the female makes subtle postural movements that align the location of her vagina with the male's point of thrusting.

An interesting element of this copulatory interaction with the male is that the percentage of time the mounting male gains intromission increases up to 80% if the female hamster is given repeated sexual experience. The behavioral goal for the female seemingly is to receive vaginal stimulation from the male. With sexual experience the female learns to better control her perineal movements to maximize the receipt of vaginal stimulation, i.e., experience increases her level of desire in future sexual interactions.

5.1.4 Behavioral paradigms for assessing sexual reward

An interpretation of the sexual desire paradigm for female hamsters is that the females find vaginal stimulation to be rewarding and thus with experience they change their behavior to receive more stimulation from the male's intromissions. In this view, mating for female rodents has rewarding consequences that maintain their interest, desire, and arousal in future encounters with males.

The primary way that sexual reward is measured in female rodents is with a conditioned place preference (CPP) apparatus [68, 69]. The CPP apparatus is often a three-chambered apparatus with two outer chambers that differ in some physical element (e.g., type of bedding on the floor and/or hue of the walls of the chamber), separated by a smaller central chamber. Females are initially placed in a center compartment and then permitted to explore the three chambers freely to determine an initial preference between the two outer chambers. After establishing the initial chamber preference, females are given repeated sexual behavior tests in one of the compartments and are placed alone in the other compartment for the same period of time and testing sessions. This allows for follow-up testing where the female again explores all of the chambers to assess an increase in preference for the chamber paired with sex. This is an example of contextual conditioning in which the sexual experiences result in a drive towards cues previously associated with sex, an endpoint suggesting sexual reward.

Female rats do not develop a CPP if the male rat is allowed to control the pacing of the sexual interaction. Females only display a place preference for sexual intercourse if they are allowed to pace the frequency and duration of sex [63, 70]. This is an adaptable behavior in that the optimal pattern of sexual interactions is both rewarding and maximizes fertility, even if these processes are neurobiologically independent.

5.2 The neurobiology of desire and reward

These behavioral tasks can be used to identify mechanisms underlying sexual interest, motivation, desire, arousal and reward. The literature to date is too vast to summarize here, so we provide a brief overview and highlight a few examples.

5.2.1 The reward circuit

The canonical reward pathway [71] in mammals (including people) has at its heart dopaminergic neurons arising in the ventral tegmental area (VTA), and projecting to the medial prefrontal cortex (PFC) and nucleus accumbens (NAc). In turn, the PFC modulates activity in the NAc. It is theorized that dopamine release in the nucleus accumbens underlies reward processing [72–74].

If this pathway underlies sexual desire and reward, for example, manipulating it should affect the behavioral paradigms we just discussed. A dramatic finding comes from studies in which the region including the NAc was damaged in female rats [75, 76]. The females were given hormones to make them sexually responsive. When placed with males, the females fought off the male's mounting attempts rather vigorously. If the male was able to mount, the female showed a normal lordosis response. These lesions seemingly eliminated sexual desire and arousal, though sparing circuits mediating the expression of the sexual response itself.

Chemically damaging the dopamine terminals in the NAc originating from the VTA, eliminated the effects of sexual experience on sexual desire in the hamster model [66]. Despite the females' repeated sexual experience, the percentage of mounts with intromission by the males was the same as in sexually inexperienced female hamsters. Again, the females showed normal levels of lordosis, but had a decreased desire for mating with the male.

As a last example, dopamine receptor antagonists were given to female hamsters prior to each of the sex conditioning tests in the CPP paradigm [68]. When given the post-test to explore the apparatus after conditioning, the females did not spend any more time in the sex behavior chamber, indicating that the dopamine receptor blocker prevented the rewarding consequences of sex.

These studies support the idea that the mesolimbic system underlies the feedforward effects of the pleasurable responses to sex in females. With decreased activity in this pathway, females become indifferent to the positive components of sexual interactions. In extreme cases, a loss of mesolimbic system input can make sex aversive and underlie the elimination of sexual desire.

5.3 Application of preclinical models to the development of therapeutics

Prior rodent studies with bremelanotide suggested that the drug enhanced sexual arousal in female rats during sexual interactions with males. In this section we review the results of those studies along with our own unpublished data on bremelanotide effects on sexual reward in female hamsters.

5.3.1 Bremelanotide increases sexual arousal

Previous behavioral studies in bilevel arena pacing chambers demonstrated that peripheral administration of bremelanotide (50, 100 or 200 μg/kg) increased proceptive behaviors indicative of sexual arousal in female rats [77, 78]. Similar effects in female rat sexual arousal were reported following systemic treatment of melanotan II, a bremelanotide analogue [79]. Injection of bremelanotide directly into the brain of female rats also increased sexual arousal and this effect was blocked with a melanocortin receptor antagonist [77].

5.3.2 Bremelanotide does not enhance sexual reward

The questionable efficacy of the FDA-approved drug Vyleesi prompted us to return to preclinical foundations to examine its effects in our female Syrian hamster model of sex reward. We aimed to determine whether sex alone or with bremelanotide would increase behavioral responding indicative of reward in the CPP apparatus.

From our prior studies we knew that 5 CPP conditioning sessions produced full sexual reward, whereas 2 sessions was minimally effective [80]. Further, by activating intracellular signaling in the NAc we could enhance the rewarding effects of 2 weeks of CPP conditioning such that the levels of conditioned reward were equivalent to that of females receiving 5 weeks of CPP [80]. Based on this positive outcome, we reasoned that bremelanotide given prior to each of 2 CPP sessions should increase sexual reward. To model the administration of bremelanotide for sexual desire in women we injected it systemically prior to the sexual conditioning session (Borland, unpublished results).

Consistent with our prior studies, the 5 CPP sessions produced maximal levels of sexual reward, with the 2 CPP sessions significantly less effective. We should note that in this study the shorter (2-week) period also increased reward. Females that had 2 CPP sessions paired with bremelanotide (regardless of dose) did not display an increase in preference for the sexually conditioned chamber (i.e., no evidence of sexual reward). To the contrary, bremelanotide actually decreased levels of sexual reward in conjunction with 2 CPP sessions. The lack of effect of bremelanotide on CPP in our hamsters is consistent with a similar absence of action on sexual reward in female rats [77].

5.3.3 Bremelanotide does not Increase MC3R or MC4R expression

To better understand the neurobiology underlying this inhibitory effect of bremelanotide, we then assessed mRNA expression of MC4R in the mesolimbic system from the hamsters in the CPP study. Interestingly, sexual experience resulted in an increase in MC4R expression in the nucleus accumbens, but not the dorsal striatum (a negative anatomical control region). Consistent with the CPP results, there was a decrease in the expression of MC4R in the nucleus accumbens for females that received bremelanotide prior to the 2 CPP sessions compared to control females.

Both MC3R and MC4R are expressed in the VTA. Neither sex nor bremelanotide treatment affected MC4R mRNA expression in the VTA. However, bremelanotide resulted in a decrease in MC3R expression in the lateral region of the VTA compared to controls. Taken together, our findings provide no evidence to support the use of bremelanotide for increasing reward derived from female sexual experiences and in fact provide evidence to support a negative effect in the reward/motivation circuit.

5.3.4 Synthesis

From the combination of studies investigating bremelanotide effects on arousal and sexual reward in female rodents, we can conclude the following: 1) In female rats bremelanotide treatment increases arousal during copulation in female rats. 2) In female rats and hamsters bremelanotide failed to increase sexual reward in CPP tests. 3) In fact, in female Syrian hamsters bremelanotide treatment not only fails to enhance sexual reward, but actually decreases sexual reward in CPP tests. 4) Finally, bremelanotide decreased MC4R expression in the nucleus accumbens and MC3R expression in the VTA.

Collectively, although bremelanotide may enhance sexual arousal in female rodents, it fails to enhance sexual reward and inhibits melanocortin neurotransmission in the reward circuit. This pattern of preclinical findings would not have supported the development of bremelanotide as a drug to promote sexual desire in women.

6. Commentary

Nappi [7] presented an expert opinion on the relative lack of drugs to treat female sexual dysfunction. She highlighted the wide range of causes for sexual dysfunction in women, as opposed to simply erectile dysfunction in men. She noted that we still have an incomplete understanding of a woman's sexuality, which is a prerequisite to developing treatments. She also pointed out that female sexual dysfunction is not a life-threatening clinical problem, so that it is important to balance the clinical effectiveness of drugs with the drug's safety for the women taking them. Finally, Nappi [7] was concerned with drugs that needed to be taken chronically (e.g., Addyi), and hoped that on-demand medications (e.g., Vyleesi) could be developed. Nappi's commentary is still very current and meaningful, and rational drug development (in her view) will only be achieved through the cooperative partnership of sexual experts, pharmaceutical companies and medical agencies [7].

6.1 A rational approach to drug development

In Section 4 we described how Addyi and Vyleesi went to clinical trials with remarkably little preclinical data supporting their effects on sexual behavior in animal models. If developing drugs to treat sexual dysfunction in women is an important endeavor, the starting point has to be investment in basic research in both the public and pharmaceutical sectors. This research should be designed to take advantage of current animal models (and develop new animal models [81]) to identify potential molecular targets for therapeutics. This is how drug development begins for essentially all diseases and is only emphasized here because this message clearly was lost in the development and marketing of drugs for HSDD in women.

6.2 Pathologizing the normal

Basson et al. [9] developed a comprehensive model of female sexuality that emphasized the complexity of a woman's sexual response. At the same time that this model is a valuable contribution to understanding female sexuality, it also highlights the individual variability in sexual responses among women, making it difficult to define what a normal response pattern is. If we cannot define a normal sexual response, then how do we define sexual dysfunction in women [82–84]. Basson et al. [82] disagree with DSM criteria that quantify numbers of sexual fantasies or whether a woman initiates sexual activity as determinants of sexual dysfunction. They assert that few or no sexual fantasies are not a pathology, nor is it pathological if a woman does not initiate sexual activity.

Based on earlier arguments, Meixel et al. [84] lay out a historical account of the many examples of the drug industry's marketing strategy of "condition branding". With condition branding, the drug company creates a medical condition to support the development of a drug. In the example of Addyi, HSDD was elevated in significance as a treatable source of distress as part of the rebranding of the drug to address the disparity in the treatment of sexual dysfunction in men and women. It is disturbing that drug-company supported continuing medical education (CME) modules were developed to "educate" clinicians about this disorder. Meixel et al. [84] note (p. 860):

"Specific marketing messages that we identified within the CME modules included the following:

1. Hypoactive sexual desire disorder is very common and underdiagnosed.

2. Hypoactive sexual desire disorder can have a profound effect on quality of life.

3. Women may not be aware that they are sick or distressed.

4. Hypoactive sexual desire disorder and distress can have other names.

5. Clinicians should initiate conversation with their patients about their sexual health.

6. Clinicians find it difficult to discuss their patients' sexual concerns and lack training and confidence in the diagnosis of sexual problems.

7. Clinicians need tools and resources to help them diagnose hypoactive sexual desire disorder.

8. Simple tools, including the decreased sexual desire screener (DSDS) and Female Sexual Function Index (FSFI) can assist clinicians in diagnosing hypoactive sexual desire disorder.

9. A major barrier to clinicians talking about hypoactive sexual desire disorder/ female sexual dysfunction is the lack of medications.

10. It is problematic that there are medicines available to treat sexual problems for men but not women."

Key elements in the continuing education modules to be noted here are that the lack (at the time) of medications for HSDD was an impediment for physicians to have discussions about sexual desire with their patients and that women may have HSDD even if they are unaware of it.

6.3 Therapeutic approaches

A starting point for therapy may lie in reassuring women that their sexual feelings are not abnormal and are shared by many other women [82]. This does not alleviate tensions and conflict in a relationship, but can more effectively set the stage for other therapeutic approaches. For example, changing a women's view of herself can aid in communication with her partner about her sexuality to alleviate interpersonal conflicts [82]. Knowing that her feelings are normal and shared will boost self-esteem and relieve personal insecurities, both of which are barriers to promoting relationship satisfaction and feeling sexually desirable. This is clearly a simplistic approach that in isolation will not be sufficient for most women [85]. Still, this is an important component of any therapeutic plan.

Given that fatigue is a key factor underlying low sexual desire in women, approaches to reduce lifestyle stress and fatigue may be helpful. Mindfulness strategies can be helpful in this regard [86–89] and have the advantage of being easy to apply and are inexpensive. Presumably other lifestyle approaches may also be beneficial when HSDD results from these types of life events.

Cognitive processes impact HSDD when women view their own behavior, rather than relationship issues, as central to their levels of sexual desire. A rather thorough review [90] supports a role of cognitive behavioral therapies in treating women with HSDD. The goals of these approaches are straightforward, aiming to increasing the rewarding experiences for women and improve relationships through cognitive restructuring and communication. As with mindfulness strategies, cognitive behavioral therapy can be conducted through online training as well as in person.

Drugs should be a last line of treatment [2, 91], and used perhaps in conjunction with behavioral therapies. The worry with drug therapies is that they necessarily carry side effects that vary in severity. This is unavoidable with any compound that affects neurotransmission, as there will be direct and indirect effects on chemical transmission that are spread throughout the central nervous system, beyond the specific circuits targeting the behaviors in question [36].

7. Conclusions

It is abundantly clear that low levels of sexual desire reduce the likelihood that women will initiate or engage in sexual activity with a partner. Even if the reduction in desire is a natural product of the amount of time in a relationship, this can still strain relationships and be a personal source of distress for women. As sexual desire has underlying psychological bases, it seems on the surface that different types of counseling and behavioral therapies would be the best approach to treatment for women for which this is a problem. Perhaps guided by the absence of approved treatments for sexual dysfunction in women, the FDA approved two drugs (Addyi and Vyleesi) to treat HSDD, despite questionable effectiveness in clinical trials. The intent to develop drugs to treat HSDD is laudable, though only if effective on their own or in conjunction with other therapies. The mistake made for current drugs is that they were not developed to treat HSDD, but rather were recast from their original developmental purpose (an antidepressant medication for Addyi and a permanent skin tanning agent for Vyleesi). If drug development for treating HSDD is to be effective in the future, it must start with a rational approach based on animal models of female sexuality. Following the basic research, a cooperative interdisciplinary effort that includes basic research on human sexuality, sex therapies, and of course pharmaceutical control will meet the challenge of drug development for HSDD and other sexual disorders in women.

We finish this chapter with a caveat. The research on models of female sexuality and the research cited in this chapter are focused on cis-gendered heterosexual women. We spoke of the individual variation in responses among these women and it should be clear that variation is dramatically amplified when we consider individuals across the range of personal sexual identities. A clear goal of future studies should be to broaden the scope of this research to address the need for gender identity-based approaches to basic research and the development of appropriate therapeutics.

Acknowledgements

Ellen Kim conducted literature searches and catalogued the articles cited in this chapter. Production of the chapter was supported by a grants from the National Institutes of Health to RLM (R01 HD100007 and R01 HD100007-03S1). JMB was supported by an NIH Training Grant (T32 DA007234) awarded to Dr. Paul Mermelstein.

RLM conceived of the focus and scope of the chapter. ALK-J and JMB, along with RLM, wrote sections of the chapter and provided editorial comments on various drafts.

Conflict of interest

The authors report no conflicts of interest, financial or otherwise, with the content of this chapter. In addition, the opinions and conclusions expressed in this chapter are those of the authors alone, and do not necessarily reflect the views of the National Institutes of Health.

Author details

Abigail L. Kohut-Jackson, Johnathan M. Borland and Robert L. Meisel*
Department of Neuroscience, University of Minnesota, Minneapolis, MN, USA

*Address all correspondence to: meisel@umn.edu

References

[1] Graham CA, Mercer CH, Tanton C, Jones KG, Johnson AM, Wellings K, et al. What factors are associated with reporting lacking interest in sex and how do these vary by gender? Findings from the third British national survey of sexual attitudes and lifestyles. BMJ Open. 2017;7:e016942. DOI: 10.1136/bmjopen-2017-016942

[2] Clayton AH, Kingsberg SA, Goldstein I. Evaluation and management of hypoactive sexual desire disorder. Sex Medicine. 2018;**6**:59-74. DOI: 10.1016/j.esxm.2018.01.004

[3] Masters WH, Johnson VE. Human Sexual Response. London: Churchill; 1966

[4] Laan E, Both S. What makes women experience desire? Feminism and Psychology. 2008;**18**:505-514. DOI: 10.1177/0959353508095533200 8

[5] Levin RJ, Both S, Georgiadis J, Kukkonen T, Park K, Yang CC. The physiology of female sexual function and the pathophysiology of female sexual dysfunction (Committee 13A). The Journal of Sexual Medicine. 2016;**13**:733-759. DOI: 10.1016/j.jsxm.2016.02.172

[6] Mark K, Herbenick D, Fortenberry D, Sanders S, Reece M. The object of sexual desire: Examining the "what" in "what do you desire?". The Journal of Sexual Medicine. 2014;**11**:2709-2719. DOI: 10.1111/jsm.12683

[7] Nappi RE. Why are there no FDA-approved treatments for female sexual dysfunction? Expert Opinion on Pharmacotherapy. 2015;**16**:1735-1738. DOI: 10.1517/14656566.2015.1064393

[8] Rantell A. Models of sexual response. In: Rantell A, editor. Sexual Function and Pelvic Floor Dysfunction. Cham: Springer; 2021. pp. 5-11

[9] Basson R, Leiblum S, Brotto L, Derogatis L, Fourcroy J, Fugl-Meyer K, et al. Revised definitions of women's sexual dysfunction. The Journal of Sexual Medicine. 2004;**1**:40-48. DOI: 10.1111/j.1743-6109.2004.10107.x

[10] Basson R. On the definition of female sexual interest/arousal disorder. Archives of Sexual Behavior. 2014;**43**:1225-1226. DOI: 10.1007/s10508-014-0324-0

[11] Stephenson KR, Meston CM. Why is impaired sexual function distressing to women? The primacy of pleasure in female sexual dysfunction. The Journal of Sexual Medicine. 2015;**12**:728-737. DOI: 10.1111/jsm.12804

[12] Kingsberg SA. Attitudinal survey of women living with low sexual desire. Journal of Womens Health. 2014;**23**:817-823. DOI: 10.1089/jwh.2014.4743

[13] Zhang H, Fan S, Yip PSF. Sexual dysfunction among reproductive-aged Chinese married women in Hong Kong: Prevalence, risk factors and associated consequences. The Journal of Sexual Medicine. 2015;**12**:738-745. DOI: 10.1111/jsm.12791

[14] Masoomie R, Elsous A, Hussein H, Taghizadeh Z, Baloushah S. Female sexual dysfunction among married women in the Gaza Strip: An internet-based survey. Annals of Saudi Medicine. 2019;**39**:319-327. DOI: 10.5144/0256-4947.2019.319

[15] Abdo CHN, Oliveira WM Jr, Moreira EDJr, Fittipaldi JAS. Prevalence of sexual dysfunctions and correlated conditions in a sample of Brazilian women—results

of the Brazilian study on sexual behavior (BSSB). International Journal of Impotence Research. 2004;**16**:160-166. DOI: 10.1038/sj.ijir.3901198

[16] Worsley R, Bell RJ, Gartoulla P, Davis SR. Prevalence and predictors of low sexual desire, sexually related personal distress, and hypoactive sexual desire dysfunction in a community-based sample of midlife women. The Journal of Sexual Medicine. 2017;**14**:675-686. DOI: 10.1016/j.jsxm.2017.03.254

[17] Stephenson KR, Meston CM. Heterosexual women's causal attributions regarding impairment in sexual function: Factor structure and associations with well-being. Archives of Sexual Behavior. 2016;**45**:1989-2001. DOI: 10.1007/s10508-016-0741-3

[18] Holloway V, Wylie K. Sex drive and sexual desire. Current Opinion in Psychiatry. 2015;**28**:424-429. DOI: 10.1097/YCO.0000000000000199

[19] Watson E, Milhausen RR, Wood J, Maitland S. Sexual motives in heterosexual women with and without sexual difficulties. Journal of Sex & Marital Therapy. 2017;**43**:110-120. DOI: 10.1080/0092623X.2015.1124303

[20] Hendrickx L, Gijs L, Janssen E, Enzlin P. Predictors of sexual distress in women with desire and arousal difficulties: Distinguishing between personal, partner, and interpersonal distress. The Journal of Sexual Medicine. 2016;**13**:1662-1675. DOI: 10.1016/j.jsxm.2016.09.016

[21] Hogue JV, Rosen NO, Bockaj A, Impett EA, Muise A. Sexual communal motivation in couples coping with low sexual interest/arousal: Associations with sexual well-being and sexual goals. PLoS One. 2019;**14**:e0219768. DOI: 10.1371/journal.pone.0219768

[22] Fleischman DS, Hamilton LD, Fessler DM, Meston CM. Disgust versus lust: Exploring the interactions of disgust and fear with sexual arousal in women. PLoS One. 2015;**10**:e0118151. DOI: 10.1371/journal.pone.0118151

[23] DePesa NS, Cassisi JE. Affective and autonomic responses to erotic images: Evidence of disgust-based mechanisms in female sexual interest/arousal disorder. Journal of Sex Research. 2017;**54**:877-886. DOI: 10.1080/00224499.2016.1252307

[24] Ferdenzi C, Delplanque S, Vorontsova-Wenger O, Pool E, Bianchi-Demicheli F, Sander D. Perception of men's beauty and attractiveness by women with low sexual desire. The Journal of Sexual Medicine. 2015;**12**:946-955. DOI: 10.1111/jsm.12795

[25] Parish SJ, Goldstein AT, Goldstein SW, et al. Toward a more evidence-based nosology and nomenclature for female sexual dysfunctions-Part II. The Journal of Sexual Medicine. 2016;**13**:1888-1906. DOI: 10.1016/j.jsxm.2016.09.020

[26] O'Loughlin JI, Basson R, Brotto LA. Women with hypoactive sexual desire disorder versus sexual interest/arousal disorder: An empirical test of raising the bar. Journal of Sex Research. 2018;**55**:734-746. DOI: 10.1080/00224499.2017.1386764

[27] Brotto LI. The DSM diagnostic criteria for hypoactive sexual desire disorder in women. Archives of Sexual Behavior. 2010;**39**:221-239. DOI: 10.1007/s10508-009-9543-12010

[28] Bradford A, Meston CM. Behavior and symptom change among women treated with placebo for sexual dysfunction. The Journal of Sexual Medicine. 2011;**8**:191-201. DOI: 10.1111/j.1743-6109.2010.02007.x

[29] Katz A. The circle of female sexual desire-Have we come a long way? Nursing for Women's Health. 2016;**20**:235-238. DOI: 10.1016/j.nwh.2016.04.002

[30] Palaniappan M, Heatherly R, Mintz LB, et al. Skills vs. pills: Comparative effectiveness for low sexual desire in women. Journal of Sex & Marital Therapy. 2018;**44**:1-15. DOI: 10.1080/0092623X.2017.1305029

[31] Weinberger JM, Houman J, Caron AT, et al. Female sexual dysfunction and the placebo effect: A meta-analysis. Obstetrics and Gynecology. 2018;**132**:453

[32] Deeks ED. Flibanserin: First global approval. Drug. 2015;**75**:1815-1822. DOI: 10.1007/s40265-015-0474-y

[33] Stahl SM, Sommer B, Allers KA. Multifunctional pharmacology of flibanserin: Possible mechanism of therapeutic action in hypoactive sexual desire disorder. The Journal of Sexual Medicine. 2011;**8**:15-27. DOI: 10.1111/j.1743-6109.2010.02032.x

[34] Borsini F, Giraldo E, Monferini E, Antonini G, Parenti M, Bietti G, et al. BIMT 17, a 5-HT2A receptor antagonist and 5-HT1A receptor full agonist in rat cerebral cortex. Naunyn-Schmiedeberg's Archives of Pharmacology. 1995;**352**:276-282. DOI: 10.1007/BF00168557

[35] Invernizzi RW, Sacchetti G, Parini S, Acconcia S, Samanin R. Flibanserin, a potential antidepressant drug, lowers 5-HT and raises dopamine and noradrenaline in the rat prefrontal cortex dialysate: Role of 5-HT(1A) receptors. British Journal of Pharmacology. 2003;**139**:1281-1288. DOI: 10.1038/sj.bjp.0705341

[36] Stahl SM. Mechanism of action of flibanserin, a multifunctional serotonin agonist and antagonist (MSAA), in hypoactive sexual desire disorder. CNS Spectrums. 2015;**20**:1-6. DOI: 10.1017/S1092852914000832

[37] Anderson R, Moffatt CE. Ignorance is not bliss: If we don't understand hypoactive sexual desire disorder, how can flibanserin treat it? The Journal of Sexual Medicine. 2018;**15**:273-283. DOI: 10.1016/j.jsxm.2018.01.001

[38] Robinson K, Cutler JB, Carris NW. First pharmacological therapy for hypoactive sexual desire disorder in premenopausal women: Flibanserin. The Annals of Pharmacotherapy. 2016;**50**:125-132. DOI: 10.1177/1060028015622182

[39] Thorp J Jr, Palacios S, Symons J, Simon J, Barbour K. Improving prospects for treating hypoactive sexual desire disorder (HSDD): Development status of flibanserin. BJOG. 2014;**121**:1328-1331. DOI: 10.1111/1471-0528.12878

[40] Chivers ML, Basson R, Brotto LA, Graham CA, Stephenson KR. Statistical and epistemological Issues in the evaluation of treatment efficacy of pharmaceutical, psychological, and combination treatments for women's sexual desire difficulties. Journal of Sex & Marital Therapy. 2017;**43**:210-217. DOI: 10.1080/0092623X.2016.1266538

[41] Holt H, Tingen J. Flibanserin (Addyi) for hypoactive sexual desire disorder in premenopausal women. American Family Physician. 2016;**93**:826-828

[42] Baid R, Agarwal R. Flibanserin: A controversial drug for female hypoactive sexual desire disorder. Industrial Psychiatry Journal. 2018;**27**:154-157. DOI: 10.4103/ipj.ipj_20_16

[43] Jin J. Flibanserin for treating low sexual desire in women. JAMA.

2015;**314**:1312. DOI: 10.1001/jama.2015.11769

[44] Snoeren EM, Veening JG, Olivier B, Oosting RS. Serotonin 1A receptors and sexual behavior in female rats: A review. Pharmacology, Biochemistry, and Behavior. 2014;**121**:43-52. DOI: 10.1016/j.pbb.2013.11.017

[45] Montejo AL, Calama J, Rico-Villademoros F, et al. A real-world study on antidepressant-associated sexual dysfunction in 2144 Outpatients: The SALSEX I study. Archives of Sexual Behavior. 2019;**48**:923-933. DOI: 10.1007/s10508-018-1365-6

[46] Kingsberg SA, Clayton AH, Portman D, et al. Bremelanotide for the treatment of hypoactive sexual desire disorder: Two randomized phase 3 trials. Obstetrics and Gynecology. 2019;**134**:899-908. DOI: 10.1097/AOG.0000000000003500

[47] Diamond LE, Earle DC, Rosen RC, Willett MS, Molinoff PB. Double-blind, placebo-controlled evaluation of the safety, pharmacokinetic properties and pharmacodynamic effects of intranasal PT-141, a melanocortin receptor agonist, in healthy males and patients with mild-to-moderate erectile dysfunction. International Journal of Impotence Research. 2004;**16**:51-59

[48] Bremelanotide. Available online: https://go.drugbank.com/drugs/DB11653 (Accessed: August 4, 2022].

[49] Spielmans GI. Re-analyzing phase III bremelanotide trials for "hypoactive sexual desire disorder" in women. Journal of Sex Research. 2021;**2021**(58):1085-1105. DOI: 10.1080/00224499.2021.1885601

[50] Allers KA, Sommer B. Paradigms for Preclinical Investigations of Female Sexual Function and Dysfunction (HSDD and FSAD). London, UK: IntechOpen; 2011. DOI: 10.5772/26773

[51] Shadiack AM, Sharma SD, Earle DC, Spana C, Hallam TJ. Melanocortins in the treatment of male and female sexual dysfunction. Current Topics in Medicinal Chemistry. 2007;7:1137-1144. DOI: 10.2174/156802607780906681

[52] Kingsberg SA, Nambiar S, Karkare S, et al. Hypoactive sexual desire disorder (HSDD) is not "female erectile dysfunction (ED)": Challenges with the characterization of HSDD in women based on a systematic literature review. Current Medical Research and Opinion. 2020;**36**:1069-1080. DOI: 10.1080/03007995.2020.1754181

[53] Anonymous. Bremelanotide (Vyleesi) for hypoactive sexual desire disorder. The Medical Letter on Drugs and Therapeutics. 2019;**61**:114-116

[54] Meisel RL, Mullins AJ. Sexual experience in female rodents: Cellular mechanisms and functional consequences. Brain Research. 2006;**1126**:56-65. DOI: 10.1016/j.brainres.2006.08.050

[55] Dunsworth H. Do animals know where babies come from? Scientific American. 2016;**314**:66-69. DOI: 10.1038/scientificamerican0116-66

[56] Agmo A, Turi AL, Ellingsen E, Kaspersen H. Preclinical models of sexual desire: Conceptual and behavioral analyses. Pharmacology, Biochemistry, and Behavior. 2004;**78**:379-404. DOI: 10.1016/j.pbb.2004.04.013

[57] Meyerson BJ, Lindström LH. Sexual motivation in the female rat. A methodological study applied to the investigation of the effect of estradiol benzoate. Acta Physiologica

Scandinavica. Supplementum. 1973;**389**:1-80

[58] Agmo A. Unconditioned sexual incentive motivation in the male Norway rat (*Rattus norvegicus*). Journal of Comparative Psychology. 2003;**117**:3-14. DOI: 10.1037/0735-7036.117.1.3

[59] Chu X, Agmo A. Sociosexual interactions in rats: Are they relevant for understanding human sexual behavior? International Journal of Psychological Research. 2016;**9**:76-95. DOI: 10.21500/20112084.2339

[60] Chu X, Zhavbert ES, Dugina JL, Kheyfets IA, Sergeeva SA, Epstein OI, et al. Sildenafil and a compound stimulating endothelial NO synthase modify sexual incentive motivation and copulatory behavior in male Wistar and Fisher 344 rats. Journal of Sexual Medicine. 2008;**5**:2085-2099. DOI: 10.1111/j.1743-6109.2008.00937.x

[61] Mendelson SD, Gorzalka BB. An improved chamber for the observation and analysis of the sexual behavior of the female rat. Physiology & Behavior. 1987;**39**:67-71. DOI: 10.1016/0031-9384(87)90345-3

[62] Mendelson SD, Pfaus JG. Level searching: A new assay of sexual motivation in the male rat. Physiology & Behavior. 1989;**45**:337-341. DOI: 10.1016/0031-9384(89)90136-4

[63] Paredes RG, Alonso A. Sexual behavior regulated (paced) by the female induces conditioned place preference. Behavioral Neuroscience. 1997;**111**:123-128. DOI: 10.1037//0735-7044.111.1.123

[64] Pfaus JG, Smith WJ, Coopersmith CB. Appetitive and consummatory sexual behaviors of female rats in bilevel chambers. I. A correlational and factor analysis and the effects of ovarian hormones. Hormones and Behavior. 1999;**35**:224-240. DOI: 10.1006/hbeh.1999.1516

[65] Pfaus JG, Smith WJ, Byrne N, Stephens G. Appetitive and consummatory sexual behaviors of female rats in bilevel chambers. II. Patterns of estrus termination following vaginocervical stimulation. Hormones and Behavior. 2000;**37**:96-107. DOI: 10.1006/hbeh.1999.1562

[66] Bradley KC, Haas AR, Meisel RL. 6-Hydroxydopamine lesions in female hamsters (*Mesocricetus auratus*) abolish the sensitized effects of sexual experience on copulatory interactions with males. Behavioral Neuroscience. 2005;**119**:224-232. DOI: 10.1037/0735-7044.119.1.224

[67] Noble RG. Sex responses of the female hamster: Effects on male performance. Physiology & Behavior. 1980;**24**:237-242. DOI: 10.1016/0031-9384(80)90080-3

[68] Meisel RL, Joppa MA, Rowe RK. Dopamine receptor antagonists attenuate conditioned place preference following sexual behavior in female Syrian hamsters. European Journal of Pharmacology. 1996;**309**:21-24. DOI: 10.1016/0014-2999(96)00389-5

[69] Oldenburger WP, Everitt BJ, de Jonge FH. Conditioned place preference induced by sexual interaction in female rats. Hormones and Behavior. 1992;**26**:214-228. DOI: 10.1016/0018-506x(92)90043-u

[70] Martinez I, Paredes RG. Only self-paced mating is rewarding in rats of both sexes. Hormones and Behavior. 2001;**40**:510-517. DOI: 10.1006/hbeh.2001.1712

[71] Salgado S, Kaplitt MG. The nucleus accumbens: A comprehensive

review. Stereotactic and Functional Neurosurgery. 2015;**93**:75-93. DOI: 10.1159/000368279

[72] Hamid AA, Pettibone JR, Mabrouk OS, Hetrick VL, Schmidt R, Vander Weele CM, et al. Mesolimbic dopamine signals the value of work. Nature Neuroscience. 2016;**19**:117-126. DOI: 10.1038/nn.4173

[73] Pessiglione M, Seymour B, Flandin G, Dolan RJ, Frith CD. Dopamine-dependent prediction errors underpin reward-seeking behaviour in humans. Nature. 2006;**442**:1042-1045. DOI: 10.1038/nature05051

[74] Schultz W. Dopamine reward prediction error coding. Dialogues in Clinical Neuroscience. 2016;**18**:23-32. DOI: 10.31887/DCNS.2016.18.1/wschultz

[75] Rivas FJ, Mir D. Effects of nucleus accumbens lesion on female rat sexual receptivity and proceptivity in a partner preference paradigm. Behavioural Brain Research. 1990;**41**:239-249. DOI: 10.1016/0166-4328(90)90111-q

[76] Rivas FJ, Mir D. Accumbens lesion in female rats increases mount rejection without modifying lordosis. Revista Española de Fisiología. 1991;**47**:1-6

[77] Pfaus JG, Shadiack A, Van Soest T, Tse M, Molinoff P. Selective facilitation of sexual solicitation in the female rat by a melanocortin receptor agonist. Proceedings of the National Academy Science USA. 2004;**101**:10201-10204. DOI: 10.1073/pnas.0400491101

[78] Pfaus J, Giuliano F, Gelez H. Bremelanotide: An overview of preclinical CNS effects on female sexual function. Journal of Sexual Medicine. 2007;**4**(Suppl. 4):269-279. DOI: 10.1111/j.1743-6109.2007.00610.x

[79] Rössler A-S, Pfaus JG, Kia HK, Bernabé J, Alexandre L, Giuliano F. The melanocortin agonist, melanotan II, enhances proceptive sexual behaviors in the female rat. Pharmacology, Biochemistry, and Behavior. 2006;**85**:514-521. DOI: 10.1016/j.pbb.2006.09.023

[80] Hedges VL, Chakravarty S, Nestler EJ, Meisel RL. Delta FosB overexpression in the nucleus accumbens enhances sexual reward in female Syrian hamsters. Genes, Brain, and Behavior. 2009;**8**:442-449. DOI: 10.1111/j.1601-183X.2009.00491.x

[81] Borland JM, Frantz KJ, Aiani LM, Grantham KN, Song Z, Albers HE. A novel operant task to assess social reward and motivation in rodents. Journal of Neuroscience Methods. 2017;**2017**(287):80-88. DOI: 10.1016/j.jneumeth.2017.06.003

[82] Basson R. Female sexual response: The role of drugs in the management of sexual dysfunction. Obstetrics and Gynecology. 2001;**98**:350-353. DOI: 10.1016/s0029-7844(01)01452-1

[83] Tiefer L. Female sexual dysfunction: A case study of disease mongering and activist resistance. PLoS Medicine. 2006;**3**(4):e178. DOI: 10.1371/journal.pmed.0030178

[84] Meixel A, Yanchar E, Fugh-Berman A. Hypoactive sexual desire disorder: Inventing a disease to sell low libido. Journal of Medical Ethics. 2015;**41**:859-862. DOI: 10.1136/medethics-2014-102596

[85] Herbenick D, Mullinax M, Mark K. Sexual desire discrepancy as a feature, not a bug, of long-term relationships: Women's self-reported strategies for modulating sexual desire. The Journal of Sexual Medicine. 2014;**11**:2196-2206. DOI: 10.1111/jsm.12625

[86] Brotto LA, Basson R. Group mindfulness-based therapy significantly improves sexual desire in women. Behaviour Research and Therapy. 2014;**57**:43-54. DOI: 10.1016/j.brat.2014.04.001

[87] Brotto L, Atallah S, Johnson-Agbakwu C, et al. Psychological and interpersonal dimensions of sexual function and dysfunction. The Journal of Sexual Medicine. 2016;**13**:538-571. DOI: 10.1016/j.jsxm.2016.01.019

[88] Paterson LQP, Handy AB, Brotto LA. A pilot study of eight-session mindfulness-based cognitive therapy adapted for women's sexual interest/arousal disorder. Journal of Sex Research. 2017;**54**:850-861. DOI: 10.1080/00224499.2016.1208800

[89] Velten J, Margraf J, Chivers ML. Brotto LA Effects of a mindfulness task on women's sexual response. Journal of Sex Research. 2018;**55**:747-757. DOI: 10.1080/00224499.2017.1408768

[90] Mestre-Bach G, Blycker GR, Potenza MN. Behavioral therapies for treating female sexual dysfunctions: A state-of-the-art review. Journal of Clinical Medicine. 2022;**11**:2794. DOI: 10.3390/jcm11102794

[91] Khajehei M, Doherty M, Tilley PJ. An update on sexual function and dysfunction in women. Archives of Women's Mental Health. 2015;**18**:423-433. DOI: 10.1007/s00737-015-0535-y

Chapter 10

The Role of Ultrasound in Women's Health

Marema Jebessa Kumsa and Zegeye Wubeshet Haile

Abstract

Ultrasound has developed into a vital medical diagnostic tool during the past 60 years. Theodore Dussik and his brother Friederich were the first to utilize ultrasound in the 1930s and 1940s to identify a brain tumor. Ultrasonography is now used for many different situations, such as disease detection, assisting with biopsy taking, monitoring previously diagnosed abnormalities, and assessing pregnancy. Unfortunately, the general public is unaware of the role of ultrasound in women's health for purposes other than pregnancy assessment. This chapter's major goal is to give a comprehensive overview of the various roles that ultrasound plays in women's health. Furthermore, this chapter aims to make the general public more aware of the importance that ultrasound plays in women's health. The authors used a wide range of sources for this work, such as books and peer-reviewed publications. The key roles of ultrasound examination in women's health include: assessment of female reproductive organs, determination of causes of infertility, assessment of pregnancy and related problems, and assessment of the breast and abdomen. The general public should be made aware of the importance of ultrasound in women's health.

Keywords: ultrasonography, female, women's health, uterine pathology, causes of infertility, breast ultrasound, abdominal ultrasound

1. Introduction

Over the past 60 years, ultrasound has become a crucial medical diagnostic tool. Ultrasound was first used in the 1930s and 1940s by the two brothers Theodore Dussik and Friederich to diagnose a brain tumor. Unfortunately, it was not widely used until the 1970s. Nowadays, ultrasonography is utilized for a variety of purposes, including disease diagnosis, guiding biopsy taking, monitoring previously identified abnormalities, and pregnancy assessment.

The evaluation of women's health with ultrasound has become routine. Particularly, it is essential in the early diagnosis of uterine and ovarian masses as well as other conditions affecting the female reproductive organs. Moreover, ultrasound is widely used for assessing pregnancy as it is radiation-free. Ultrasound is used to determine the location of the gestational sac, determine gestational age, determine the number of fetuses, assess the fetus, monitor its growth, evaluate fetal well-being, determine fetal presentation, estimate fetal weight, and detect abnormalities of the fetus to identify the fetus [1–4]. Ultrasound diagnosis of obstetric complications helps to reduce maternal morbidity. Due to its radiation-free nature, ultrasound is extensively used for fetal scanning, fetal growth monitoring, and fetal anomaly detection.

In addition, ultrasound is essential for assessing breast lesions and abdominal organs in female patients. Screening for breast cancer reduces breast cancer-related mortality. The Global Breast Cancer Initiative employs three key strategies: health promotion and early detection, timely diagnosis, and comprehensive breast cancer management [5]. Ultrasound has emerged as a primary supplemental screening modality, especially in women with dense breasts.

Ultrasonographic assessment of the female pelvis and early detection of abnormalities are critical in providing timely and comprehensive treatment. Similarly, early detection [discovery, finding] of breast and other malignancies aids in comprehensive care provision. The importance of ultrasonography in women's health is covered in this chapter. The chapter focused on the usefulness of sonography in evaluating the female reproductive system, pregnancy and related problems, and the breast and abdomen. The authors believe it will offer a comprehensive understanding of the roles of ultrasound in women's health.

2. Role of ultrasound in the assessment of female reproductive organs

Ultrasound imaging can be utilized to assess pelvic lesions, uterine abnormalities, ovarian lesions, and pelvic pain [6–8]. Trans-abdominal or trans-vaginal sonographic scanning methods can be employed to evaluate the female pelvis.

Ultrasound is used to examine normal female reproductive organs [9]. Similarly, it is used to assess the physiological changes in the female reproductive system. For example, the normal endometrial cavity measured up to 1.6 cm in the middle of the menstrual cycle during the premenopausal period and up to 0.5 cm during the postmenopausal period [8].

In suspected pelvic lesion, clinical assessments of female reproductive organs were difficult due to poor clinical characterization of lesion with physical examination alone [10]. Even though histopathology has been considered as a gold standard in the assessment of female pelvic lesions, the radiological imaging transformed the assessment of the lesion, characterization, guiding surgical plan, and follow-up assessments [11]. Ultrasonography and MRI are the most frequently used radiological imaging modalities in the assessment of female pelvic organs [10]. This section has discussed the role of ultrasound to diagnose lesions, abnormalities, and infertility-related problems in the female pelvic organs.

2.1 Sonographic assessment of female reproductive organs' malformations

Uterine malformations are developmental abnormalities of the female reproductive tract and occur due to various changes in the normal development of the Müllerian ducts. These malformations can result from underdevelopment, a fusion defect, or a resorption defect in the Müllerian duct [12–14]. The ASRM Müllerian Anomalies Classification 2021 classifies Müllerian anomalies into the nine categories [15]. The ASRM identified the malformations by descriptive terminology: Müllerian agenesis, cervical agenesis, unicornuate uterus, uterus didelphys, bicornuate uterus, septate uterus, longitudinal vaginal septum, transverse vaginal septum, and complex

Malformation	Clinical symptoms	Management	Purpose of treatment	Obstetric outcomes
Müllerian agenesis—Mayer-Rokitansky-Küster-Hauser Syndrome [19]	Primary amenorrhea	Surgical management	To enable satisfactory sexual intercourse with the construction of a neovagina.	Uterine factor infertility
Unicornuate uterus [20–22]	Dysmenorrhea, chronic pelvic pain, and hematometra leading to endometriosis and infertility.	The rudimentary horn can be resected in those with intractable severe dysmenorrhea, dyspareunia, and chronic pelvic pain related to endometriosis. Surgery is also recommended for patients with a functional rudimentary horn containing an endometrial cavity to prevent a complicated or dangerous pregnancy within the horn.	Symptom relief, to prevent complicated pregnancy within rudimentary horn.	First-trimester miscarriage, preterm birth
Bicornuate uterus [23, 24]	Intra- and postmenstrual dysmenorrhea, pelvic tumor, postmenstrual spotting	Surgical management with a Strassmann metroplasty	To avoid adverse obstetric outcome	Predisposed to both first- and second-trimester miscarriages
Uterus didelphys uterus	Hematocolpos, pyocolpos, hematometra, hematosalpinx	Surgical management with a Strassmann metroplasty	To improve recurrent pregnancy loss	Recurrent pregnancy loss

Table 1.
Uterine malformations.

anomalies. Acién, M. and Acién, P. (2022) proposed a system for classifying female genitourinary anomalies according to their embryologic origin, with six groups: (1) agenesis or hypoplasia of an entire urogenital ridge, (2) mesonephric anomalies, (3) isolated Müllerian anomalies, (4) gubernaculum dysfunctions, (5) anomalies of the urogenital sinus, and (6) combinations of malformations [16, 17].

Imaging techniques are being adopted to diagnose uterine abnormalities, which have a significant effect on optimizing women's health. Ultrasound, especially 3D ultrasound, is a preferred method for detecting uterine abnormalities. Contrast-enhanced 3D sonography is currently recognized as the gold standard diagnostic technique [18]. Finding the anomalies makes it easier to identify related problems and allows for proper management. In **Table 1**, the anomalies and related problems are depicted.

2.2 Sonographic assessment of female pelvic lesions

Ultrasound is the imaging choice when evaluating a pelvic lesion or an undefined pelvic pain in patients. It is used to evaluate the location, size, number, and appearance of the lesions. Once the pelvic lesion has been identified by ultrasound, it is also important to track mass growth over time [8].

Leiomyomas (myomas, fibroids) are the most common uterine lesions in premenopausal women and usually detected by sonography [8, 9]. Uterine fibroids are benign tumors arising from uterine smooth muscle cells with varying amounts of the fibrous tissue. Most women having fibroids are asymptomatic. However, if the fibroid is submucosal, menorrhagia may occur, and subfertility may occur due to either the mass effect or narrowed fallopian tube, or interfere with implantation. Pain, urinary, and bowel symptoms may be experienced. In addition, fibroids also cause fetal malposition and premature uterine contraction in pregnant women [9]. Fibroids are estrogen dependent, so that they regress after the menopause. In addition, ultrasound is used to assess cervical and ovarian lesions.

2.2.1 Sonographic assessment of uterine lesions

Ultrasonography is used to identify uterine leiomyomas and hence used to guide the treatment. They have variable sonographic appearances. On sonography, an enlarged uterus with or without irregular outline, a well-defined hypoechoic round mass within uterus, or areas of mixed echogenicity [25] is observed. And there is distortion of the endometrial outline, if there is submucosal lesion. Fibroids also undergo degeneration and calcify. Ultrasonography also localizes the fibroids as: submucosal, intramural, subserosal, or pedunculated. The location of the lesions is very important to plan treatment.

The other uterine lesion detected by ultrasonography is adenomyosis. Adenomyosis is defined as the presence of endometrial tissue within the uterine myometrium [26, 27]. It causes dysmenorrhea, menorrhagia, urinary tract dysfunction and affects fertility [28].

Ultrasound is used to diagnose adenomyosis. Adenomyosis appeared on ultrasound as an enlarged uterus, often with an asymmetric anterior and posterior myometrial walls [29]. In addition, myometrial heterogeneity caused by endometrial implants and myometrial cysts is evident on ultrasound [27].

2.2.2 Endometrial abnormalities

Whether a woman presents with or without abnormal uterine bleeding, ultrasound is helpful in identifying endometrial abnormalities. Ultrasonography is considered the gold standard for determining endometrial thickness and diagnosing benign or malignant endometrial lesions [30, 31]. It helps in the assessment of the Asherman syndrome, hematometra, endometritis, endometrial hyperplasia, endometrial polyp, and endometrial cancer.

Asherman syndrome is manifested as intrauterine adhesions caused by trauma to a gravid uterine cavity, trauma to non-gravid endometrium, infection, Müllerian duct malformations (especially septate uterus), and genetic predisposition [32]. The symptoms of Asherman syndrome include menstrual abnormalities (amenorrhea and hypomenorrhea), infertility, recurrent pregnancy loss, and spontaneous miscarriage.

Sonohysterography, which combines transvaginal sonography with intrauterine injection of saline solution, has been shown to be superior to transvaginal ultrasonography in the detection of intrauterine adhesions. The visualization of echogenic areas within the saline-filled cavity denotes the presence of intrauterine adhesions [33].

Ultrasonography is also a choice of imaging to detect hematometra. Hematometra is a collection or retention of blood in the uterus most commonly due to an imperforate hymen or transverse vaginal septum. Ultrasonography effectively evaluates hematometra [23]. It is also used to evaluate the resolution of hematometra after treatment [34].

Ultrasonography is also used to evaluate uterine infections. Uterine infections usually occur in the puerperium, postoperatively, or after septic abortion. Pyometra within endometrial cavity is seen with a cervical stenosis due to cervical mass, following radiotherapy or as a result of complication of endometritis.

Another endometrial abnormality evaluated by ultrasound is endometrial hyperplasia, the proliferation of the endometrial gland. It causes abnormal uterine bleeding, postmenopausal bleeding, and infertility. Transvaginal sonography is an appropriate diagnostic tool in premenopause and postmenopause women presenting with abnormal uterine bleeding, especially in detecting endometrial hyperplasia [11].

Endometrial polyps are also detected by ultrasound. They are focal growths of the uterine mucosa and consist of endometrial glands, stroma, and blood vessels. Even though they may be asymptomatic, polyps are commonly identified during investigations for abnormal uterine bleeding and infertility [7]. Sonohysterography is used to detect polyps [25].

A malignant adenocarcinoma arising from the endometrium, endometrial carcinoma, is also assessed using ultrasound. It is a common malignancy affecting women worldwide [35]. The most significant risk factors for endometrial carcinomas are age, race, metabolic syndrome, unopposed estrogen exposure, and genetic predispositions [36]. It clinically manifests with postmenopausal uterine bleeding. Ultrasound shows non-specific thickening of the endometrium and this can be indistinguishable from hyperplasia or polyps. There may be a disruption in irregular endometrial surface.

2.2.3 Sonographic assessment of cervical pathologies

Ultrasound also plays a great role in the evaluation of cervical lesions. Ultrasound is used to diagnose nabothian cysts and cervical carcinoma. Nabothian cysts (retention cysts) are formed from the occlusion of the cervical glands, which lie close to the endocervical canal. They may be single or multiple. Nabothian cysts typically contain simple fluid and are asymptomatic. Uncommonly, nabothian cysts may be complicated by hemorrhage or infection or grow to large size [37]. Cervical cancer is a common gynecologic malignancy among women. It is the fourth for both incidence and mortality in Global Cancer Statistics 2018 [38]. Cervical cancer is the leading cause of cancer-related deaths in women, especially among women living in lower-income countries [39]. Its clinical presentation includes abnormal uterine bleeding (especially after intercourse) and vaginal discharge. Ultrasound is used to detect enlarged cervix, hypoechoic mass with or without hydro- or hematometra, and its complications like hydronephrosis.

2.2.4 Sonographic assessment of ovaries

Ultrasound is the imaging of choice for the assessment of the ovaries. Ultrasound is used to assess normal ovarian changes due to age and menstrual cycles, physiological ovarian cysts, cystic ovarian lesions, solid ovarian lesions, and vascular ovarian abnormalities [6, 8].

2.2.4.1 Physiologic ovarian cyst

The majority of ovarian cysts in premenopausal women are physiologic cysts. These cysts include follicular cysts and corpus luteal cysts. A follicular cyst develops if ovulation does not occur and follicular growth continues because of the lack of the luteinizing hormone surge and excessive stimulation by follicular stimulating hormone. On the other hand, corpus luteal cyst formed after an egg is detached from a dominant ovarian follicle. Follicular cyst appeared well-defined, thin-walled, anechoic, and homogeneous internal echogenicity on ultrasound. Corpus luteal cyst appeared as thick-walled cyst demonstrating peripheral color Doppler signal. The corpus luteum may bleed internally as a result of vascularization of the inner granulosa layer following ovulation forming a hemorrhagic corpus luteum. These cysts frequently resolved spontaneously [40].

All functional cysts may undergo hemorrhagic changes, most frequently seen in corpus luteal cysts. Ultrasound is also used to evaluate hemorrhagic ovarian cysts [6]. Women with hemorrhagic ovarian cysts frequently present with acute onset of pelvic pain. Hemorrhagic ovarian cysts show a spectrum of findings because of the variable sonographic appearances of blood, amount of hemorrhage, and time of the hemorrhage [41].

Sonography is used in the assessment of polycystic ovarian syndrome. It is a multifaceted endocrinologic disorder of ovarian dysfunction and the common cause of infertility and a higher rate of early pregnancy loss [42]. On sonography, polycystic ovarian syndrome appeared as bilaterally enlarged ovaries containing multiple small follicles and increased stromal echogenicity.

2.2.4.2 Cystic ovarian lesion

Ultrasound is used to diagnose cystic ovarian lesions. Most ovarian tumors are cystic: serous cystadenoma, dermoid cyst, mucinous cystadenoma, polycystic ovarian syndrome, surface epithelial cyst, and theca lutein cyst [6, 43, 44].

The sonographic features of the cystic ovarian lesions are non-specific. But some of the cystic ovarian lesions have more specific sonographic features [8]. For instance, dermoid cyst appeared as a cystic mass with echogenic nodules projecting into lumen, posterior sound attenuation, fine internal echogenic lines, and a fluid-fluid level on sonography. While serous cystadenoma appeared as an usually large, thin-walled, and unilocular cyst, it may contain thin septations [44]. Mucinous cystadenoma appeared as a multilocular cyst with thin septations.

2.2.4.3 Solid ovarian lesions

Solid ovarian tumors are divided as epithelial, gem cells, and sex cord-stromal. Some of solid ovarian tumors include Brenner tumor, dysgerminoma, fibroma, and granulosa cell tumor. Ovarian cancer can be treated with a very good prognosis if detected in the early stages, but not after it has advanced. Ultrasound is used to identify ovarian tumors. Transvaginal ultrasound is capable of identifying changes in ovarian size and structure, and thereby detects early ovarian malignancies [45]. Transvaginal ultrasound combined with Doppler blood flow imaging and power

Doppler is used to evaluate blood flow to ovarian tumors and to identify patterns of flow associated with ovarian neoplasia.

2.2.4.4 Vascular ovarian abnormalities

Ultrasound is also helpful in the assessment of ovarian vascular abnormalities such as: ovarian torsion. It is caused by either partial or complete rotation of the ovary over its pedicle and is commonly associated with adnexal mass [8]. Its clinical presentation is acute onset of pelvic pain. Its timely diagnosis is very essential to prevent loss of ovary. A surgical emergency is a choice of management. On ultrasound, the torsed ovary appears asymmetrically enlarged, round, heterogeneous, free fluid and may be a coexisting adnexal mass. On Doppler study, either decreased or absent arterial and venous flow to the ovary is observed.

2.2.5 Sonographic assessment of fallopian tubes

Ultrasound is used to assess the fallopian tubes [44]. Assessing fallopian tubes may help to diagnose hydrosalpinx, pyosalpinx, salpingitis, and tubo-ovarian abscess. Hydrosalpinx appears on ultrasound as thin-walled anechoic tubular adnexal mass without internal vascular flow [8, 46]. And pyosalpinx appears on ultrasound as complex tubular adnexal mass with irregular margins and sound attenuation, while tubo-ovarian abscess appears as complex multilocular adnexal mass with ill-defined wall margins [8, 44].

3. Role of sonography in the assessment of infertility

Infertility is suggested when conception does not occur within 1 year. It can be caused either by male or female reproductive abnormalities. Ultrasound is used in the assessment of some of the causes of infertility that arise from female reproductive abnormalities. Some of the causes of infertility diagnosed by ultrasound are: pelvic inflammatory disease (PID), fibroids, polycystic ovarian syndrome, uterine malformations, endometriosis, endometrial pathologies, para-ovarian cyst, peritoneal inclusion cyst, Krukenberg tumor, and endometriosis [7, 23, 43, 47, 48].

Ultrasound is used to assess the structural anatomy of the uterus and endometrium [8, 44, 49]. Uterus is assessed for any congenital anomalies and abnormalities. A septate uterus has a high incidence of infertility [8, 12, 15, 17, 18]. Saline infusion sonograms with or without 3D assessment are used to assess the uterine cavity for any abnormalities and can also be used for tubal patency assessment [50]. Ultrasound is used to assess endometrium for the presence of polyps and intrauterine adhesions (Asherman's syndrome) [8, 32, 33, 51]. Polycystic ovarian syndrome contributes to female infertility secondary to anovulation and its sonographic findings are discussed above [44].

Pelvic inflammatory disease is an infection of the upper genital tract, usually related to *Neisseria gonorrhoeae* or chlamydia. It is a term used to describe a group of infections affecting the uterus, fallopian tubes, and ovaries. Adolescent females are in a higher-risk group, and thus, PID should be considered in sexually active females with pelvic pain. On ultrasound, pelvic scan may appear normal, and uterus may be enlarged and more hyperechoic, may contain a small amount of fluid in the endometrial canal, and may have indistinct margins, fluid-filled and dilated fallopian tubes (pyosalpinx), ovarian enlargement with tiny cysts, and tubo-ovarian abscess (heterogeneous adnexal mass) [8].

Ultrasound is also utilized in the assessment of endometriosis. It is the result of functional endometrium located outside the uterus causing painful periods, chronic pelvic pain, pain during and/or after sexual intercourse, painful bowel movements, painful urination, fatigue, depression or anxiety, and abdominal bloating and nausea [48, 52–54]. In addition to the above, endometriosis can cause infertility. Infertility occurs due to the probable effects of endometriosis on the pelvic cavity, ovaries, fallopian tubes, or uterus [55].

Endometriosis remains difficult to diagnose. Although further study is required to determine their accuracy, transvaginal ultrasonography and MRI show some hope in the diagnosis of endometriosis [56]. Particularly, ultrasound is helpful in the diagnosis of ovarian endometrioma, adhesions, and deep nodular forms of endometriosis.

4. The role of ultrasound in the assessment of pregnancy

Since 1978, ultrasound has been used in clinical obstetrics. With technological advancements, resolution has improved, allowing for far better imaging of the fetus. This, together with recent discoveries in the field of screening for pregnancy problems, has led to a change in the clinical application of ultrasonography in the management of routine low-risk pregnant women [57].

The use of obstetric ultrasound in pregnant women is considered a safe and reliable method [5–60]. Its utilization in pregnancy is crucial, as it allows for early detection of various fetal abnormalities, assessment of fetal biometry, and ultimately improves the quality of antenatal care and pregnancy outcomes [58, 61, 62]. The World Health Organization (WHO) recommends all pregnant women get at least one obstetric US before 24 weeks of gestational age (GA) [63].

The use of ultrasound in obstetrics can be either elective or reactive. Elective or planned use of ultrasound implies scanning to detect potential problems in an otherwise seemingly uncomplicated pregnancy (screening), whereas reactive use is the application of ultrasound to help in the management of a clinical problem such as suspected fetal growth restriction [57].

Planned use of ultrasound includes: pregnancy dating, assessment of multiple pregnancies, placental location, amniotic fluid volume, and screening (of chromosomal aneuploidy, congenital heart defects, neural tube defects, pre-eclampsia and intra-uterine growth restriction, and preterm delivery) [4, 8, 44].

Reactive use of ultrasound includes: assessment of fetal growth (small for gestational age, large for gestational age, reduced fetal movements, antepartum hemorrhage, ruptured membranes, and prolonged pregnancy) [61, 64, 65].

4.1 Ultrasound imaging in the first trimester

First-trimester ultrasonography is a common procedure performed within the first 14-week post-conception [63]. It may be used as part of the standard prenatal evaluation or to interpret other problematic signs and symptoms. It can be done trans-abdominally (with the transducer placed over the abdomen) or trans-vaginally (the transducer is narrow and placed in the vagina). Both procedures can be done at the same time in some cases [66].

4.1.1 Indications

First-trimester ultrasonography can be done for a variety of reasons. Pelvic pain, suspected ectopic pregnancy, suspected twin pregnancy, vaginal bleeding, suspected trophoblastic disease, assessment for fetal growth abnormalities, nuchal translucency measurement, evaluation of pelvic masses or uterine abnormalities, and as an adjunct to chorionic villus sampling are common indications [64].

Additionally, asymptomatic patients in the first trimester may also be scheduled for a regular ultrasound if resources are available to determine an accurate gestational age [67].

The main objectives of ultrasound examination in the first trimester are establishing pregnancy location, confirmation of viability (cardiac activity in the embryo/fetus), assessment of gestational age (pregnancy dating), detection of signs of early pregnancy failure, assessment of basic anatomy after 11 weeks, and assessment of the existence of multifetal gestations [66].

4.2 The role of ultrasound in reducing maternal mortality in the first trimester

Ultrasound plays a significant role in reducing maternal and perinatal mortality. The common first-trimester conditions that can result in maternal mortality are ectopic pregnancy, abortion, and gestational trophoblastic diseases (GTDs), due to the possibility of severe hemorrhage, shock, or sepsis [51]. To diagnose these early trimester disorders correctly, ultrasound imaging is of utmost value. Therefore, it is critical to rule out early pregnancy pathology in any woman of reproductive age who presents with amenorrhea, unusual bleeding, and/or discomfort utilizing diagnostic ultrasound imaging and beta-human chorionic gonadotropin (HCG).

Ultrasound imaging also plays a crucial role in perinatal mortality reduction by identifying indicators of chromosomal aberrations and structural problems in the fetus to enable early intervention or close monitoring.

4.3 Ultrasound imaging in the second trimester

The second trimester is the most common time for a routine prenatal ultrasound. In many countries, the mid-trimester ultrasound (also known as the second-trimester anatomy scan) is a routine examination used to check fetal anatomy and diagnose any congenital malformations [68].

An ultrasound scan performed between 18 and 22 weeks of gestation provides information to the pregnant woman and her care provider about many aspects of her pregnancy. It is commonly used to assess the number of fetuses, viability, gestational age, anatomical survey, placental location, amniotic fluid, and maternal pelvic organs [69].

4.3.1 The role of ultrasound in reducing maternal mortality in the second trimester

Between 18 and 24 weeks of gestation, ultrasound imaging of the second trimester is commonly carried out. To examine the fetal and maternal structures for abnormalities that could cause maternal and/or perinatal mortality, ultrasound imaging is used.

Fetal anatomy, fetal biometry, amniotic fluid volume, the placenta, the mother's cervix, and uterine and umbilical artery Doppler velocimetry are among the features assessed. The goal is to rule out results connected to preterm labor, IUGR, pre-eclampsia, and fetal chromosomal abnormalities [70].

To optimize pregnancy outcomes, early detection of pre-eclampsia and intrauterine growth restriction using ultrasound imaging in the second trimester are critical and they are significant causes of maternal and newborn mortality that must be identified as early as possible.

4.4 Ultrasound imaging in the third trimester

Ultrasound is commonly used during the third trimester of pregnancy in patients who present asymptomatically or with symptoms. Ultrasound can be used to identify fetal and maternal pathology as well as to follow the progression of a pregnancy.

In the third trimester, ultrasound is indicated for the evaluation and determination of fetal anatomy, fetal anomalies, gestational age, fetal growth, fetal presentation, suspected multiple gestations, placental location, cervical insufficiency, and pelvic mass [71].

4.4.1 The role of ultrasound in reducing maternal mortality in the third trimester

Third-trimester pregnancy complications, such as antepartum hemorrhage, hypertensive disorders, thromboembolism, chorioamnionitis, heart disease, anemia (sickle cell disease), rupture of uterine scar, can all result in maternal death [51].

Ultrasound imaging plays a key role in the assessment of fetal development and health, presentation, placental position, and ultrasound-guided operations are all important factors to consider when deciding whether to carry out an intervention to improve survival rates [65].

Hypertensive disorders are one of the leading causes of maternal deaths globally. These disorders include gestational hypertension, pregnancy-induced hypertension that can progress to pre-eclampsia (mild or severe) and eclampsia, chronic hypertension, chronic hypertension with superimposed pre-eclampsia and/or superimposed eclampsia, and chronic hypertension with superimposed eclampsia [72].

Due to the precise date of gestational age provided by ultrasound imaging, especially when performed in the first trimester, it is helpful to prevent maternal and neonatal death. To enable early intervention when necessary, ultrasound is also utilized to monitor fetal growth and health.

4.5 The role of ultrasound in intrapartum care

A woman in labor is typically evaluated and managed based on clinical findings. The digital assessment of cervical dilatation and fetal head station and position plays a major role in the diagnosis of labor arrest and decisions about the timing or kind of intervention. However, a clinical examination of the head station and position is unreliable and subjective, particularly when the caput succedaneum makes it difficult to feel the sutures and fontanels [73]. The use of ultrasound has been proposed to aid in the management of labor [74].

Intrapartum ultrasound (ultrasound in labor) is a relatively new concept that has emerged in the last 10 years and is getting more popular in developed nations as a component of the assessment of labor progress [75]. It can be performed using a trans-abdominal approach mainly to determine fetal head and spine positions, fetal heart rate, amniotic fluid, and presentation [76], or a transperineal approach, for the assessment of head station and position at low stations [77]. It could also be used to monitor labor progress and, possibly, predict how the labor will turn out [78].

Indication for ultrasound evaluation in labor includes:

- Slow progress or arrest of labor in the first stage.
- Slow progress or arrest of labor in the second stage.
- Ascertainment of fetal head position and station before or when performing instrumental vaginal delivery.
- Objective assessment of fetal head malpresentation and amniotic fluid volume.

4.6 The postpartum ultrasound scan

The postpartum period begins immediately after the delivery of the infant and placenta and lasts for approximately 6–8 weeks, as the reproductive tract anatomically and physiologically returns to the non-pregnant state [79]. Postpartum complications involving the uterus occur in approximately from 8 to 10% of cases. Immediate and late postpartum hemorrhage, puerperal sepsis, and septic pelvic thromboembolism are still potentially fatal conditions [80]. According to WHO data, severe bleeding after childbirth—postpartum hemorrhage (PPH)—is the leading cause of maternal mortality worldwide. Each year, about 14 million women experience PPH resulting in about 70,000 maternal deaths globally [81].

Ultrasound assessment of the postpartum uterus plays an important role in the evaluation of a large proportion of symptomatic puerperal women. It is a preferred imaging modality for excluding the retained placental tissue. Proper application of postpartum ultrasound may allow for more accurate identification of women requiring surgical intervention, resulting in reduced patient morbidity and clinical workload [82].

Common indications for postpartum ultrasound are as follows: Referral to ultrasound may be indicated for a variety of reasons, including suspected retained products of conception or pelvic sepsis, which frequently presents with excessive or erratic bleeding, and primary postpartum hemorrhage (PPH).

5. Ultrasonography assessment of breast

Breast ultrasound is a type of imaging exam that employs sound waves to produce pictures of the internal structures of the breast. It is an important imaging modality commonly utilized for the detection and characterization of lesions in the breast including breast cancer screening [83].

Breast ultrasound is a safe, rapid, widely available, low-cost imaging modality that does not require ionizing radiation and non-invasive procedure without any complications of the procedure itself [83, 84]. Ultrasound (US) is both an adjunct and a complement breast exam and used to help with the diagnosis of breast masses or other abnormalities found during a physical exam, or mammography, or magnetic resonance imaging (MRI) [85–87]. However, in symptomatic women with a lump or localized pain in the breast, ultrasound is a good initial technique for examination.

The following are common indications for breast ultrasound [83, 88]:

- Evaluation and characterization of breast-related complaints and other palpable masses.
- Analyses of abnormalities seen on mammography or breast magnetic resonance imaging.
- A palpable lump discovered during a clinical breast examination.
- Breast implant rupture suspicion is used to distinguish between intracapsular and extracapsular ruptures.
- Percutaneous breast biopsy with needle guidance.
- Patients who underwent follow-up after neoadjuvant chemotherapy.

Ultrasound can also be utilized as an adjuvant breast cancer screening technique in women with dense breast tissue and a negative mammography. These breast US applications have broadened the spectrum of sonographic features currently examined, even permitting the identification of a non-invasive disease, a significant advancement beyond the early basic cyst-versus-solid assessment.

6. Abdominal ultrasound

Most people, aside from women when they hear ultrasound, associate it with pregnancy and how it is used in monitoring the development of a baby in the womb. However, ultrasound can be used to diagnose and help in the treatment of many health issues related to women. Abdominal ultrasound imaging is performed to evaluate kidneys, liver, gallbladder, bile ducts, pancreas, spleen, and abdominal aorta and other blood vessels of the abdomen [8].

Ultrasound is used to help diagnose a variety of conditions, such as abdominal pain or distention, assessment of liver condition, gall stones, enlarged abdominal organ, kidney problems, vascular problems like an abdominal aortic aneurysm, and provide guidance for biopsies [41, 44]. Abdominal ultrasound may also help to pinpoint the cause of an unexplained abdominal pain [89]. Doppler ultrasound also helps to see and evaluate: blockages to blood flow, narrowing of vessels, tumors and congenital vascular malformations, reduced or absent blood flow to various organs, and increased blood flow [9, 90].

7. Conclusion

Ultrasonography plays a significant role in women's health, in the assessment of female reproductive organs and related malformation/lesions, in the determination of infertility, in the assessment of breast, and abdominal examinations. It also plays an important role during antenatal period in determining fetal biometry, in assessing pregnancy and related problems, and in reducing maternal mortality. In general, the addition of ultrasound examination in the evaluation of women's health plays a vital role.

Conflict of interest

The authors declare no conflict of interest.

Author details

Marema Jebessa Kumsa* and Zegeye Wubeshet Haile
Addis Ababa University, Addis Ababa, Ethiopia

*Address all correspondence to: marema.jabessa@aau.edu.et

References

[1] Bricker L, Garcia J, Henderson J, Mugford M, Neilson J, Roberts T, et al. Ultrasound screening in pregnancy: A systematic review of the clinical effectiveness, cost-effectiveness and women's views. Health Technology Assessment. 2000;**4**:1-193

[2] Whitworth M, Bricker L, Mullan C. Ultrasound for fetal assessment in early pregnancy. Cochrane Database of Systematic Reviews. 2015;**2015**:CD007058

[3] Blue NR, Beddow ME, Savabi M, Katukuri VR, Mozurkewich EL, Chao CR. A comparison of methods for the diagnosis of fetal growth restriction between the Royal College of Obstetricians and Gynaecologists and the American College of Obstetricians and Gynecologists. Obstetrics & Gynecology. 2018;**131**:835-841

[4] WHO antenatal care recommendations for a positive pregnancy experience. Maternal and fetal assessment update: imaging ultrasound before 24 weeks of pregnancy. Geneva: World Health Organization; 2022. Licence: CC BY-NC-SA 3.0 IGO

[5] Global Breast Cancer Initiative Implementation Framework: assessing, strengthening and scaling-up of services for the early detection and management of breast cancer. Geneva: World Health Organization; 2023. Licence: CC BY-NC-SA 3.0 IGO

[6] Smorgick N, Maymon R. Assessment of adnexal masses using ultrasound: A practical review. International Journal of Women's Health. 2014;**6**:857-863

[7] Al Chami A, Saridogan E. Endometrial polyps and subfertility. The Journal of Obstetrics and Gynecology of India. 2017;**67**:9-14

[8] Norton ME, Scoutt LM, Feldstein VA, Callen PW. Callen's Ultrasonography in Obstetrics and Gynecology. Philadelphia: Elsevier; 2017

[9] Hagen-Ansert SL. Textbook of Diagnostic Sonography-E-Book. 8th ed. Elsevier Health Sciences; 2018

[10] Kishan TV, Kumar GP, Reddy TV. Role of ultrasonography and magnetic resonance imaging in evaluation of female pelvic masses from reproductive organs with histopathological correlation. International Journal of Radiology and Imaging. 2021;**4**:30-37

[11] Shokouhi B. Role of transvaginal ultrasonography in diagnosing endometrial hyperplasia in pre- and post-menopause women. Nigerian Medical Journal. 2015;**56**:353

[12] Acién P, Acién M, Sánchez-Ferrer M. Complex malformations of the female genital tract. New types and revision of classification. Human Reproduction. 2004;**19**:2377-2384

[13] Acién P. Embryological observations on the female genital tract. Human Reproduction. 1992;7:437-445

[14] Grimbizis GF, Campo R. Congenital malformations of the female genital tract: The need for a new classification system. Fertility and Sterility. 2010;**94**:401-407. DOI: 10.1016/j.fertnstert.2010.02.030

[15] Pfeifer SM, Attaran M, Goldstein J, Lindheim SR, Petrozza JC, Rackow BW, et al. ASRM müllerian anomalies classification 2021. Fertility and Sterility. 2021;**116**:1238-1252

[16] Acién M, Acién P. Classification of Müllerian anomalies: Is a consensus possible? Case Reports Women's Heal. 2022;**34**:e00413

[17] Acie MI, Acie P. The history of female genital tract malformation classifications and proposal of an updated system. 2011;**17**:693-705

[18] Amaral PP, Ambrósio P, Condeço R. Congenital malformations of the female genital tract: A review of available classification systems. International Society for Gynecologic Endoscopy. 2022;**3**:44-56

[19] Frank RT. The formation of an artificial vagina without operation. American Journal of Obstetrics & Gynecology. 1938;**35**:1053-1055

[20] Li Y, Phelps A, Zapala MA, Mackenzie JD, Mackenzie TC, Courtier J. Magnetic resonance imaging of Müllerian duct anomalies in children. Pediatric Radiology. 2016;**46**:796-805

[21] Duhan N, Kadian YS, Dahiya K, Yadav K, Rattan KN. Reproductive issues in müllerian anomalies. Journal of Gynecologic Surgery. 2012;**28**:127-133

[22] Chan YY, Jayaprakasan K, Tan A, Thornton JG, Coomarasamy A. Reproductive outcomes in women with congenital uterine anomalies: A systematic review. Ultrasound Obstet Gynecol. 2011;**37**:371-382

[23] Rackow BW, Arici A. Reproductive performance of women with müllerian anomalies. Current Opinion in Obstetrics & Gynecology. 2007;**19**:229-237

[24] Letterie GS. Management of congenital uterine abnormalities. Reproductive BioMedicine Online. 2011;**23**:40-52

[25] Wozniak A, Wozniak S. Ultrasonography of uterine leiomyomas. Przegląd Menopauzalny. 2017;**16**:113-117

[26] Habiba M, Benagiano G, Brosens I. The pathophysiology of adenomyosis. Uterine Adenomyosis. 2015;**4**:45-70

[27] Bergeron C, Amant F, Ferenczy A. Pathology and physiopathology of adenomyosis. Best Practice & Research. Clinical Obstetrics & Gynaecology. 2006;**20**:511-521

[28] Ekin M, Cengiz H, Öztürk E, Kaya C, Yaşar L. Genitourinary symptoms in patients with adenomyosis. International Urogynecology Journal and Pelvic Floor Dysfunction. 2013;**24**:509-512

[29] Cunningham RK, Horrow MM, Smith RJ, Springer J. Adenomyosis on US Radiographics. Radio Graphics. 2018;**8**:1576-1589

[30] Giannella L, Mfuta K, Setti T, Boselli F, Bergamini E, Cerami LB. Diagnostic accuracy of endometrial thickness for the detection of intra-uterine pathologies and appropriateness of performed hysteroscopies among asymptomatic postmenopausal women. European Journal of Obstetrics, Gynecology, and Reproductive Biology. 2014;**177**:29-33. DOI: 10.1016/j.ejogrb.2014.03.025

[31] Van Den Bosch T, Verbakel JY, Valentin L, Wynants L, De Cock B, Pascual MA, et al. Typical ultrasound features of various endometrial pathologies described using international endometrial tumor analysis (IETA) terminology in women with abnormal uterine bleeding. Ultrasound in Obstetrics & Gynecology. 2021;**57**:164-172

[32] Yu D, Wong YM, Cheong Y, Xia E, Li TC. Asherman syndrome-one century later. Fertility and Sterility. 2008;**89**:759-779

[33] Manchanda R, Rathore A, Carugno J, Della Corte L, Tesarik J, Török P, et al. Classification systems of Asherman's syndrome. An old problem with new directions. Minimally Invasive Therapy and Allied Technologies. 2021;**30**:304-310. DOI: 10.1080/13645706.2021.1893190

[34] Di Spiezio SA, Di Carlo C, Salerno MC, Sparice S, Bifulco G, Guida M, et al. Use of office hysteroscopy to empty a very large hematometra in a young virgin patient with mosaic Turner's syndrome. Fertility and Sterility. 2007;**87**:417.e1-417.e3

[35] Song Y, Yang J, Liu Z, Shen K. Preoperative evaluation of endometrial carcinoma by contrast-enhanced ultrasonography. BJOG: An International Journal of Obstetrics & Gynaecology. 2009;**116**:294-299

[36] Passarello K, Kurian S, Villanueva V. Endometrial cancer: An overview of pathophysiology, management, and care. Seminars in Oncology Nursing. 2019;**35**:157-165. DOI: 10.1016/j.soncn.2019.02.002

[37] Fleischer AC, Kepple DM. Benign conditions of the uterus, cervix and endometrium. In: Nyberg DA, Hill LM, Böhm-Velez M, Mendelson EB, editors. Transvaginal Ultrasound. St. Louis: Mosby Inc; 1992. pp. 21-24

[38] Bray F, Ferlay J, Soerjomataram I, Siegel RL, Torre LA, Jemal A. Global cancer statistics 2018: GLOBOCAN estimates of incidence and mortality worldwide for 36 cancers in 185 countries. CA: a Cancer Journal for Clinicians. 2018;**68**:394-424

[39] International Agency for Research on Cancer [Internet]. Available from: https://gco.iarc.fr/ [Accessed: February 15, 2023]

[40] Romiti A, Moro F, Ricci L, Codeca C, Pozzati F, Viggiano M, et al. Using IOTA terminology to evaluate fetal ovarian cysts: Analysis of 51 cysts over 10 years. Ultrasound in Obstetrics & Gynecology. 2022;**61**(3):408-414

[41] Bhargava SK, Kumar A, Agarwal V. Sonographic spectrum of hepatic tumors. Ultrasound International. 2002;**8**:127-133

[42] Eden JA, Warren P. A review of 1019 consecutive cases of polycystic ovary syndrome demonstrated by ultrasound. Australasian Radiology. 1999;**43**:41-46

[43] Buttram VC, Gomel V, Siegler A, DeCherney A, Gibbons W, March C. The American fertility society classifications of adnexal adhesions, distal tubal occlusion, tubal occlusion secondary to tubal ligation, tubal pregnancies, Mullerian anomalies and intrauterine adhesions. Fertility and Sterility. 1988;**49**:944-955. DOI: 10.1016/S0015-0282(16)59942-7

[44] Rumack CM, Levine D. Diagnostic ultrasound. 5th ed. Philadelphia: Elsevier Health Sciences; 2017

[45] DiSantis DJ, Scatarige JC, Kemp G, Given FT, Hsiu JG, Cramer MS. A prospective evaluation of transvaginal sonography for detection of ovarian disease. American Journal of Roentgenology. 1993;**161**:91-94

[46] Benacerraf BR, Abuhamad AZ, Bromley B, Goldstein SR, Groszmann Y, Shipp TD, et al. Consider ultrasound first for imaging the female pelvis. American Journal of Obstetrics & Gynecology. 2015;**212**:450-455

[47] Felker EA. Uterus didelphys and pregnancy. Journal of Diagnostic Medical Sonography. 2004;**20**:131-133

[48] Moro F, Leombroni M, Testa AC. Ultrasound imaging in endometriosis. Obstetrics and Gynecology Clinics of North America. 2019;**46**:643-659

[49] Stephenson SR. Diagnostic medical sonography: Obstetrics and gynecology. 3rd ed. Philadelphia: Lippincott Williams & Wilkins; 2012

[50] Rashid SQ, Chou YH, Tiu CM. Ultrasonography of uterine Leiomyomas. Journal of Ultrasound in Medicine. 2016;**24**:3-12. DOI: 10.1016/j.jmu.2015.12.006

[51] Cheng Y-L, Lee C-Y, Huang Y-L, Buckner CA, Lafrenie RM, Dénommée JA, et al. The role of obstetric ultrasound in reducing maternal and perinatal mortality. In: Ultrasound Imaging–Medical Applications. Rijeka, Croatia: InTech; 2011. pp. 207-234

[52] Woodward PJ, Sohaey R, Mezzetti TP. From the archives of the AFIP. Endometriosis: Radiologic-pathologic correlation. Radiographics. 2001;**21**:193-216

[53] Zondervan KT, Becker CM, Missmer SA. Endometriosis. The New England Journal of Medicine. 2020;**382**:1244-1256

[54] Agarwal SK, Chapron C, Giudice LC, Laufer MR, Leyland N, Missmer SA, et al. Clinical diagnosis of endometriosis: A call to action. American Journal of Obstetrics and Gynecology. 2019;**220**:354.e1-354.e12. DOI: 10.1016/j.ajog.2018.12.039

[55] Endometriosis [Internet]. Available from: https://www.who.int/news-room/fact-sheets/detail/endometriosis [Accessed: February 19, 2023]

[56] Nisenblat V, Bossuyt PMM, Farquhar C, Johnson N, Hull ML. Imaging modalities for the non-invasive diagnosis of endometriosis. Cochrane Database of Systematic Reviews. 2016;**2016**:CD009591

[57] Roberts N, Thilaganathan B. The role of ultrasound in obstetrics. Obstetrics, Gynaecology and Reproductive Medicine. 2007;**17**:79-85

[58] Abduljabbar HS, Jabal NA Bin, Hussain FA, Alqabbaa RM, Marwani FA, Alghamdi SA, et al. Knowledge, Attitudes and Practice about Obstetric Ultrasonography among Women Attending a University Hospital: A Cross-Sectional Study. Open Journal of Obstetrics and Gynecology. 2020;**10**:1763-1775

[59] Bashour H, Hafez R, Abdulsalam A. Syrian women's perceptions and experiences of ultrasound screening in pregnancy: Implications for antenatal policy. Reproductive Health Matters. 2005;**13**:147-154

[60] Wanyonyi SZ, Mariara CM, Vinayak S, Stones W. Opportunities and challenges in realizing universal access to obstetric ultrasound in sub-Saharan Africa. Ultrasound International Open. 2017;**3**:E52-E59

[61] WHO recommendations on antenatal care for a positive pregnancy experience. Geneva: World Health Organization; 2016

[62] Yetwale A, Kabeto T, Biyazin T, Fenta B. Prenatal ultrasound utilization and its associated factors among pregnant women in Jimma town public health institutions, Ethiopia. Health Services Research and Managerial Epidemiology. 2022;**9**:1-8

[63] Lee WA, Nelson G, Grogan SP. Sonography 1st Trimester Assessment,

Protocols, and Interpretation. Treasure Island (FL): StatPearls Publishing; 2022

[64] Mei JY, Afshar Y, Platt LD. First-trimester ultrasound. Clinical Obstetrics and Gynecology. 2019;**46**:829-852

[65] Eik-Nes SH, Salvesen KÅ, Økland O, Vatten LJ. Routine ultrasound fetal examination in pregnancy: The "ålesund" randomized controlled trial. Ultrasound in Obstetrics & Gynecology. 2000;**15**:473-478

[66] Murugan VA, Murphy BO, Dupuis C, Goldstein A, Kim YH. Role of ultrasound in the evaluation of first-trimester pregnancies in the acute setting. Ultrasonography. Korean Society of Ultrasound in Medicine. 2020;**39**:178

[67] Butt K, Lim K. SOGC clinical practice guideline No. 303: Determination of gestational age by ultrasound. Journal of Obstetrics and Gynaecology Canada. 2014;**36**:171-181

[68] Jabaz D, Abed M. Sonography 2nd Trimester Assessment, Protocols, and Interpretation. Treasure Island (FL): StatPearls Publishing; 2021

[69] Cargill Y, Morin L, Bly S, Butt K, Denis N, Gagnon R, et al. Content of a complete routine second trimester obstetrical ultrasound examination and report. Journal of Obstetrics and Gynaecology Canada. 2009;**31**:272-275

[70] Tunçalp P-RJP, Lawrie T, Bucagu M, Oladapo OT, Portela A, et al. WHO recommendations on antenatal care for a positive pregnancy experience—Going beyond survival. BJOG An International Journal of Obstetrics and Gynaecology. 2017;**124**:860-862

[71] AIUM. Practice parameter for the performance of detailed second- and third-trimester diagnostic obstetric ultrasound examinations. Journal of Ultrasound in Medicine. 2019;**38**:3093-3100

[72] Kenny LC. Hypertensive disorders of pregnancy. Obstetrcs by Ten Teachers. 20th ed. New York: CRC Press; 2017. pp. 133-146

[73] Akmal S, Tsoi E, Nicolaides KH. Intrapartum sonography to determine fetal occipital position: Interobserver agreement. Ultrasound in Obstetrics & Gynecology. 2004;**24**:421-424

[74] Ghi T, Eggebø T, Lees C, Kalache K, Rozenberg P, Youssef A, et al. ISUOG practice guidelines: Intrapartum ultrasound. Ultrasound in Obstetrics & Gynecology. 2018;**52**:128-139

[75] Lau W-L, Yt V, Mbbs C, Hui Mbbs W, Lam W-. Role of intrapartum ultrasound in modern obstetrics. Hong Kong Journal of Gynaecology, Obstetrics and Midwifery. 2017;**17**:134-140

[76] Blasi I, D'Amico R, Fenu V, Volpe A, Fuchs I, Henrich W, et al. Sonographic assessment of fetal spine and head position during the first and second stages of labor for the diagnosis of persistent occiput posterior position: A pilot study. Ultrasound in Obstetrics & Gynecology. 2010;**35**:210-215

[77] Youssef A, Maroni E, Ragusa A, De Musso F, Salsi G, Iammarino MT, et al. Fetal head-symphysis distance: A simple and reliable ultrasound index of fetal head station in labor. Ultrasound in Obstetrics & Gynecology. 2013;**41**:419-424

[78] Tutschek B, Torkildsen EA, Eggebø TM. Comparison between ultrasound parameters and clinical examination to assess fetal head station in labor. Ultrasound in Obstetrics & Gynecology. 2013;**41**:425-429

[79] Vardar Z, Dupuis CS, Goldstein AJ, Siddiqui E, Vardar BU, Kim YH. Pelvic ultrasonography of the postpartum uterus in patients presenting to the emergency room with vaginal bleeding and pelvic pain. Ultrasonography. 2022;**41**(4):782-795

[80] Hansmann M, Bernhard-Joachim Hackelöer AS. Postpartum ultrasound. ultrasound diagnosis in obstetrics and gynecology. Berlin: Springer; 1986. pp. 347-348

[81] WHO Postpartum Haemorrhage Summit [Internet]. Available from: https://www.who.int/news-room/events/detail/2023/03/07/default-calendar/who-postpartum-haemorrhage-summit [Accessed: February 19, 2023]

[82] Üçyiğit A, Johns J. The Postpartum Ultrasound Scan. Ultrasound. Vol. 24. London, England: SAGE Publications Sage UK; 2016. pp. 163-169

[83] Sung JS. High-quality breast ultrasonography imaging -image quality. Radiologic Clinics of North America. 2014;**52**:519-526

[84] Malherbe K, Tafti D. Breast Ultrasound. Treasure Island (FL): StatPearls Publishing; 2022

[85] Esmaeili M, Ayyoubzadeh SM, Ahmadinejad N, Ghazisaeedi M, Nahvijou A, Maghooli K. A decision support system for mammography reports interpretation. Health Information Science and Systems. 2020;**8**:1-8

[86] Hooley RJ, Scoutt LM, Philpotts LE. Breast ultrasonography: State of the art. Radiology. Sep 2013;**268**(3):642-659

[87] Berg WA. Reducing unnecessary biopsy and follow-up of benign cystic breast lesions. Radiology. 2020;**295**:52-53

[88] Lee JM, Arao RF, Sprague BL, Kerlikowske K, Lehman CD, Smith RA, et al. Performance of Screening Ultrasonography as an Adjunct to Screening Mammography in Women Across the Spectrum of Breast Cancer Risk. JAMA Internal Medicine. 2019;**179**:658-667

[89] Ross A, Leleiko NS. Acute abdominal pain differential diagnosis mapped to location of abdominal pain. Paediatrics Reviews. 2010;**31**:135-144

[90] Moradia M. Revealing the hidden facts in ultrasound. Journal of Advanced Medical and Dental Sciences Research. 2015;**3**:86-89

Chapter 11

Perspectives on the Pathogenesis and Complications of PE

Sathiya Ramasamy, Sumathi Saravanan and Jayanthi Rajendran

Abstract

Preeclampsia is a multisystem disorder characterized by hypertension and proteinuria after 20 weeks of gestation. Globally, it is the leading cause of fetal and maternal morbidity and mortality. Nearly 8–10% of women develop hypertension during pregnancy worldwide. Although the actual pathogenesis of PE has not been fully understood, the only cure for the disease is delivery. So, the growing evidence suggests that improper spiral artery remodeling creates placental hypoxia and leads to altered immune response followed by endothelial dysfunction, the release of angiogenic and antiangiogenic factors, and various other vasoactive factors into the maternal circulation. Reliable biochemical markers are needed for the diagnosis of PE at the earliest. MMPs are differentially expressed as a result of the trophoblast invasion's distinct temporal features. Early in the gestational period, MMPs create the conditions for the ensuing incursion to the placental bed. Endothelial dysfunction is the cause of the clinical sign of the mother such as impairment of the hepatic endothelium causing the HELLP syndrome to develop, impairment of the cerebral endothelium causing refractory neurological problems, or even eclampsia. Also, this chapter reveals the various maternal consequences like HELLP syndrome, Seizure, future cardiovascular events, and end-organ dysfunction; fetal complications include premature delivery, respiratory distress, IUGR, etc.

Keywords: preeclampsia, pathogenesis, risk factors, endothelial dysfunction, complications

1. Introduction

Preeclampsia (PE), a multisystem illness, includes hypertension, proteinuria, abnormal maternal biochemical findings either with intrauterine growth restriction, and decreased amniotic fluid volume [1]. PE starts after 20 weeks of pregnancy with vascular dysfunction. Delivering both the fetus and placenta has been the only method of treatment so far, however, this causes more premature births and stunted child growth [2].

Compared to developed countries, women in developing nations had 14 times higher risk of dying from maternal complications. Around 289,000 women globally perished in 2013 as a result of pregnancy problems, and 99% of them were residents of underdeveloped nations. PE alone claims the lives of roughly 12% of mothers worldwide [3]. According to World Health Organization (WHO) estimates, PE occurs seven times more frequently in underdeveloped nations than in wealthy nations. PE is more common in developing nations than in developed ones, with rates ranging from 1.8 to 16.7% [3].

Even though the cause of PE is yet unknown, it is believed that factors such as poor decidualization, inadequate cytotrophoblast invasion, endothelial dysfunction, and unsuitable immunological responses to the allogenic fetus may play a role in the illness [4]. If left untreated, PE involves conditions like stroke, kidney damage, hypoxemia, liver failure, and eclampsia [5]. These processes are linked by an excess release of various biochemical factors, into the maternal circulation, and a common downstream impairment of spiral artery remodeling [4]. This chapter will describe the molecular pathways involved in the pathophysiology and complications of PE.

2. Pathogenesis of PE

The pathogenesis of PE is caused by a variety of causes, including the shallow invasion of cytotrophoblasts, restricted spiral artery remodeling, involvement of immunologic factors, genetical, involvement of microRNAs, etc.

2.1 PE's placental roots

2.1.1 Differentiation of trophoblasts

About 6 days after conception (a.c.)., at the stage of the blastocyst, the trophoblast is the first cell lineage to differentiate Two distinct trophoblast pathways, the villous and the extravillous pathway, are formed as a result of further differentiation processes. The early syncytiotrophoblast is created at the moment of implantation and grows in size as a result of a mechanism that continuously supplies it with mononucleated cytotrophoblast cells [6]. Villous trophoblast cells begin to form at around day 12 post-conception when the cytotrophoblast cells begin to break through the syncytiotrophoblastic mass and move in the direction of the first branches that extend into the intervillous space. The cytotrophoblast cells have reached the mother's side of the syncytiotrophoblast mass only at day 15 a.c. Mononucleated trophoblast cells make their initial contact with the maternal decidual stroma at this stage. Therefore, the subtype of extravillous trophoblast cells is only developed in week 5 post menstruation [7].

The trophoblast lineage develops in week 1 post-conception, whereas the differentiation of the two paths (villous and extravillous) takes place in week 3 post-conception. Regarding the placental origins of prenatal diseases like PE and Intrauterine growth restriction (IUGR), this time variation may be significant [2, 7].

The very early changes in the serum marker concentrations show that PE appears to start developing at the beginning of placentation, possibly even around implantation [8].

1. The trophoblast cell lineage may suffer a serious deficit if the very first differentiation of the lineage is compromised during development from morula to blastocyst. This could lead to IUGR and PE or even more serious consequences including spontaneous abortions.

2. The same dramatic effect as stated above may occur if the insult occurs a little while later when the blastocyst trophoblast divides into the first cytotrophoblast and syncytiotrophoblast

3. If only the development of the extravillous trophoblast pathway is subsequently impacted, this may lead to pure IUGR, which has all the hallmark features such as unsuccessful invasion and aberrant uterine artery Doppler.

4. PE, which has its classic symptoms such as the production of syncytiotrophoblast membrane fragments and a maternal inflammatory response, may occur if only the villous route is impacted.

PE has been well recognized as a result of the realization that early-onset and late-onset PE have different pathophysiologies. Early pregnancy maternal spiral artery transformation was reduced in early-onset, commonly known as placental PE [9]. This is linked to the gross and molecular diseases of the placental tissues as well as placental malperfusion. Increased soluble fms-like Tyrosine kinase-1 (sFLT-1) production and decreased Placental growth factor (PlGF) are caused by the placenta being under oxidative stress, which reflects the biomarker patterns. There is little indication of decreased arterial conversion in late-onset PE, also known as maternal PE, and placental perfusion is maintained or even improved. As a result, there is only a minor degree of placental stress, and the placenta secretes sFLT-1 and PlGF at levels that are close to the normal range [10].

The pathogenesis of early-onset PE begins with aberrant blood vessel development in the mother's spiral arteries. Major adaptive changes, such as spiral artery remodeling in the uterus of the pregnant woman, occur throughout a typical pregnancy to lower maternal blood vessel resistance and subsequently raise uteroplacental perfusion [11]. The placenta receives high-capacitance, low- pressure blood flow as a result of these changes in the spiral arteries, which are crucial for embryonic nourishment [12]. Through trophoblast invasion and the removal of the smooth muscle in the blood vessel wall, spiral artery remodeling is accomplished.

2.2 Immune maladaptation

The PE clinical syndrome, a systemic inflammatory response, and malfunction of maternal peripheral endothelium cells are all caused by placental stress. Reduced blood flow to maternal organs is accompanied by physiological findings such as vasospasm, activation of the coagulation cascade, and decreased plasma volume before the onset of clinical illness [10]. Although there may be hyperplasia of the underlying cytotrophoblast cells, some of them also go through apoptosis or cellular aging. These lesions are connected to the release of trophoblastic debris, which is not surprising [10].

The development of hypertension is facilitated by the excessive release of placental factors such as syncytialtrophoblastic knots/debris, sFlt-1, and the soluble receptor for a vascular endothelial growth factor (VEGF) into the maternal circulation as a result of placental ischemia. These factors together increase oxidative stress. These angiogenic factors are also important inflammatory mediators that support PE-related maternal inflammation (**Figure 1**). Villous cytotrophoblasts secrete inflammatory cytokines such as interleukins (ILs)-1, -2, -4, -6, -8, -10, -12, and -18, transforming growth factor (TGF)-1, IFN- inducible protein 10/IP-10, tumor necrosis

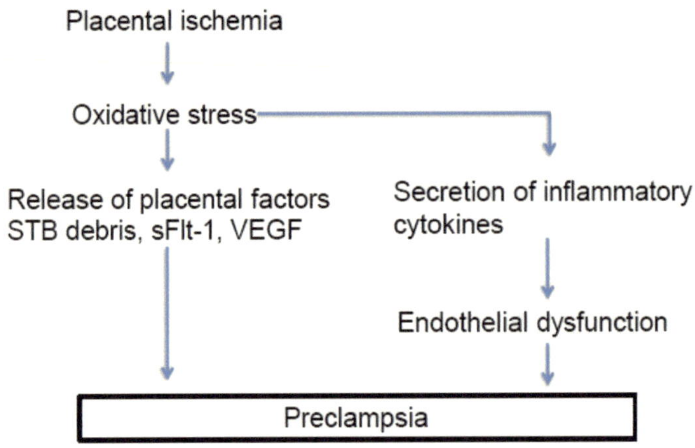

Figure 1.
The diagram depicts the distinct pathways leading to PE. Placental tension causes a release of various placental factors and inflammatory cytokines.

factor (TNF)-, interferon (IFN)-, monocyte chemotactic protein (MCP)-1, intercellular adhesion molecule [8, 13], which contribute in the development of PE.

2.3 Endothelial dysfunction

Endothelial dysfunction is the cause of the clinical sign of mother such as impairment of the hepatic endothelium causing HELLP (Hemolysis, Elevated Liver enzymes, and Low Platelet count) syndrome to develop, impairment of the cerebral endothelium causing refractory neurological problems, or even eclampsia [14]. Vascular endothelial growth factor depletion in podocytes increases the ability of endotheliosis to obstruct the basement membrane's slit diaphragms, contributing to decreased glomerular filtration and proteinuria. The promotion of microangiopathic hemolytic anemia by endothelial dysfunction leads to edema, especially in the lower limbs or lungs, while vascular hyperpermeability brought on by low blood albumin induces edema [9].

2.4 Role of matrix metalloproteinases

Matrix metalloproteinases (MMPs) comprise a group of zinc in the catalytic field of enzyme and calcium-dependent endoproteases, it is well-known to degrade several components of the extracellular matrix (ECM) at physiological pH. It is categorized into collagenases, gelatinases, stromelysins, matrilysins, membrane-type MMPs, and others according to their structure, unique substrate, and subcellular localization [15]. MMPs have numerous tissue distribution, secreted specifically with the aid of pro-inflammatory, uteroplacental tissue including lymphocytes, fibroblasts, vascular smooth muscle, endothelial cells, cytotrophoblasts, neutrophils, and osteoblasts [14]. It is actively involved in extracellular matrix remodeling in physiological and also in some pathological conditions like vascular disorders, cancer, rheumatoid arthritis, neurological, cancer, reproductive changes as well as in chronic inflammation [11, 16].

MMPs are differentially expressed as a result of the trophoblast invasion's distinct temporal features. Early in the gestational period, MMPs create the conditions for the ensuing incursion to the placental bed. MMP-2 has a major function during implantation and MMP-9 during the invasion. In PE, the trophoblast will generate less MMP-9 and MMP-9 inhibition or gene silencing, which will impair trophoblast invasion in vitro. As a result, dysregulated secretion of these enzymes may interfere with physiological trophoblast invasion [15]. Studies demonstrate that during the first trimester of pregnancy, a low concentration of placental MMPs may have an impact on the remodeling of the spiral arteries, leading to a poorly perfused fetoplacental unit. The vasoconstriction, altered vascular reactivity, and endothelial damage caused by various MMPs may be the cause of the vascular dysfunction seen at the late stage of PE [11, 14, 15]. Due to these factors, MMPs have emerged as potent indicators for identifying pregnant women at risk for PE and as viable biological targets for the treatment of this disease.

2.5 Angiogenic and antiangiogenic markers

PE can be described as a two-stage process, with the preclinical phase beginning early in pregnancy (first trimester) and being defined by aberrant placentation, and the symptomatic phase following (occurring after 20 weeks gestation) and being characterized by the maternal syndrome of hypertension and multiorgan dysfunction [17]. In a healthy pregnancy, the placental bed and uterine circulation dramatically vascularize to allow for the circulation of blood between the mother and the fetus. Uterine vasculature includes vasculogenesis, angiogenesis, and maternal spiral artery remodeling [9]. The molecules that control angiogenesis and vessel remodeling must be carefully balanced for these processes to occur. Ischemia and damage to the placenta are caused by deficiencies in appropriate vascularization and vascular remodeling [2]. When a placenta is aberrant, more antiangiogenic substances, such as sFLT1 and soluble endoglin (sENG), are created and released into the maternal system [4].

3. Indicators of PE risk

National Institute for Health and Care Excellence (NICE) recommendations 2019 [18] classify a woman at high risk of PE if there is a history of hypertensive disease during a previous pregnancy or a maternal disease including chronic kidney disease, autoimmune diseases, diabetes, or chronic hypertension (**Table 1**). Women are at moderate risk if they are nulliparous, ≥40 years of age, have a body mass index (BMI) ≥ 35 kg/m [2], have a family history of PE, a multifoetal pregnancy, or have a pregnancy interval of more than 10 years [3]. These risk factors are echoed in the largest meta-analysis of clinical risk factors to date conducted by Bartsch et al. [8], who analyzed over 25 million pregnancies from 92 studies. The presence of one high-risk factor, or two or more moderate risk factors, is used to help guide aspirin prophylaxis, which is effective in reducing the risk of PE if administered before 16 weeks of pregnancy [9, 10]. There are additional clinical factors that significantly increase PE risk, including raised mean arterial blood pressure before 15 weeks gestation [11], polycystic ovarian syndrome [12–14], sleep-disordered breathing [15], and various infections such as periodontal disease, urinary tract infections [16], and *Helicobacter pylori* [17, 18]. In terms of obstetric history, vaginal bleeding for at least 5 days during pregnancy increases PE risk [11], as does the use of oocyte donation, which has a higher risk of PE in comparison to In Vitro Fertilization (IVF) without oocyte donation or natural conception [19–21].

High-risk factors	Moderate risk	Other clinical factors
Previous history of PE	>40 years of age	Increased mean arterial
Chronic kidney disease	BMI ≥35 kg/m	pressure before 15wks of
Autoimmune diseases	Family history of PE	gestation
Diabetes	Multifoetal pregnancy	Polycystic ovarian
Chronic hypertension	Lengthy	syndrome (PCOD)
Pre-gestational diabetes	interconceptional period	Sleep-disordered
	(> 5 years)	breathing
	Assisted Reproduction	Infections (*H. Pylori*,
		Urinary tract infections
		(UTI)
		Vaginal bleeding

Table 1.
Risk factors of PE [10, 18, 19].

4. Screening and early diagnosis of PE

PE frequently has no symptoms, making it challenging to predict the syndrome. A terminal crisis, such as eclampsia or HELLP syndrome, which necessitates an immediate termination of pregnancy, is frequently heralded by symptoms like epigastric discomfort or excruciating headache [10]. Circulating biomarkers or a Doppler ultrasonography analysis of the uteroplacental circulation can both identify PE that is either impending or already present [2]. This may be helpful for the early-onset form of the condition but not the late-onset form. To allow for therapies like aspirin prophylaxis, which must be started early to be effective, it is crucial to screen for PE in the first trimester of pregnancy [20]. In the Fetal Medicine Foundation (FMF) approach, the additional evaluation of biochemical and biophysical parameters, including monitoring the mean arterial blood pressure, the uterine artery Doppler analysis, as well as assessing biomarkers like the placental protein A (PAPP-A) and PlGF, can identify up to 75% of women who are destined to develop PE, requiring delivery 37 weeks of gestation [20].

A known risk factor for PE is being overweight or obese. According to much research, PE potentiates the normal disruption of the connection between adiposity and serum leptin concentrations, which is then furthered by rising BMI [21–23]. In response to hypoxic conditions, the levels of leptin rise in the vascular compartment and are used as an indicator of placental ischemia. The under-perfused placenta may receive more nutrients as a result of this feedback mechanism [23].

5. Complications of PE

Hypertension during pregnancy increases the risk of PE with unfavorable maternal, fetal, and neonatal consequences [24]. Moreover, the risk of PE needs to be separated from the patient's inherent risk, which could only be shown when PE is under stress. To enhance the health of women around the world, this information

Maternal outcome	Fetal outcome
Hypertension	**IUGR**
Diabetes mellitus	Respiratory distress
Antepartum and postpartum	Preterm delivery
hemorrhage	Stillbirth
Pulmonary edema	Necrotizing enterocolitis
Placental abruption	
Coagulopathy	
Future cardiovascular risk	
Renal disorder	
Hepatic failure	
CNS damage	
Seizure	
Death	

Table 2.
Maternal and fetal outcome due to adverse effects of PE [9, 25–27].

will help create new treatments, interventions, and screening suggestions [12]. There are several placenta-related consequences of the diseases, including placental insufficiency, placental abruption, intrauterine growth restriction, premature birth, and intrauterine fetal death (**Table 2**). Thrombocytopenia disseminated intravascular coagulation, acute pulmonary edema, cerebrovascular diseases, and chronic hypertension were additional systemic complications of the disorders whose risk increases by three to twenty-five times compared to women without hypertension (**Table 2**) [28]. Short-term maternal problems of PE include HELLP syndrome, eclampsia, retinal detachment, and cerebrovascular hemorrhage. However, as was already said, PE is now known for its long-term effects, which can appear up to 15 years after childbirth [12].

Worldwide, PE and eclampsia are responsible for 10–15% of maternal mortality. Eclampsia is the primary cause of death in underdeveloped nations, but PE-related complications are more common in industrialized nations. In as many as 3% of severe PE instances, pulmonary edema, a rare but dangerous issue, leads to problems [25]. Eclampsia case fatality ratios range from 0 to 1.8% in high-income countries to 17.7% in middle-income nations like India, which reflects the disparity in maternal health-care quality. In Sweden, there were no maternal deaths attributable to eclampsia in a year, whereas an Indian hospital reported 11 eclampsia-related fatalities [28].

A prospective cohort study in 2022 found a higher level of unfavorable maternal outcomes was seen in the PE group in the Sidama region compared to the normotensive group [29]. PE patients experienced greater rates of maternal death, ICU admission, postpartum hemorrhage, antepartum hemorrhage, and blood transfusion than normotensive patients, also an Indian study reported placental abruption and coagulopathy were the most frequent consequences [25]. The commonest perinatal outcome is preterm birth followed by IUGR, stillbirth, and newborn ended up with early neonatal death [24–26, 30].

6. Conclusions

A complex clinical condition called PE harms nearly all of a pregnant woman's essential organs. The early and late-onset variants are currently the most likely ends of the spectrum. The early onset form is mostly caused by faulty placentation in the first few weeks of pregnancy, which shares an underlying pathophysiology with other placental abnormalities, including reduced fetal growth. In contrast, late-onset PE causes increased oxidative stress followed by maternal malperfusion and demand in fetal-placental function. The last 10 years have seen significant progress in the study of preeclampsia as evidenced by the discovery of a wide array of novel biomarkers that allow early diagnosis of the disease and prediction of the outcome after a half-century of struggling to understand the molecular basis of the disease.

Acknowledgements

To make this study possible, the authors would like to thank Prof. S. Seetesh Ghose, Dean-MGMCRI, Prof. N. Ananthakrishnan, Dean-Faculty, Prof. S.R. Rao, Vice President-Research, Sri Balaji Vidyapeeth, and Prof. SC Parija, Hon'ble Vice-Chancellor, Sri Balaji Vidyapeeth.

Conflict of interest

The authors declare that there is no conflict of interest.

Author details

Sathiya Ramasamy[1*], Sumathi Saravanan[2] and Jayanthi Rajendran[2]

1 Department of Biochemistry, Mahatma Gandhi Medical College and Research Institute (MGMCRI), Sri Balaji Vidyapeeth (Deemed to be University), Puducherry, India

2 Department of Biochemistry, MGMCRI, Puducherry, India

*Address all correspondence to: sathiyar1889@gmail.com

References

[1] Sibai BM. Evaluation and management of severe PE before 34 weeks gestation. American Journal of Obstetrics & Gynecology. 2011;**205**:191-198

[2] Jena MK, Sharma NR, Petitt M, et al. Pathogenesis of PE and therapeutic approaches targeting the placenta. Biomolecules. 2020;**10**:953

[3] Mou AD, Barman Z, Hasan M, et al. Prevalence of PE and the associated risk factors among pregnant women in Bangladesh. Scientific Reports. 2021;**11**:21339

[4] Khalil G. PE: Pathophysiology and the maternal-fetal risk. Available from: https://clinmedjournals.org/articles/jhm/journal-of-hypertension-and-management-jhm-3-024.php?jid=jhm. [Accessed 3 December 2022]

[5] Phipps E, Prasanna D, Brima W, et al. PE: Updates in pathogenesis, definitions, and guidelines. CJASN. 2016;**11**:1102-1113

[6] Fisher SJ. Why is placentation abnormal in PE? American Journal of Obstetrics and Gynecology. 2015;**213**:S115-S122

[7] Huppertz B. Placental origins of PE. Hypertension. 2008;**51**:970-975

[8] Murthi P, Pinar AA, Dimitriadis E, et al. Inflammasomes—A molecular link for altered immunoregulation and inflammation mediated vascular dysfunction in PE. International Journal of Molecular Sciences. 2020;**21**:1406

[9] Armaly Z, Jadaon JE, Jabbour A, et al. PE: Novel mechanisms and potential therapeutic approaches. Frontiers in Physiology. 2018;**9**:1-15. Available from: https://www.frontiersin.org/articles/10.3389/fphys.2018.00973. [Accessed 27 December 2022]

[10] Burton GJ, Redman CW, Roberts JM, et al. PE: pathophysiology and clinical implications. BMJ. 2019;**366**:12381

[11] Beaudeux J-L, Giral P, Bruckert E, et al. Matrix metalloproteinases, inflammation and atherosclerosis: Therapeutic perspectives. Clinical Chemistry and Laboratory Medicine. 2004;**42**:121-131

[12] Turbeville HR, Sasser JM. PE beyond pregnancy: Long-term consequences for mother and child. American Journal of Physiology-Renal Physiology. 2020;**318**:F1315-F1326

[13] Harmon AC, Cornelius DC, Amaral LM, et al. The role of inflammation in the pathology of PE. Clinical Science (London, England: 1979). 2016;**130**:409

[14] Wang X, Khalil RA. Matrix metalloproteinases, vascular remodeling, and vascular disease. Advances in Pharmacology. 2018;**81**:241-330

[15] Sosa SEY, Flores-Pliego A, Espejel-Nuñez A, et al. New Insights into the Role of Matrix Metalloproteinases in PE. International Journal of Molecular Sciences. 20 Jul 2017;**18**(7):1448. 22. DOI: 10.3390/ijms18071448

[16] Lopez-Avila V, Spencer JV. Methods for detection of matrix metalloproteinases as biomarkers in cardiovascular disease. Clinical Medicine Cardiology. 2008;**2**:CMC.S484

[17] Rana S, Burke SD, Karumanchi SA. Imbalances in circulating angiogenic

factors in the pathophysiology of PE and related disorders. American Journal of Obstetrics and Gynecology. 2022;**226**:S1019-S1034

[18] Overview — Hypertension in pregnancy: Diagnosis and management — Guidance — NICE. Available from: https://www.nice.org.uk/guidance/ng133. [Accessed 17 December 2022]

[19] Fox R, Kitt J, Leeson P, et al. PE: Risk factors, diagnosis, management, and the cardiovascular impact on the offspring. Journal of Clinical Medicine. 2019;**8**:1625

[20] Sroka D, Verlohren S. Short term prediction of PE. Maternal-Fetal Medicine. 2021;**3**:107

[21] de Knegt VE, Hedley PL, Kanters JK, et al. The role of leptin in fetal growth during PE. International Journal of Molecular Sciences. 2021;**22**:4569

[22] Veiga de ECA, Korkes HA, Salomão KB, et al. Association of LEPTIN and other inflammatory markers with PE: A systematic review. Front Pharmacol. 10 Aug 2022;**13**:966400. Available from: https://www.frontiersin.org/articles/10.3389/fphar.2022.966400. [2022, Accessed 21 December 2022]

[23] Devarajachar R, Rangareddy H. Role of leptin in PE. International Journal of Reproduction, Contraception, Obstetrics and Gynecology. 2021;**10**:814-817

[24] Belay Tolu L, Yigezu E, Urgie T, et al. Maternal and perinatal outcome of PE without severe feature among pregnant women managed at a tertiary referral hospital in urban Ethiopia. PLoS One. 2020;**15**:e0230638

[25] Nankali A, Malek-khosravi S, Zangeneh M, et al. Maternal complications associated with Severe PE. Journal of Obstetrics and Gynaecology of India. 2013;**63**:112-115

[26] Khan B, Yar RA, Khan KA, et al. PE incidence and its maternal and neonatal outcomes with associated risk factors. Cureus. 6 Nov 2022;**14**(11):e31143. DOI: 10.7759/cureus.31143

[27] Abraham AJM, Bobby Z, Chaturvedula L, et al. Maternal adverse outcomes in hypertensive disorders of pregnancy and their association with serum adiponectin and redox markers. Fetal and Pediatric Pathology. 2022;**41**:1-17

[28] Nakimuli A, Nakubulwa S, Kakaire O, et al. The burden of maternal morbidity and mortality attributable to hypertensive disorders in pregnancy: A prospective cohort study from Uganda. BMC Pregnancy and Childbirth. 2016;**16**:205

[29] Jikamo B, Adefris M, Azale T, et al. The effect of PE on adverse maternal outcomes in Sidama region, Ethiopia: A prospective open cohort study. Scientific Reports. 2022;**12**:19300

[30] Kongwattanakul K, Saksiriwuttho P, Chaiyarach S, et al. Incidence, characteristics, maternal complications, and perinatal outcomes associated with PE with severe features and HELLP syndrome. International Journal of Women's Health. 2018;**10**:371-377

Section 4

The Relation between Reproductive System and General Health

Chapter 12

Ovarian Factors of Cardiovascular Disease: The Way to Go?

Igor V. Lakhno

Abstract

The function of the female reproductive system is critically dependent on the general health of a woman. However, the activity of ovaries has its projection on metabolic processes, vascular tone, and endothelial function. Hyperandrogenicity in polycystic ovarian disease is a trigger for adiposity, diabetes type II, and atherogenic vasculopathy. The increased level of testosterone persists to stay even after menopause. The data on hormonal changes during menopause is discussed. Hormone replacement therapy did not demonstrate an evident beneficial effect on the cardiovascular system. The possible therapeutic strategy for improved cardiovascular health during the transitional year of life is presented. The use of diet, L-arginine, and xylitol could be a reasonable option in the management of perimenopausal women.

Keywords: menopause, estrogens, testosterone, cardiovascular disease, lifestyle modification, hormone replacement therapy, L-arginine, xylitol

1. Introduction

Cardiovascular disease (CVD) takes a special place among all challenges and issues of humankind. This fact is due to a wide range of risk factors for increased blood pressure (BP), numerous pathogenic mechanisms in the scenario of arterial hypertension, as well as age and gender features of this pathology. The autonomic and endocrine regulation of BP has certain differences in female and male persons. Since the functioning of the female reproductive system has an obvious hierarchical organization, it is necessary to consider the main mechanisms of regulation that ensure the participation of the ovaries in the processes of homeostasis. The hypothesis of "fetal programming" explains the role of the antenatal period in the development of diseases during adulthood [1]. However, the manifestation of systemic atherogenic vasculopathy before menopause is minor. Therefore, hypoestrogenicity could be a trigger for CVD in women.

The continual search for the regulation of the female reproductive system contributed to the discovery of a number of fundamental methods of diagnosis. Stockard and Papanicolaou described changes in the vaginal mucous layer depending on the phase of the menstrual cycle, which was known as a hormonal colpocytology in 1917 [2]. Rock and Bartlett proposed the use of endometrial biopsy for the detection of the phase of the ovarian cycle in 1937 [3]. Netter used this method and demonstrated the relationship between the endometrium changes and the phase of the ovarian cycle [4]. Allen and Doisy found the effect of follicular fluid extract on the morphological changes of the vaginal mucosal layer in female mice in 1923 [5]. Corner and Allen isolated progesterone in the same year. They definitely indicated the site of production of estrogens (Graafian follicles) and progesterone (corpus luteum) in 1929 [6]. A new milestone in the study of the functional properties of the ovaries was the research performed by the Swedish scientist Bent Falck in 1959. Bent Falck delivered a report "The use of micrografts to determine the site of estrogen production in the ovaries of rats" at the medical faculty of the University of Lund. He evidently supported that estrogen and androgen secretion occurs only in transplants containing cells of the theca interna and interstitial cells together with granulosa or corpus luteum cells (the so-called "two-cell theory") [3].

The research of the gynecologists from Chicago Irving Stein and Michael Leventhal "Amenorrhea associated with bilateral polycystic ovaries" was of great theoretical and practical value. According to the primary source, polycystic ovary syndrome (PCOS) is "menstrual irregularity, including amenorrhea, infertility, hirsutism, somewhat delayed development of the mammary glands, and obesity." The authors found that ovarian resection improved the condition of patients and led to the restoration of a normal menstrual cycle [7]. PCOS is extremely widespread in the modern female population and leads to significant short- and long-term consequences, such as hyperandrogenism, insulin resistance, impaired carbohydrate metabolism, obesity, chronic inflammation, endothelial malfunction, dyslipidemia, and arterial hypertension. These pathological processes are involved in the pathogenic pathways of diabetes mellitus (DM) type 2, coronary heart disease, and brain stroke [8]. The lack of ovulation and ovarian hyperandrogenicity are typical for patients with PCOS. The presentation of metabolic disorders in this population allows us to think about the relationship between hyperadrenogenicity and disturbed carbohydrate metabolism in women with PCOS [9].

The impaired follicle maturation is one of the mechanisms of hyperandrogenicity in women with PCOS. The follicles do not reach the preovulatory level. This is due to the low concentration of FSH, which does not elevate enough to the necessary threshold level for the aromatase activation and the synthesis of estrogens. The activity of the androgen fraction dominates. The anti-Müllerian hormone (AMH) reduces the sensitivity of granulosa cells to FSH. AMH is a glycoprotein and belongs to transforming growth factor-β. The concentration of AMH in women with PCOS is three times higher than in healthy persons [10]. Obesity, insulin resistance, and hyperandrogenicity have been shown to play a significant role in elevated AMH in some studies [11, 12].

The history of PCOS lasts for about 40 thousand years according to the theory of Aziz [13]. The unbeneficial living conditions of people during the Paleolithic period led to the suppression of fertility and the accumulation of fat. The wave of migration of primitive people from Africa to Europe showed the need to survive in conditions of cold winters and food shortages. The storage of additional energy supply was achieved by an increase in the insulin level and excessive development of adipose tissue. Declining fertility also increased the chances of survival for women at that time. Therefore, PCOS contributed to the preservation of humanity and is an endocrinopathy of the surviving descendants of insulin-resistant ancestors.

2. The role of ovaries in general health

2.1 Recent advances in PCOS

The etiology of PCOS is still unknown. The occurrence of this pathology could be associated with hereditary reasons. However, the specific genes related to PCOS are not found. Barker's theory of fetal programming captures the effect of excessive androgen levels on the fetus that contribute to metabolic disorders in adult life. This is due to reprogramming at the genetic level and subsequently causes the manifestation of oligo-anovulation, polycystic morphology of the ovaries, and insulin resistance [14]. The risk of metabolic syndrome X, DM type 2, and CVD was twice as high in women with PCOS relative to the general population [15]. The negative effect of testosterone on the fetus was found in an experimental animal model. The increased incidence of metabolic disorders similar to PCOS was found [16]. However, the human embryo is protected from excess maternal androgen levels by a combination of high concentrations of androgen-binding proteins and significant aromatase activity in the placenta. Placental aromatases take part in the transformation of maternal androgens into estrogens (mainly estriol). Nowadays, it has already been proven that maternal hyperandrogenicity can cause hyperproduction of fetal sebaceous glands, which persists during the neonatal period. Thus, fetal programming associated with high androgen concentration may be a significant etiological factor of PCOS.

The main branches in the pathogenesis of PCOS are insulin resistance and chronic inflammation. Women with PCOS have an increased risk of metabolic syndrome X and CVD. The odds ratio (OR) of CVD in women with PCOS is 1.3–2.0 in several meta-analyses [17]. Premenopausal age is an additional factor that increases the risk of systemic vasculopathy. Obesity is known to be associated with insulin resistance and inflammation. Thin women with PCOS do not have an increased risk of DM type 2, but the risk of CVD is currently being investigated [18]. All women with PCOS are recommended to be screened for the markers of metabolic syndrome. However, the study of lipid profiles in young patients is not often informative and has no influence on treatment strategy. The most important prognostic markers for the development of CVD are elevated blood pressure, hyperglycemia, and dyslipidemia. The risk of CVD can be reduced under the influence of drug therapy. At the same time, the fasting insulin level remained stable under the influence of combined oral contraceptives (COC). However, the use of COCs causes an increase in thrombin concentration and the risk of thromboembolic complications. Thus, COC use increases the chances of CVD [19].

A recent study found that the relative risk (RR) of arterial hypertension and dyslipidemia in women with PCOS was 1.7. CVD in obese women in this study was 2.4 [20]. It was also found that more than 30% of patients with PCOS had blood pressure $\geq$ 130/85 mmHg. Women with PCOS also had signs of hypertension, dyslipidemia, hyperglycemia, and hyperinsulinemia in the Chinese study [21]. In total, 18% of women with PCOS had an elevated level of triglycerides (>1.7 mmol/l). It has been confirmed that insulin resistance contributes to CVD. When BP increases, lipid profile and pancreatic β-cell function deteriorate in women with PCOS in the process of aging. It is also very important that the body mass index (BMI) was very different in patients with different phenotypes. Phenotype A is featured by hyperandrogenism, anovulation, and polycystic ovarian morphology. The last sign is absent in women with phenotype B. Phenotype C is the so-called "ovulatory" PCOS (characterized by hyperandrogenism and polycystic ovarian morphology). Phenotype D is called "non-androgenic" PCOS (ovulatory dysfunction and polycystic ovarian morphology). Recently, it has been established that the level of AMH reflects the severity of PCOS. The most difficult is the combination of phenotype A with a high level of AMH. However, there is no clear correlation between AMH concentration and insulin resistance. One Chinese study found that AMH is a valuable prognostic marker for insulin resistance [22].

Hypertrophied adipocytes are known to have a significant number of genes involved in inflammation and cytokines production. The presence of tissue hypoxia may contribute to the accumulation of macrophages and other immune cells in adipose tissue. Inflammation in adipose tissue causes a disturbed hepatic carbohydrate metabolism and reduces the sensitivity of skeletal muscles to insulin. All patients with PCOS have elevated levels of inflammatory markers: IL-6 and C-reactive protein (C-RP). Proinflammatory cytokines: TNF-α, IL-6, and IL-1β have a paracrine effect that contributes to insulin resistance. It is also known that an elevated blood level of pro-inflammatory cytokines is involved in the development of atherosclerosis and CVD [23]. IL-18, TNF-α, IL-6, and C-RP are the main markers of inflammation occurring in women with PCOS. It is quite interesting that both thin and fat women have increased levels of pro-inflammatory substances that contribute to the development of insulin resistance, atherosclerosis, and hypertension. It has been known for more than 10 years that women with PCOS have elevated levels of C-RP. This dependence increases with age and body weight growth. It can be considered that a high concentration of C-RP is a marker of increased risk of CVD in women with PCOS. IL-6 is also considered a risk indicator of atherosclerosis, coronary heart disease, and hypertension. IL-6 is known as a potential inducer of C-RP synthesis by hepatocytes. The increase in the concentration of C-RP supports the severe atherosclerotic process, and the risk of myocardial infarction and stroke [24]. IL-6 and C-RP levels are elevated in women with PCOS and insulin resistance. Since leukocytes are located in visceral adipose tissue and these cells are a source of pro-inflammatory cytokines, it can be assumed that insulin resistance is a factor contributing to the excessive activity of leukocytes. The correlation between C-RP, IL-6, and body mass index (BMI) was found. It is possible that the use of C-RP testing is an important addition to the traditional CVD risk screening in women with PCOS. The elevated proinflammatory cytokines may be an early marker of insulin resistance and atherosclerosis. There are also other known markers of inflammation in women with PCOS. Chemerin affects metabolic risk factors and blood pressure. The level of this novel adipokine is increased in women with hyperandrogenicity. The elevated levels of visfatin were found to be associated with beta-cell damage in type 2 DM. The visfatin level is elevated and correlates with body mass index, insulin resistance, and hyperinsulinemia in patients with hyperandrogenicity [25]. The increased concentrations of vaspin, leptin, and resistin were also found. However, the level of irisin ("hormone of physical activity") is reduced in this category of patients. This myokine improves cognitive impairment [26]. Therefore, menopause contributes to the development of metabolic syndrome X.

Adrenomedullin, natriuretic peptide, and copeptin were found to participate in the regulation of fluid balance and hemodynamic processes by modulating vascular tone and diuresis. These substances may play a significant role in the pathogenesis of arterial hypertension in women with PCOS [27]. Adrenomedullin is known to be produced by smooth muscle cells and endothelial cells and is distributed throughout the body. It is also considered an adipokine because it can be produced by adipose tissue. Adrenomedullin secretion increases in response to inflammation, hypoxia, and insulin resistance in CVD and DM type 2. It is known that natriuretic peptide is released from cardiomyocytes in case of heart failure and as a result of adrenergic stimulation. Natriuretic peptide causes vasodilatation, stimulates natriuresis, and suppresses the activity of the renin-angiotensin-aldosterone system, reducing the effects of adrenomimetic substances. Natriuretic peptide stimulates lipolysis. An increase in the concentration of this substance is observed in CVD and heart failure [28]. However, obesity and insulin resistance have been shown to decrease natriuretic peptide levels in a large cohort study. The release of copetin captures vasopressin activation. Copeptin is more stable to measure than vasopressin and also reflects osmolality. Copeptin has certain prospects as a marker of myocardial infarction in combination with troponin. It has been established that an increase in the concentration of copeptin in heart failure worsens the prognosis. Copeptin also increases with obesity [29]. The significant value of studying the level of adrenomedullin, natriuretic peptide, and copeptin for predicting CVD in PCOS has been established.

2.2 Menopause in PCOS

A high risk of CVD in women with PCOS is typical for patients with obesity, arterial hypertension, dyslipidemia, impaired carbohydrate tolerance, and a family history of CVD. An increased BMI plays the most important role among all risk factors for arterial hypertension. The risk of systemic vasculopathy and kidney disease is very high in women with metabolic syndrome X [30]. Therefore, all patients with PCOS in addition to a gynecological examination should be examined by a general practitioner, a cardiologist, an endocrinologist, and a neurologist. This is the basis of an interdisciplinary approach to the management of women with PCOS. This strategy provides an individual CVD prevention program. Thus, the prevention of CVD in women with PCOS includes screening for metabolic syndrome X (BMI, BP, lipid profile, and carbohydrate metabolism) even in young and thin women. There is evidence that metabolic disorders in PCOS are associated with IL-6 gene polymorphisms and can be corrected with lifestyle changes and metformin use.

The majority of middle-aged women suffer not only from decreased levels of estrogen but also testosterone insufficiency. The use of testosterone is a possible therapeutic option for women during their transitional period. However, the declined level of testosterone is associated with suppressed libido and, therefore, is known as a reason for sexual dysfunction [31]. However, hyperandrogenicity in women with PCOS persists even after menopause and elevates cardiometabolic risks [32]. The topical or systemic use of estriol or estradiol could stimulate the proliferation of vaginal epithelium and interfere with vulvovaginal aging. But estrogens have no influence on libido. Since the prescription of testosterone preparations is out of label in the majority of cases, the possible risks and adverse effects of testosterone in female organisms should be discussed. The lack of information about dosage, forms, and duration of testosterone administration is linked to insufficient research data.

Nowadays, the vaginal use of hyaluronic acid becomes very popular. The application of hyaluronic acid gel was found to decrease vaginal dryness, itching, and bleeding, and improve sexual function in women of the transitional period [33]. Therefore, hyaluronic acid is an alternative for hormone treatment of atrophic vaginitis.

The main target population for testosterone use is transgender individuals. These persons could be the model for the investigation of systemic male steroid application in female organisms. The problem is that these patients are younger than perimenopausal women. However, the available experience demonstrates all possible advances and complications of testosterone clinical use [34]. The prescription of testosterone is logical only in case of vaginal atrophy. Testosterone is known to increase hemoglobin levels due to its potency to stimulate bone marrow and elevate the production of erythropoietin in kidneys. Several studies showed that testosterone increased hemoglobin levels in patients with unexplained anemia [32]. Androgens and estrogen are involved in inflammatory pathways. Sexual steroids have immunosuppressive and anti-inflammatory activity. Testosterone was found to modulate renal perfusion and, therefore, could produce an acute kidney injury. The elevation of creatinine was found in transgender individuals in the process of testosterone administration [35]. Thus, the possible nephrotoxic action of testosterone must be kept in mind. The effect of testosterone on cognitive function and mood is not completely known. The impact of this substance on muscle strength, body fat, and mineral bone density is not evident. Systemic use of testosterone in perimenopausal women was found to increase acne but not related to hair loss. Oral testosterone therapy is associated with an adverse lipid profile and, therefore, should be avoided in women with cardiometabolic risks [36]. However, transdermal use of androgens is possible therapeutical management for women with decrease in testosterone.

2.3 Current approaches and interventions improving cardiovascular health in menopausal women

The first step in lifestyle modification is a diet, regular physical training, and cessation of smoking. It has been proven that the loss of excess weight in patients with PCOS leads to an improvement of the lipid profile, normalization of carbohydrate metabolism, reduction of hyperandrogenism, and restoration of ovulation. It is necessary to reduce body weight by 20% for women with morbid obesity [37].

Pharmacotherapy includes drugs that increase insulin sensitivity, and lower cholesterol, BP, and body weight. Metformin has the longest history of use for the treatment of insulin resistance. Due to its multipotent effect, this drug is often called the "aspirin of the XXI century." Metformin is prescribed as the first line of therapy, especially when the patient refuses to lose weight. The drug should be taken during meals because, on an empty stomach, it can cause symptoms of irritation of the gastrointestinal tract (sometimes it can cause diarrhea). Metformin does not have a significant effect on body weight but improves the lipid profile. It was also found that the use of metformin contributes to a decrease in the level of C-RP and prevention of atherogenic vasculopathy. However, the main indications for prescribing metformin are insulin resistance and hyperinsulinemia. Several studies have been conducted that proved the same antiandrogenic effect of metformin and the combined oral contraceptive with cyproterone acetate [38]. The level of side effects of the combined oral contraceptive such as increased body weight, increased BP, depression, headache, and chest pain was significantly higher. However, combined oral contraceptives are more effective in regulating the menstrual cycle compared to metformin.

There has been a growing interest in the use of vitamin D_3 as a factor that improves insulin resistance, chronic inflammation, and oxidative stress in patients with PCOS for the past decades. Several studies *in vitro* showed a decrease in the synthesis of pro-inflammatory cytokines and an increase in the concentrations of anti-inflammatory substances [39]. At the same time, the anti-inflammatory effect of vitamin D_3 has been confirmed in some clinical studies. A recent meta-analysis presented data from seven clinical trials of vitamin D_3 in women with PCOS. Vitamin D_3 supplementation in women with PCOS reduced C-RP and malondialdehyde levels, and increased antioxidant capacity in this meta-analysis [40].

If the level of low-density lipoprotein is more than 160 mg/dl, and the concentration of very low-density lipoprotein is more than 190 mg/dl, pharmaceutical correction with a drug that lowers the cholesterol level should be started. Statins are the most often used. Many studies have shown that statins decrease low-density lipoprotein levels, and testosterone concentrations, reduce insulin resistance, and improve endothelial function. Antihypertensive drugs should be prescribed when blood pressure rises above 140/90 mm Hg. The level of BP about 120/80 should be considered the optimal one that prevents the incidence of complications. The experience of the drug application for weight loss sibutramine in women with PCOS is known [41]. It was established that sibutramine reduces body weight and the concentration of insulin, testosterone, and triglycerides. However, the level of evidence for these results is insufficient for inclusion in recommendations for women with PCOS. The use of inositol and resveratrol, as well as naltrexone, is promising. The first two of these drugs have a positive effect on carbohydrate metabolism and increase the antioxidant potential [42]. Naltrexone is a centrally acting drug, and its use, although it does not yet have a sufficient evidence base, could be the initial step in a neuroendocrine approach to the treatment of PCOS. The experience of gastric banding is also known, which contributes to the normalization of metabolic processes, and correction of BP in women with obesity refractory to pharmacotherapy.

Unfortunately, HRT is not recognized as an efficient method for metabolic syndrome X prevention [43]. Since metabolic disorders reduce the active working capacity and life period in general, it is necessary to develop a therapeutic strategy focused on their negative impact on a woman's health prevention or reduction. Women with a normal weight before the onset of menopause should be recommended to increase physical activity, and obese patients should be asked for a diet [44]. Diet was found to be associated with a reduction in incident cardiovascular and coronary adverse events, as well as heart failure. The daily consumption of 400 g of vegetables for 3 weeks was found in one study to improve lipid metabolism and glycemic control in obese menopausal women [45]. The Mediterranean diet may help in the primary prevention of bone, metabolic, and cardiovascular diseases in the postmenopausal period [46]. Interestingly, CVD risk in postmenopausal women appears to be sensitive to a change to a low-fat dietary pattern and, among healthy women, includes both coronary heart disease benefit and brain stroke risk [47]. The existing experience of wellness anti-aging programs indicates the use of medical nutrition and physical education. However, the issue of emotional and physical comfort in the process of weight loss remains open.

The state of moderate ketosis is known to reduce the patient's appetite in the process of medical diet therapy [48]. However, ketosis leads to the predominance of anaerobic glycolysis, the accumulation of lactate, and lipid peroxidation tissue products. This supports oxidative stress and adversely affects hepatic lipid metabolism. Increased ketogenesis is dangerous for people with DM and requires adjustment of insulin dose or a sulfonylurea drug. How can these deviations be prevented? The obvious prospect is the use of xylitol preparations, which are not an insulin-dependent source of energy and could prevent the transition from the Krebs cycle to other metabolic pathways.

Xylitol is known as a source of energy to achieve balance with an excellent anti-catabolic effect. Xylitol can reduce constipation, DM, obesity, and other diseases. This polyol has a stimulating effect on digestion and immune system. The level of xylitol was found to be used as a predictor of the prospect of weight loss without surgical interventions in patients with morbid obesity [49]. After the use of xylitol, the glycemia level stays constant, and the processes of gluconeogenesis prevail over glycolysis. The long-term experience of using xylitol in the food industry supports its anti-inflammatory and antibacterial effects. It is capable of counteracting the etiological microbial factors of gingivitis, pneumonia, and media otitis. The dose-dependent antimicrobial effect of xylitol is known. Xylitol can compensate for NADH deficiency in patients with hemolytic anemia. There is also evidence that xylitol can reduce the proliferation of cancer cells. Xylitol enhances the processes of lipolysis, contributing to the reduction of adipose tissue, and has a therapeutic effect on dyslipidemia. It protects the heart, liver, kidneys, and pancreas from the negative effects of oxidative stress. Xylitol promotes a better metabolism of calcium and phosphorus and prevents the occurrence of osteoporosis after bilateral oophorectomy in experimental animals. Xylitol was found to have a beneficial effect on gut microbiota and increased the absorption of phytoestrogens in another experimental study. These findings could support its possible use for the prevention and treatment of osteoporosis.

Prevention of endothelial malfunction is one of the main tasks of women in menopause management. Formerly, HRT was found to have a protective effect on endothelium [50]. But this effect is critically dependent on NO-system. Estrogen-mediated effects, including increasing nitric oxide bioavailability and attenuating oxidative stress and inflammation, contribute to preserving cardiovascular health. The level of nitric oxide was found to be decreased in women of transitional age. The lack of this vasodilating agent induces vasculopathy. HRT is known to contribute to the restoration of the lipid profile, increase the activity of nitric oxide synthase, and release this powerful vasodilator from the endothelium. The level of nitric oxide synthase is the key to the vasorelaxant effect of estradiol. Since L-arginine is a substrate for the synthesis of nitric oxide, its use could be a promising option for women obtaining HRT. The application of L-arginine could provide anti-inflammatory, metabolic, and vasoactive effects [51]. L-arginine deficiency possibly plays a key role in the progress of endothelial malfunction after menopause. A combination of aerobic exercise and regular L-arginine intake contributed to decreased blood pressure (BP) and inflammatory markers in older women [52].

2.4 "Life extension" is an innovative intervention in antiaging medicine

The development of a therapeutic and preventive strategy including HRT, physical activity, diet therapy, and the use of xylitol and L-arginine preparations could make a favor in improving the quality of life of women over 45 years old. Xylitol solution with micronutrients should be administered in the form of infusions from the first days of the reduction diet once for 5 days. Administration of L-arginine should be started intravenously at 200 ml once a day for a week, and then be continued in oral form for another 3 weeks. The results of 1-month and 3-month programs, including physical training, diet, xylitol, and L-arginine, were already reported [53, 54]. The findings showed a real prospect of such a strategy for life extension. But the emphasis should be done.

A total of 71 perimenopausal women were enrolled in the study. Thirty-six patients with or without periods from Group II received sequential or continuous combined HRT. Thirty-five women of transitional age (Group III) additionally to HRT received a diet, L-arginine infusions of 200.0 ml once daily for a week, 20 ml of oral L-arginine solution for 3 weeks, and also xylitol solution 200.0 ml once daily during the 5 days were included in Group III. A low-carbohydrate and mild-fat diet (less than 26% carbohydrates or less than 130 gm/day) was used in the study. The distribution of the nutrients was 20% carbohydrates, 40% fat, and 40% protein. This diet featured a low glycemic index, slow ketogenesis, and anti-atherogenic effects [55]. Thirty-five healthy reproductive-aged women were included in Group I (control).

The obtained results showed that obesity plays an important role in the pathogenesis of climacteric syndrome. The findings of the study demonstrated a moderate positive correlation between BMI and diastolic BP, BMI, and Cooperman's score, BMI and glucose level, BMI and C-RP (**Figure 1**). The reduction of BMI was found in patients from Group III (**Figure 2**). The declining Cooperman's score in these patients

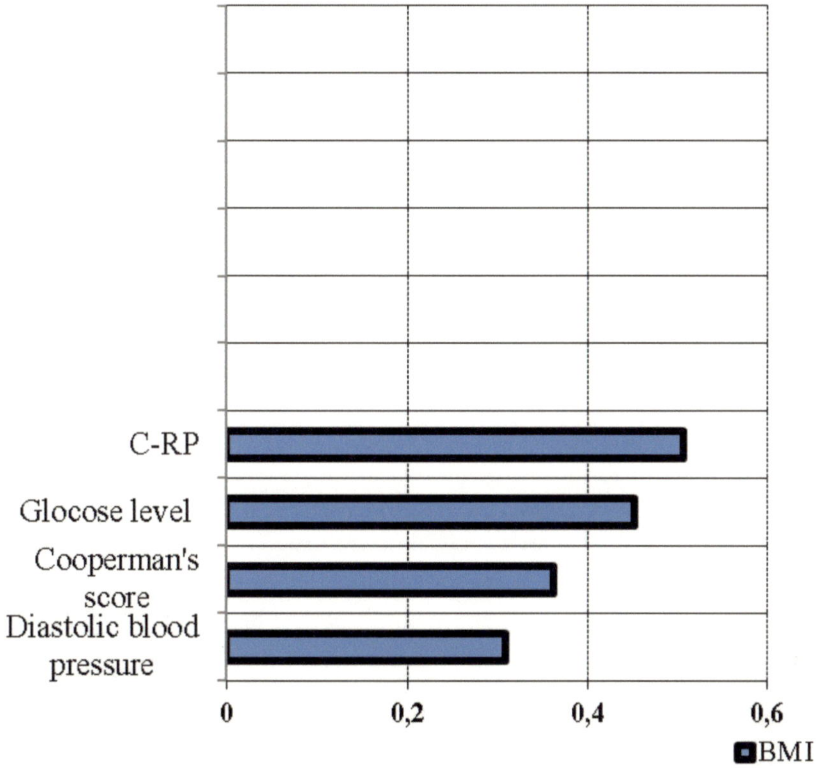

Figure 1.
The correlation between BMI and diastolic BP, BMI and Cooperman's score, BMI and glucose level, and BMI and C-RP.

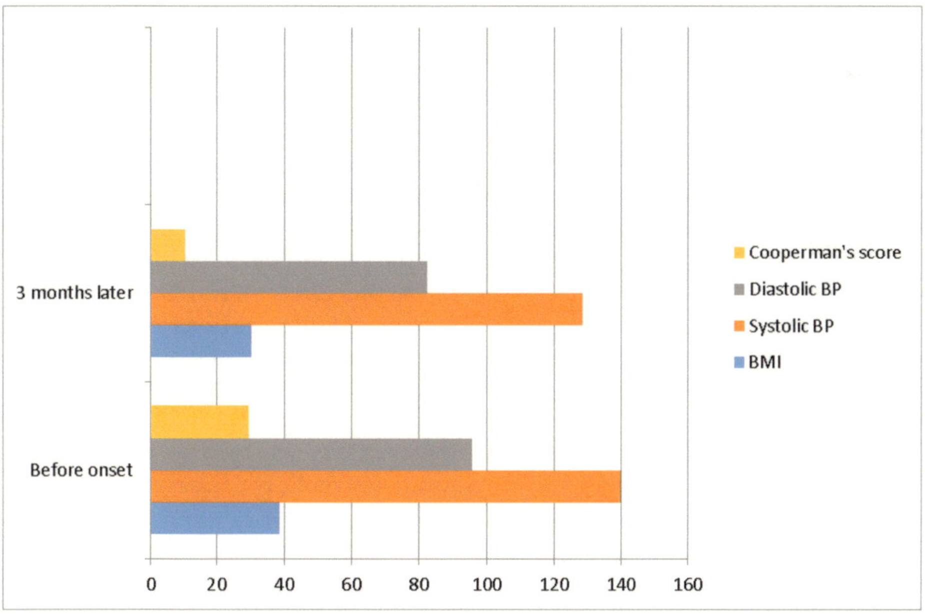

Figure 2.
The changes in BMI, systolic BP, diastolic BP, and Cooperman's score in group III.

C-RP before and after 3 months program

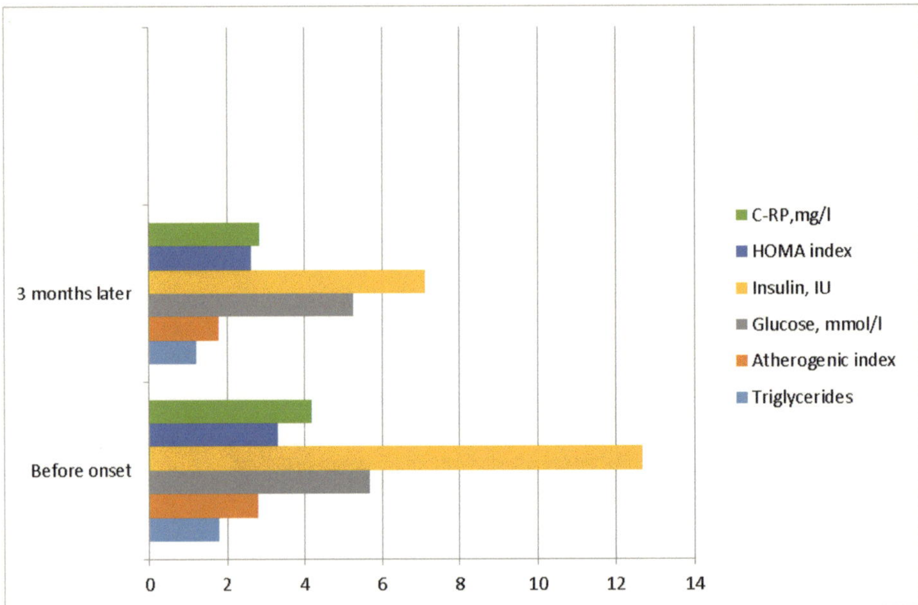

Figure 3.
The level of triglycerides, atherogenic index, glucose, insulin, HOMA index, and C-RP before and after 3-month program.

supported the opinion of the use of diet in the treatment of early menopausal disorders. The reduction of BP was possibly associated with improved metabolic profile of patient in Group III (**Figure 3**). But the effect could be also associated with autonomic tone restoration by reducing sympathetic regulation. The decrease of atherogenicity, improved carbohydrate metabolism, and complete history of chronic inflammation were found in perimenopausal women (**Figure 3**). These findings support available data on the relationship between insulin resistance, atherogenicity, and systemic inflammation.

Since the effect of HRT on BP is multifactorial, the use of estrogens is not definitely postulated. Some studies showed the increased risk of complications of CVD in elderly women who obtained HRT [56]. The proposed 3-month program demonstrated its positive vasoactive effect. This method of management for perimenopausal women has a positive synergistic with estradiol effect on endothelium. Thus, L-arginine donation could be thought of as an efficient intervention for an improved cardiovascular health in perimenopausal women. Thus, the use of diet, L-arginine, and xylitol could be an important supplement to HRT. The findings emphasize the possible options for the prevention of atherogenicity. Weight gain and increased BMI was the main factor for insulin resistance, atherogenicity, and menopausal disorders. The use of diet, xylitol, and L-arginine improved metabolic processes and reduced menopausal disorders [53, 54].

Weight gain was the main factor for insulin resistance, atherogenicity, and menopausal disorders. The use of diet, xylitol, and L-arginine improved metabolic processes and reduced menopausal disorders.

BMI in perimenopausal women was responsible for BP, menopausal Cooperman's score, carbohydrate metabolism, and inflammatory response. The use of a 3-month program including diet, xylitol, and L-arginine solutions contributed to the reduction of Cooperman's score, chronic inflammation, and restoration of lipid and carbohydrate metabolism. This program could help us to make another step in the march toward improved women's health in their perimenopausal years.

3. Conclusion

Menopause is still in transition from conventional strategies to anti-aging medicine. Healthy aging could be provided only in case of the absence of serious diseases. CVD is a "destiny" for the postmenopausal women. The continual search in the field could help to provide completely safe and efficient interventions for longevity and stamina.

Author details

Igor V. Lakhno
Kharkiv National Medical University, Ukraine

*Address all correspondence to: igorlakhno71@gmail.com

References

[1] Hoyer D, Żebrowski J, Cysarz D, Gonçalves H, Pytlik A, Amorim-Costa C, et al. Monitoring fetal maturation-objectives, techniques and indices of autonomic function. Physiological Measurement. 2017;**38**(5):R61-R88. DOI: 10.1088/1361-6579/aa5fca

[2] Stockard CR, Papanicolaou GN. The existence of a typical oestrous cycle in the Guinea-pig with a study of its histological and physiological changes. The American Journal of Anatomy. 1917;**22**:225

[3] Longo LD. Classic pages in obstetrics and gynecology. Anatomical variations in the female pelvis and their effect in labor with a suggested classification. William Edgar Caldwell and Howard Carmen Moloy. American journal of obstetrics and gynecology, vol. 26, pp. 479-505, 1933. American Journal of Obstetrics and Gynecology. 1977;**127**(7):798

[4] Netter A, Henry R. Le dosage des oestrogènes dans les liquides de kystes Para-utérins; hypothèse de la lymphocrine ovarienne [ratio of estrogens in the fluid contents of Para-uterine cysts; hypothesis of ovarian lymphocrinia]. Annales d'endocrinologie. 1950;**11**(6):630-633

[5] Allen E, Doisy EA. Landmark article sept 8, 1923. An ovarian hormone. Preliminary report on its localization, extraction and partial purification, and action in test animals. By Edgar Allen and Edward A. Doisy. Journal of the American Medical Association. 1983;**250**(19):2681-2683. DOI: 10.1001/jama.250.19.2681

[6] Corner GW, Allen WM. Physiology of the corpus luteum. 1929. American Journal of Obstetrics and Gynecology. 2005;**193**(4):1574. discussion 1575. DOI: 10.1016/j.ajog.2005.02.116

[7] Leventhal ML. The stein-Leventhal syndrome. American Journal of Obstetrics and Gynecology. 1958;**76**(4):825-838

[8] Marciniak A, Nawrocka Rutkowska J, Brodowska A, Wiśniewska B, Starczewski A. Cardiovascular system diseases in patients with polycystic ovary syndrome - The role of inflammation process in this pathology and possibility of early diagnosis and prevention. Annals of Agricultural and Environmental Medicine. 2016;**23**(4):537-541. DOI: 10.5604/12321966.1226842

[9] Diamanti-Kandarakis E. Insulin resistance in PCOS. Endocrine. 2006;**30**(1):13-17. DOI: 10.1385/ENDO:30:1:13

[10] Jiang L, Ruan X, Li Y, Gu M, Cheng J, Wang Y, et al. Diagnostic value of anti-Müllerian hormone combined with androgen-levels in Chinese patients with polycystic ovary syndrome. Gynecological Endocrinology. 2023;**39**(1):2206927. DOI: 10.1080/09513590.2023.2206927

[11] Bakeer E, Radwan R, El Mandoury A, El Rahman AA, Gad M, El Maksoud SA. Anti-Müllerian hormone as a diagnostic marker in Egyptian infertile polycystic ovary syndrome females: Correlations with vitamin D, total testosterone, dyslipidemia and anthropometric parameters. Journal of Medical Biochemistry. 2018;**37**(4):448-455. DOI: 10.1515/jomb-2017-0068

[12] Wiweko B, Indra I, Susanto C, Natadisastra M, Hestiantoro A. The correlation between serum AMH and

HOMA-IR among PCOS phenotypes. BMC Research Notes. 2018;**11**(1):114. DOI: 10.1186/s13104-018-3207-y

[13] Azziz R. Introduction: Determinants of polycystic ovary syndrome. Fertility and Sterility. 2016;**106**(1):4-5. DOI: 10.1016/j.fertnstert.2016.05.009

[14] Homburg R, Gudi A, Shah A, Layton MA. A novel method to demonstrate that pregnant women with polycystic ovary syndrome hyper-expose their fetus to androgens as a possible stepping stone for the developmental theory of PCOS. A pilot study. Reproductive Biology and Endocrinology. 2017;**15**(1):61. DOI: 10.1186/s12958-017-0282-1

[15] Teede HJ, Tay CT, Laven J, Dokras A, Moran LJ, Piltonen TT, et al. Recommendations from the 2023 international evidence-based guideline for the assessment and management of polycystic ovary syndrome†. Human Reproduction. 2023;**38**(9):1655-1679. DOI: 10.1093/humrep/dead156

[16] Gurule S, Sustaita-Monroe J, Padmanabhan V, Cardoso R. Developmental programming of the neuroendocrine axis by steroid hormones: Insights from the sheep model of PCOS. Frontiers in Endocrinology (Lausanne). 2023;**14**:1096187. DOI: 10.3389/fendo.2023.1096187

[17] van der Ham K, Koster MPH, Velthuis BK, Budde RPJ, Fauser BCJM, Laven JSE, et al. Change in androgenic status and Cardiometabolic profile of middle-aged women with polycystic ovary syndrome. Journal of Clinical Medicine. 2023;**12**(16):5226. DOI: 10.3390/jcm12165226

[18] Ollila MM, Arffman RK, Korhonen E, Morin-Papunen L, Franks S, Junttila J, et al. Women with PCOS have an increased risk for cardiovascular disease regardless of diagnostic criteria-a prospective population-based cohort study. European Journal of Endocrinology. 2023;**189**(1):96-105. DOI: 10.1093/ejendo/lvad077

[19] Glintborg D, Sidelmann JJ, Altinok ML, Mumm H, Andersen M. Increased thrombin generation in women with polycystic ovary syndrome: A pilot study on the effect of metformin and oral contraceptives. Metabolism. 2015;**64**(10):1272-1278. DOI: 10.1016/j.metabol.2015.06.011

[20] Glintborg D, Rubin KH, Nybo M, Abrahamsen B, Andersen M. Cardiovascular disease in a nationwide population of Danish women with polycystic ovary syndrome. Cardiovascular Diabetology. 2018;**17**(1):37. DOI: 10.1186/s12933-018-0680-5

[21] Yang H, Chen Y, Liu C. Triglyceride-glucose index is associated with metabolic syndrome in women with polycystic ovary syndrome. Gynecological Endocrinology. 2023;**39**(1):2172154. DOI: 10.1080/09513590.2023.2172154

[22] Li J, Chen S, Qin R, Liu X, Fan L, Wei M, et al. Talin1 regulates glucose metabolism and endometrial receptivity via GLUT-4 in patients with polycystic ovary syndrome and insulin resistance. Gynecological Endocrinology. 2023;**39**(1):2231085. DOI: 10.1080/09513590.2023.2231085

[23] Bril F, Ezeh U, Amiri M, Hatoum S, Pace L, Chen YH, et al. Adipose tissue dysfunction in polycystic ovary syndrome. The Journal of Clinical Endocrinology and Metabolism. 2023:dgad356. DOI: 10.1210/clinem/dgad356 [Ahead of print]

[24] Wong ND, Budoff MJ, Ferdinand K, Graham IM, Michos ED, Reddy T, et al. Atherosclerotic cardiovascular disease risk assessment: An American society for preventive cardiology clinical practice statement. American Journal of Preventive Cardiology. 2022;**10**:100335. DOI: 10.1016/j.ajpc.2022.100335

[25] Pan X. Metabolic characteristics of obese patients with polycystic ovarian syndrome: A meta-analysis. Gynecological Endocrinology. 2023;**39**(1):2239934. DOI: 10.1080/09513590.2023.2239934

[26] Luo Y, Qiao X, Xu L, Huang G. Irisin: Circulating levels in serum and its relation to gonadal axis. Endocrine. 2022;**75**(3):663-671. DOI: 10.1007/s12020-022-02981-5

[27] Frøssing S, Nylander M, Kistorp C, Skouby SO, Faber J. Effect of liraglutide on atrial natriuretic peptide, adrenomedullin, and copeptin in PCOS. Endocrine Connections. 2018;**7**(1):115-123. DOI: 10.1530/EC-17-0327

[28] Al Rifai M, Taffet GE, Matsushita K, Virani SS, De Lemos J, Khera A, et al. Age-related differences in the contribution of systolic blood pressure and biomarkers to cardiovascular disease risk prediction: The atherosclerosis risk in communities (ARIC) study. The American Journal of Cardiology. 2023;**204**:295-301. DOI: 10.1016/j.amjcard.2023.07.118

[29] Polak K, Czyzyk A, Simoncini T, Meczekalski B. New markers of insulin resistance in polycystic ovary syndrome. Journal of Endocrinological Investigation. 2017;**40**(1):1-8. DOI: 10.1007/s40618-016-0523-8

[30] Liu R, Li M, Wang P, Yu M, Wang Z, Zhang GZ. Preventive online and offline health management intervention in polycystic ovary syndrome. World Journal of Clinical Cases. 2022;**10**(10):3060-3068. DOI: 10.12998/wjcc.v10.i10.3060

[31] Bernstein SR, Kelleher C, Khalil RA. Gender-based research underscores sex differences in biological processes, clinical disorders and pharmacological interventions. Biochemical Pharmacology. 2023;**215**:115737. DOI: 10.1016/j.bcp.2023.115737

[32] Johansen N, Lindén Hirschberg A, Moen MH. The role of testosterone in menopausal hormone treatment. What is the evidence? Acta Obstetricia et Gynecologica Scandinavica. 2020;**99**(8):966-969. DOI: 10.1111/aogs.13819

[33] Buzzaccarini G, Marin L, Noventa M, Vitagliano A, Riva A, Dessole F, et al. Hyaluronic acid in vulvar and vaginal administration: Evidence from a literature systematic review. Climacteric. 2021;**24**(6):560-571. DOI: 10.1080/13697137.2021.1898580

[34] Davis SR, Baber R, Panay N, Bitzer J, Perez SC, Islam RM, et al. Global consensus position statement on the use of testosterone therapy for women. The Journal of Clinical Endocrinology and Metabolism. 2019;**104**(10):4660-4666. DOI: 10.1210/jc.2019-01603

[35] Uzel K, Lakhno I, Eminli I. Comparison of the effects of testosterone on pre- and PostHysterectomy findings in transgender individuals. International Medical Journal. 2021;**28**(4):407-410

[36] Renke G, Tostes F. Cardiovascular safety and benefits of testosterone implant therapy in postmenopausal women: Where are we? Pharmaceuticals (Basel). 2023;**16**(4):619. DOI: 10.3390/ph16040619

[37] Patel SS, Truong U, King M, Ferland A, Moreau KL, Dorosz J, et al.

Obese adolescents with polycystic ovarian syndrome have elevated cardiovascular disease risk markers. Vascular Medicine. 2017;**22**(2):85-95. DOI: 10.1177/1358863X16682107

[38] Alesi S, Forslund M, Melin J, Romualdi D, Peña A, Tay CT, et al. Efficacy and safety of anti-androgens in the management of polycystic ovary syndrome: A systematic review and meta-analysis of randomised controlled trials. EClinicalMedicine. 2023;**63**:102162. DOI: 10.1016/j.eclinm.2023.102162

[39] Nudy M, Xie R, O'Sullivan DM, Jiang X, Appt S, Register TC, et al. Association between coronary artery vitamin D receptor expression and select systemic risks factors for coronary artery atherosclerosis. Climacteric. 2022;**25**(4):369-375. DOI: 10.1080/13697137.2021.1985992

[40] Xue Y, Xu P, Xue K, Duan X, Cao J, Luan T, et al. Effect of vitamin D on biochemical parameters in polycystic ovary syndrome women: A meta-analysis. Archives of Gynecology and Obstetrics. 2017;**295**(2):487-496. DOI: 10.1007/s00404-016-4247-y

[41] Legro RS, Dodson WC, Kris-Etherton PM, Kunselman AR, StetterCM, WilliamsNI, et al. Randomized controlled trial of preconception interventions in infertile women with polycystic ovary syndrome. The Journal of Clinical Endocrinology and Metabolism. 2015;**100**(11):4048-4058. DOI: 10.1210/jc.2015-2778

[42] Myers SH, Russo M, Dinicola S, Forte G, Unfer V. Questioning PCOS phenotypes for reclassification and tailored therapy. Trends in Endocrinology and Metabolism. 2023;**S1043-2760**(23):00158-00153. DOI: 10.1016/j.tem.2023.08.005

[43] Bermingham KM, Linenberg I, Hall WL, Kadé K, Franks PW, Davies R, et al. Menopause is associated with postprandial metabolism, metabolic health and lifestyle:The ZOE PREDICT study. eBioMedicine. 2022;**85**:104303. DOI: 10.1016/j.ebiom.2022.104303

[44] Proietto J. Obesity and weight management at menopause. Australian Family Physician. 2017;**46**(6):368-370

[45] Sari IK, Utari DM, Kamoshita S, et al. Increasing vegetable intake 400 g/day to control body weight and lipid profile in overweight hyperlipidemia menopausal women. Journal of Public Health Research. 2020;**9**(3):1733. DOI: 10.4081/jphr.2020.1733

[46] Rangel-Huerta OD, Pastor-Villaescusa B, Gil A. Are we close to defining a metabolomic signature of human obesity? A systematic review of metabolomics studies. Metabolomics. 13 Jun 2019;**15**(6):93. DOI: 10.1007/s11306-019-1553-y. PMID

[47] Prentice RL, Aragaki AK, Van Horn L, Thomson CA, Beresford SA, Robinson J, et al. Low-fat dietary pattern and cardiovascular disease: Results from the Women's Health Initiative randomized controlled trial. The American Journal of Clinical Nutrition. 2017;**106**(1):35-43. DOI: 10.3945/ajcn.117.153270

[48] Hirahatake KM, Jiang L, Wong ND, Shikany JM, Eaton CB, Allison MA, et al. Diet quality and cardiovascular disease risk in postmenopausal women with type 2 diabetes mellitus: The Women's Health Initiative. Journal of the American Heart Association. 2019;**8**(19):e013249. DOI: 10.1161/JAHA.119.013249

[49] Benahmed AG, Gasmi A, Arshad M, et al. Health benefits of xylitol. Review Applied Microbiology and

Biotechnology. 2020;**104**(17):7225-7237. DOI: 10.1007/s00253-020-10708-7

[50] Somani YB, Pawelczyk JA, De Souza MJ, et al. Aging women and their endothelium: Probing the relative role of estrogen on vasodilator function review. American Journal of Physiology. Heart and Circulatory Physiology. 2019;**317**(2):H395-H404. DOI: 10.1152/ajpheart.00430.2018

[51] Klawitter J, Hildreth KL, Christians U, et al. A relative L-arginine deficiency contributes to endothelial dysfunction across the stages of the menopausal transition. Physiological Reports. 2017;**5**(17):e13409

[52] Puga GM, Novais IP, Katsanos CS, et al. Combined effects of aerobic exercise and l-arginine ingestion on blood pressure in normotensive postmenopausal women: A crossover study. Randomized Controlled Trial Life Science. 2016;**151**:323-329. DOI: 10.1016/j.lfs.2016.02.091

[53] Lakhno I. State of metabolic processes and ways to improve them in premenopausal women due to the life extension strategy. Reproductive Endocrinology. 2021;**61**:51-54. DOI: 10.18370/2309-4117.2021.61.51-54

[54] Lakhno I, Korovai S, Struk T, Pak S. The pathogenic pathways of cardiovascular disease in perimenopausal women. Menopause Review/Przegląd Menopauzalny. 2023;**22**(2):59-63. DOI: 10.5114/pm.2023.127902

[55] Silva TR, Oppermann K, Reis FM, Spritzer PM. Nutrition in menopausal women: A narrative review. Nutrients. 2021;**13**(7):2149. DOI: 10.3390/nu13072149

[56] Taylor JE, Baig MS, Helmy T, Gersh FL. Controversies regarding postmenopausal hormone replacement therapy for primary cardiovascular disease prevention in women. Cardiology in Review. 2021;**29**(6):296-304. DOI: 10.1097/CRD.0000000000000353